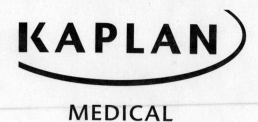

USMLE®
STEP 1
Lecture Notes
2016

Pathology

© 2016 by Kaplan, Inc.

Published by Kaplan Medical, a division of Kaplan, Inc.
750 Third Avenue
New York, NY 10017

Printed in the United States of America

10 9 8 7 6 5 4 3 2 1

Course ISBN: 978-1-5062-0030-9

Retail ISBN: 978-1-5062-0045-3

Kaplan Publishing print books are available at special quantity discounts to use for sales promotions, employee premiums, or educational purposes. For more information or to purchase books, please call the Simon & Schuster special sales department at 866-506-1949.

EDITORS

John Barone, M.D.

Anatomic and Clinical Pathologist
Beverly Hills, CA

Manuel A. Castro, M.D., AAHIVS

Diplomate of the American Board of Internal Medicine
Certified by the American Academy of HIV Medicine
Wilton Health Center (Private Practice)
Wilton Manors, FL

Nova Southeastern University
Clinical Assistant Professor of Medicine
Fort Lauderdale-Davie, FL

LECOM College of Osteopathy
Clinical Assistant Professor of Medicine
Bradenton, FL

The editors would like to acknowledge
Henry Sanchez, M.D. (UCSF, San Francisco) and **Heather Hoffmann, M.D.**
for their invaluable contributions.

These volumes of Lecture Notes represent the most-likely-to-be-tested material on the current USMLE Step 1 exam.

We want to hear what you think. What do you like about the Notes? What could be improved? Please share your feedback by e-mailing us at **medfeedback@kaplan.com**.

Best of luck on your Step 1 exam!

Kaplan Medical

Contents

Fundamentals of Pathology

Learning Objectives

❏ Define etiology, pathogenesis, morphology, and clinical significance of disease

❏ List techniques for staining pathologic specimens

OVERVIEW OF PATHOLOGY

Definitions

- The study of the essential nature of disease, including symptoms/signs, pathogenesis, complications, and morphologic consequences including structural and functional alterations in cells, tissues, and organs

- The study of all aspects of the disease process focusing on the pathogenesis leading to classical structural changes (gross and histopathology) and molecular alterations

The **etiology** (cause) of a disease may be genetic or environmental. The **pathogenesis** of a disease defines the temporal sequence and the patterns of cellular injury that lead to disease. **Morphologic** changes of the disease process include both gross changes and microscopic changes. The **clinical significance** of a disease relates to its signs and symptoms, disease course including complications, and prognosis.

Methods Used

Gross examination of organs on exam questions has 2 major components: identifying the organ and identifying the pathology. Useful gross features include consideration of size, shape, consistency, and color.

Microscopic examination of tissue

- In light microscopic examination of tissue, **hematoxylin and eosin (H&E)** is considered the gold standard stain and is used routinely in the initial microscopic examination of pathologic specimens.

Table 1-1. Structures Stained by Hematoxylin and Eosin

Hematoxylin	Eosin
Stains blue to purple	Stains pink to red
• Nuclei	• Cytoplasm
• Nucleoli	• Collagen
• Bacteria	• Fibrin
• Calcium	• RBCs
	• Thyroid colloid

The common denominator of the features shown in Table 1-1 is that hematoxylin binds nucleic acids and calcium salts, while eosin stains the majority of proteins (both extracellular and intracellular).

- **Other histochemical stains** (chemical reactions): Prussian blue (stains iron), Congo red (stains amyloid), acid fast (Ziehl-Neelsen, Fite) (stains acid-fast bacilli), periodic acid-Schiff (PAS, stains high carbohydrate content molecules), Gram stain (stains bacteria), trichrome (stains cells and connective tissue), and reticulin (stains collagen type III molecules).

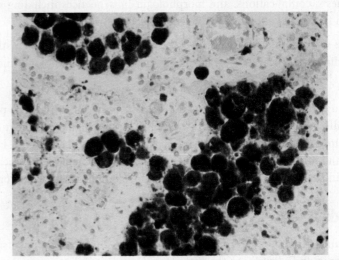

© Katsumi M. Miyai, M.D., Ph.D.; Regents of the University of California. Used with permission.

Figure 1-1. Prussian Blue Stain Showing Hemosiderin, Which Results from RBC Breakdown Within Macrophages

- **Immunohistochemical (antibody) stains** include cytokeratin (stains epithelial cells), vimentin (stains cells of mesenchymal origin except the 3 muscle types; stains many sarcomas), desmin (stains smooth, cardiac, and skeletal myosin), prostate specific antigen, and many others.

Ancillary techniques include **immunofluorescence microscopy (IFM)**, typically used for renal and autoimmune disease, and **transmission electron microscopy (EM)**, used for renal disease, neoplasms, infections, and genetic disorders.

Molecular techniques include protein electrophoresis, Southern and Western blots, polymerase chain reaction (PCR), and cytogenetic analysis (karyotyping, in situ hybridization studies).

Chapter Summary

- Pathology is the study of disease and concerns itself with the etiology, pathogenesis, morphologic changes, and clinical significance of different diseases.

- Gross examination of organs involves identifying pathologic lesions by evaluating abnormalities of size, shape, consistency, and color.

- Tissue sections stained with hematoxylin (nucleic acids and calcium salts) and eosin (most proteins) are used for routine light microscopic examination.

- Additional techniques that pathologists use to clarify diagnoses include histochemical stains, immunohistochemical stains, immunofluorescence microscopy, transmission electron microscopy, and molecular techniques.

Cellular Injury and Adaptation | 2

Learning Objectives

❏ Explain causes of cellular injury

❏ Demonstrate understanding of cellular changes during injury and cell death

❏ Answer questions about cellular adaptive responses to injury

❏ Describe cellular alterations during injury

CAUSES OF CELLULAR INJURY

Hypoxia is the most common cause of injury; it occurs when lack of oxygen prevents the cell from synthesizing sufficient ATP by aerobic oxidation. Major mechanisms leading to hypoxia are ischemia, cardiopulmonary failure, and decreased oxygen-carrying capacity of the blood (e.g., anemia). **Ischemia**, due to a loss of blood supply, is the most common cause of hypoxia, and is typically related to decreased arterial flow or decreased venous outflow (e.g., atherosclerosis, thrombus, thromboembolus).

Pathogens (viruses, bacteria, parasites, fungi, and prions) can injure the body by direct infection of cells, production of toxins, or host inflammatory response.

Immunologic dysfunction includes hypersensitivity reactions and autoimmune diseases.

Congenital disorders are inherited genetic mutations (e.g., inborn errors of metabolism).

Chemical injury can occur with drugs, poisons (cyanide, arsenic, mercury, etc.), pollution, occupational exposure (CCl_4, asbestos, carbon monoxide, etc.), and social/lifestyle choices (alcohol, smoking, IV drug abuse, etc.)

Physical forms of injury include trauma (blunt/penetrating/crush injuries, gunshot wounds, etc.), burns, frostbite, radiation, and pressure changes.

Nutritional or vitamin imbalance

- **Inadequate calorie/protein intake** can cause marasmus (decrease in total caloric intake), and kwashiorkor (decrease in total protein intake).

- **Excess caloric intake** can cause obesity (second leading cause of premature preventable death in the United States) and atherosclerosis.

- **Vitamin deficiencies** can be seen with vitamin A (night blindness, squamous metaplasia, immune deficiency), vitamin C (scurvy), vitamin D (rickets and osteomalacia), vitamin K (bleeding diathesis), vitamin B12 (megaloblastic anemia, neuropathy, and spinal cord degeneration), folate (megaloblastic anemia and neural tube defects), and niacin (pellagra [diarrhea, dermatitis, and dementia]).

- **Hypervitaminosis** is less commonly a problem but can result in tissue specific abnormalities.

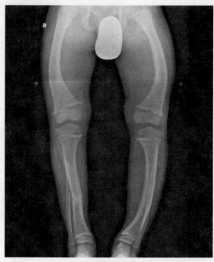

© Dr. Angela Byrne, Radiopaedia.org.
Used with permission.

Figure 2-1. Radiograph of a Child with Rickets Shows Bowed Legs

CELLULAR CHANGES DURING INJURY

Cellular responses to injury include adaptation (hypertrophy or atrophy, hyperplasia or metaplasia), reversible injury, and irreversible injury and cell death (necrosis, apoptosis, or necroptosis).

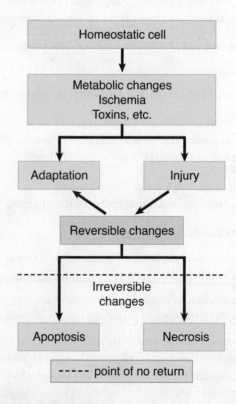

Figure 2-2. Cellular Response to Stress and Injurious Stimuli

The **cellular response to injury depends on several important factors**, including the type of injury, duration (including pattern) of injury, severity and intensity of injury, type of cell injured, the cell's metabolic state, and the cell's ability to adapt.

The **critical intracellular targets that are susceptible to injury** are DNA, production of ATP via aerobic respiration, cell membranes, and protein synthesis.

Important mechanisms of cell injury are as follows:

- Damage to DNA, proteins, lipid membranes, and circulating lipids (LDL) can be caused by oxygen-derived free radicals, including superoxide anion ($O_2^{\bullet-}$), hydroxyl radical ($OH^\bullet$), and hydrogen peroxide (H_2O_2).

- ATP depletion: Several key biochemical pathways are dependent on ATP. Disruption of Na^+/K^+ or Ca^{++} pumps cause imbalances in solute concentrations. Additionally, ATP depletion increases anaerobic glycolysis that leads to a decrease in cellular pH. Chronic ATP depletion causes morphological and functional changes to the ER and ribosomes.

- Increased cell membrane permeability: Several defects can lead to movement of fluids into the cell, including formation of the membrane attack complex via complement, breakdown of Na+/K+ gradients (i.e., causing sodium to enter or potassium to leave the cell), etc.

- Influx of calcium can cause problems because calcium is a second messenger, which can activate a wide spectrum of enzymes. These enzymes include proteases (protein breakdown), ATPases (contributes to ATP depletion), phospholipases (cell membrane injury), and endonucleases (DNA damage).

- Mitochondrial dysfunction causes decreased oxidative phosphorylation and ATP production, formation of mitochondrial permeability transition (MPT) channels, and release of cytochrome c (a trigger for apoptosis).

Note

Protective Factors against free radicals include:

- Antioxidants
  Vitamins A, E, and C
- Superoxide dismutase
  Superoxide → hydrogen peroxide
- Glutathione peroxidase
  Hydroxyl ions or hydrogen peroxide → water
- Catalase
  Hydrogen peroxide → oxygen and water

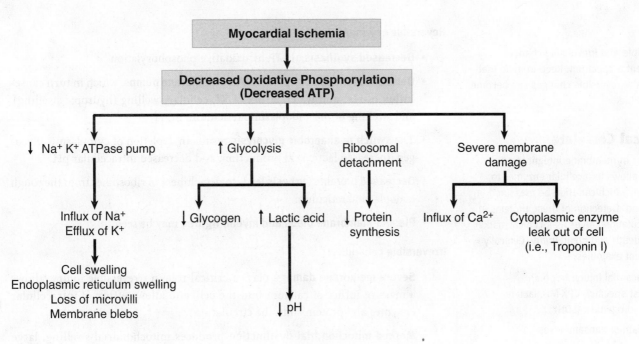

Figure 2-3. Classic Example of Cellular Injury Caused by Hypoxia

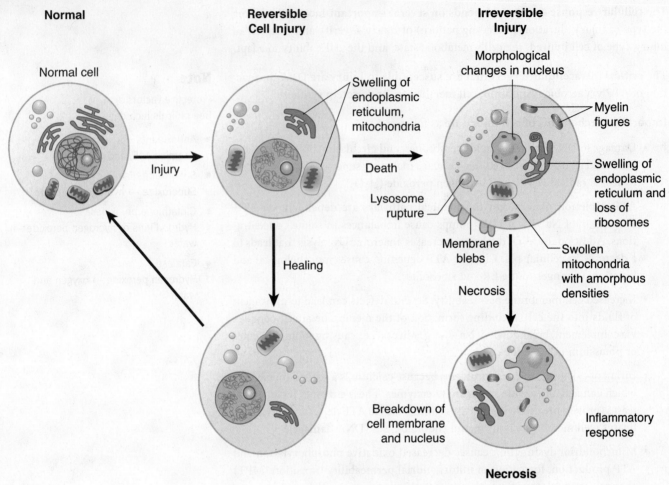

Figure 2-4. Cell Injury

Note

Reversible and irreversible changes represent a spectrum. Keep in mind that any of the reversible changes can become irreversible.

Clinical Correlate

The loss of membrane integrity (cell death) allows intracellular enzymes to leak out, which can then be measured in the blood. Detection of these proteins in the circulation serves as a clinical marker of cell death and organ injury. Clinically important examples:

- Myocardial injury: troponin (most specific), CPK-MB, lactate dehydrogenase (LDH)
- Hepatitis: transaminases
- Pancreatitis: amylase and lipase
- Biliary tract obstruction: alkaline phosphatase

Reversible cell injury:

- **Decreased synthesis of ATP** by oxidative phosphorylation.

- **Decreased function of Na+K+ ATPase membrane pumps**, which in turn causes influx of Na$^+$ and water, efflux of K$^+$, cellular swelling (hydropic swelling), and swelling of the endoplasmic reticulum.

- The **switch to anaerobic glycolysis** results in depletion of cytoplasmic glycogen, increased lactic acid production, and decreased intracellular pH.

- **Decreased protein synthesis** leads to detachment of ribosomes from the rough endoplasmic reticulum.

- **Plasma-membrane blebs and myelin figures** may be seen.

Irreversible cell injury:

- **Severe membrane damage** plays a critical role in irreversible injury, allows a massive influx of calcium into the cell, and allows efflux of intracellular enzymes and proteins into the circulation.

- **Marked mitochondrial dysfunction** produces mitochondrial swelling, large densities seen within the mitochondrial matrix, irreparable damage of the oxidative phosphorylation pathway, and an inability to produce ATP.

- **Rupture of the lysosomes** causes release of lysosomal digestive enzymes into the cytosol and activation of acid hydrolases followed by autolysis.

- **Nuclear changes** can include pyknosis (degeneration and condensation of nuclear chromatin), karyorrhexis (nuclear fragmentation), and karyolysis (dissolution of the nucleus).

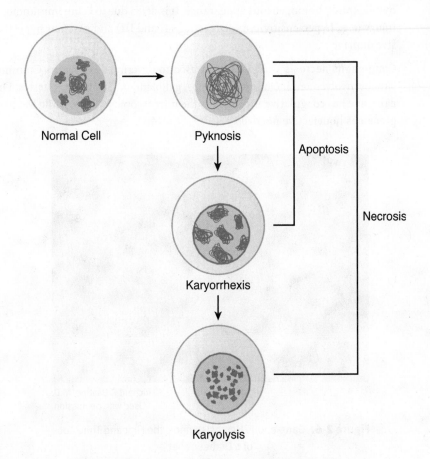

Normal Cell   Pyknosis

Apoptosis

Necrosis

Karyorrhexis

Karyolysis

Figure 2-5. Nuclear Changes in Irreversible Cell Injury

CELL DEATH

Morphologic types of necrosis (cell death in living tissue, often with an inflammatory response) are as follows:

- **Coagulative necrosis**, the most common form of necrosis, is most often due to ischemic injury (infarct). It is caused by the denaturing of proteins within the cytoplasm. Microscopic examination shows loss of the nucleus but preservation of cellular shape. Coagulative necrosis is common in most organs, including the heart, liver, and kidney, but not the brain.

- **Liquefaction necrosis** results from cellular destruction by hydrolytic enzymes, leading to autolysis (release of proteolytic enzymes from injured cells) and heterolysis (release of proteolytic enzymes from inflammatory cells). Liquefaction necrosis occurs in abscesses, brain infarcts, and pancreatic necrosis.

- **Caseous necrosis** is a combination of coagulation and liquefaction necrosis. The gross appearance is soft, friable, and "cheese-like." Caseous necrosis is characteristic of granulomatous diseases, including tuberculosis.

Note

Liquefaction by leukocyte enzymes is called suppuration, and the resultant fluid is called pus.

Bridge to Biochemistry

Damage to fat cells releases triglycerides. The triglycerides are broken down by the action of lipases to fatty acids. The fatty acids may associate with calcium and form calcium soaps (saponification).

Note

Necrotic tissue within the body evokes an inflammatory response that removes the dead tissue and is followed by healing and tissue repair. Necrotic debris may also undergo dystrophic calcification.

- **Fat necrosis** is caused by the action of lipases on adipocytes and is characteristic of acute pancreatitis. On gross examination fat necrosis has a chalky white appearance.

- **Fibrinoid necrosis** is a form of necrotic connective tissue that histologically resembles fibrin. On microscopic examination fibrinoid necrosis has an eosinophilic (pink) homogeneous appearance. It is often due to acute immunologic injury (e.g., hypersensitivity type reactions II and III) and vascular hypertensive damage.

- **Gangrenous necrosis** is a gross term used to describe dead tissue. Common sites of involvement include lower limbs, gallbladder, GI tract, and testes. Dry gangrene has coagulative necrosis for the microscopic pattern, while wet gangrene has liquefactive necrosis.

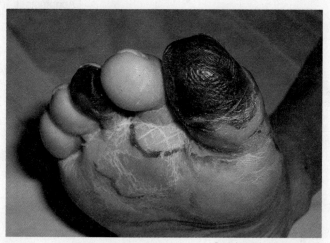

© Richard P. Usatine, M.D.
Used with permission.

Figure 2-6. Gangrenous Necrosis Affects the First and Third Toes of a Diabetic Foot

Clinical Correlate

- If the cells in the interdigital space fail to undergo apoptosis, the fetus will be born with webbed hands and/or webbed feet, a condition known as *syndactyly*.

- Another example is the hormone-dependent apoptosis prior to menstruation; programmed cell death plays a role in endometrial gland morphological changes.

Apoptosis is a specialized form of programmed cell death without an inflammatory response. It is an active process regulated by proteins that often affects only single cells or small groups of cells.

- In **morphologic appearance,** the cell shrinks in size and has dense eosinophilic cytoplasm. Next, nuclear chromatin condensation (pyknosis) is seen that is followed by fragmentation of the nucleus (karyorrhexis). Cytoplasmic membrane blebs form next, leading eventually to a breakdown of the cell into fragments (apoptotic bodies). Phagocytosis of apoptotic bodies is by adjacent cells or macrophages.

- **Stimuli for apoptosis** include cell injury and DNA damage, lack of hormones, cytokines, or growth factors, and receptor-ligand signals such as Fas binding to the Fas ligand and tumor necrosis factor (TNF) binding to TNF receptor 1 (TNFR1).

- **Apoptosis is regulated by proteins.** The protein bcl-2 (which inhibits apoptosis) prevents release of cytochrome c from mitochondria and binds pro-apoptotic protease activating factor (Apaf-1). The protein p53 (which stimulates apoptosis) is elevated by DNA injury and arrests the cell cycle. If DNA repair is impossible, p53 stimulates apoptosis.

- **Execution of apoptosis** is mediated by a cascade of caspases (cysteine aspartic acid proteases). The caspases digest nuclear and cytoskeletal proteins and also activate endonucleases.

- **Physiologic examples of apoptosis** include embryogenesis (organogenesis and development), hormone-dependent apoptosis (menstrual cycle), thymus (selective death of lymphocytes).

- **Pathologic examples of apoptosis** include viral diseases (viral hepatitis [Councilman body]), graft-versus-host disease, and cystic fibrosis (duct obstruction and pancreatic atrophy).

Serum enzyme markers of cell damage include aspartate aminotransferase (AST) (liver injury), alanine aminotransferase (ALT) (liver injury), creatine kinase (CK-MB) (heart injury), and amylase and lipase (pancreatic injury; amylase also rises with salivary gland injury).

Clinical Correlate

Graft-versus-host disease (GVHD) is an example of apoptosis which occurs in allogeneic hematopoietic stem cell transplant recipients. The transplanted marrow has cytotoxic T-cells which recognize the new host proteins (usually HLA) as foreign. Organs typically involved include the skin, mucosa, liver, and GI tract. The histologic hallmark of GVHD is apoptosis.

CELLULAR ADAPTIVE RESPONSES TO INJURY

In general, cellular adaptation is a potentially reversible change in response to the environment.

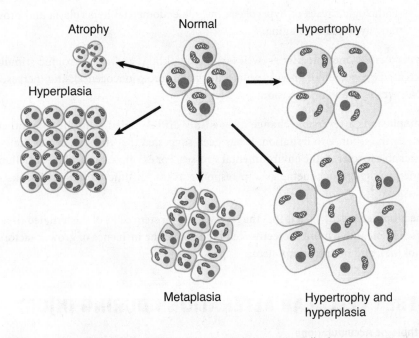

Figure 2-7. Cellular Adaptive Responses to Cell Injury

Atrophy is a decrease in cell/organ size and functional ability. Causes of atrophy include decreased workload/disuse (immobilization); ischemia (atherosclerosis); lack of hormonal or neural stimulation, malnutrition, and aging.

Light microscopic examination shows small shrunken cells with lipofuscin granules. Electron microscopy shows decreased intracellular components and autophagosomes.

Hypertrophy is an increase in cell size and functional ability due to increased synthesis of intracellular components.

Causes of hypertrophy include:

- Increased mechanical demand can be physiologic (striated muscle of weight lifters) or pathologic (cardiac muscle in hypertension).

- Increased endocrine stimulation plays a role in puberty (growth hormone, androgens/estrogens, etc.), gravid uterus (estrogen), and lactating breast (prolactin and estrogen).

Hypertrophy is mediated by growth factors, cytokines, and other trophic stimuli and leads to increased expression of genes and increased protein synthesis.

Hypertrophy and hyperplasia often occur together.

Clinical Correlate

Residence at high altitude, where oxygen content of air is relatively low, leads to compensatory hyperplasia of red blood cell precursors in the bone marrow and an increase in the number of circulating red blood cells (secondary polycythemia).

Hyperplasia is an increase in the number of cells in a tissue or organ. Some cell types are unable to exhibit hyperplasia (e.g., nerve, cardiac, skeletal muscle cells).

- Physiologic causes of hyperplasia include compensatory mechanisms (e.g., after partial hepatectomy), hormonal stimulation (e.g., breast development at puberty), and antigenic stimulation (e.g., lymphoid hyperplasia).

- Pathologic causes of hyperplasia include endometrial hyperplasia and prostatic hyperplasia of aging.

Hyperplasia is mediated by growth factors, cytokines, and other trophic stimuli; increased expression of growth-promoting genes (proto-oncogenes); and increased DNA synthesis and cell division.

Clinical Correlate

Barrett's esophagus is a classic example of metaplasia. The esophageal epithelium is normally squamous, but it undergoes a change to intestinal epithelium (columnar) when it is under constant contact with gastric acid.

Metaplasia is a reversible change of one fully differentiated cell type to another, usually in response to irritation. It has been suggested that the replacement cell is better able to tolerate the environmental stresses. For example, bronchial epithelium undergoes squamous metaplasia in response to the chronic irritation of tobacco smoke.

The proposed mechanism is that the reserve cells (or stem cells) of the irritated tissue differentiate into a more protective cell type due to the influence of growth factors, cytokines, and matrix components.

OTHER CELLULAR ALTERATIONS DURING INJURY

Pathologic Accumulations

- **Lipids** that can accumulate intracellularly include triglycerides (e.g., fatty change in liver cells), cholesterol (e.g., atherosclerosis, xanthomas), and complex lipids (e.g., sphingolipid accumulation).

- **Proteins** can accumulate in proximal renal tubules in proteinuria and can form Russell bodies (intracytoplasmic accumulation of immunoglobulins) in plasma cells.

- **Glycogen storage diseases** (*See* Genetic Disorders chapter.)

- **Exogenous pigments** include anthracotic pigmentation of the lung (secondary to the inhalation of carbon dust), tattoos, and lead that has been ingested (e.g., gingival lead line, renal tubular lead deposits).

Endogenous pigments

- **Lipofuscin** is a wear-and-tear pigment that is seen as perinuclear yellow-brown pigment. It is due to indigestible material within lysosomes and is common in the liver and heart.

- **Melanin** is a black-brown pigment derived from tyrosine found in melanocytes and substantia nigra.

- **Hemosiderin** is a golden yellow-brown granular pigment found in areas of hemorrhage or bruises. Systemic iron overload can lead to hemosiderosis (increase in total body iron stores without tissue injury) or hemochromatosis (increase in total body iron stores with tissue injury). Prussian blue stain can identify the iron in the hemosiderin.

- **Bilirubin** accumulates in newborns in the basal ganglia, causing permanent damage (kernicterus).

Hyaline change is a nonspecific term used to describe any intracellular or extracellular alteration that has a pink homogenous appearance (proteins) on H&E stains.

- Examples of **intracellular hyaline** include renal proximal tubule protein reabsorption droplets, Russell bodies, and alcoholic hyaline.

- Examples of **extracellular hyaline** include hyaline arteriolosclerosis, amyloid, and hyaline membrane disease of the newborn.

Pathologic forms of calcification

- **Dystrophic calcification** is the precipitation of calcium phosphate in dying or necrotic tissues. Examples include fat necrosis (saponification), psammoma bodies (laminated calcifications that occur in meningiomas and papillary carcinomas of the thyroid and ovary), Mönckeberg medial calcific sclerosis in arterial walls, and atherosclerotic plaques.

- **Metastatic calcification** is the precipitation of calcium phosphate in normal tissue due to hypercalcemia (supersaturated solution). The many causes include hyperparathyroidism, parathyroid adenomas, renal failure, paraneoplastic syndrome, vitamin D intoxication, milk-alkali syndrome, sarcoidosis, Paget disease, multiple myeloma, metastatic cancer to the bone. The calcifications are located in the interstitial tissues of the stomach, kidneys, lungs, and blood vessels.

Chapter Summary

- Causes of cellular injury include hypoxia, pathogens, hypersensitivity reactions, autoimmune diseases, congenital disorders, chemical injury, physical injury, and nutritional imbalance.

- The response of cells to an insult depends on both the state of the cell and the type of insult. The response can range from adaptation to reversible injury to irreversible injury with cell death.

- Intracellular sites and systems particularly vulnerable to injury include DNA, ATP production, cell membranes, and protein synthesis.

- Reversible cell injury is primarily related to decreased ATP synthesis by oxidative phosphorylation, leading to cellular swelling and inadequate protein synthesis. Irreversible cell injury often additionally involves severe damage to membranes, mitochondria, lysosomes, and nucleus.

- Death of tissues (necrosis) can produce a variety of histologic patterns, including coagulative necrosis, liquefaction necrosis, caseous necrosis, fibrinoid necrosis, and gangrenous necrosis, often with an inflammatory response.

- Apoptosis is a specialized form of programmed cell death that can be regulated genetically or by cellular or tissue triggers without an inflammatory response.

- Cellular adaptive responses to injury include atrophy, hypertrophy, hyperplasia, and metaplasia. Other cellular alterations secondary to injury include pathologic accumulations (lipids, proteins, pigments), hyaline change, and pathologic calcification.

Inflammation 3

Learning Objectives

❏ Solve problems concerning acute and chronic inflammation

❏ Describe tissue responses to infectious agents

ACUTE INFLAMMATION

Acute inflammation is an immediate response to injury or infection, which is part of innate immunity.

- Short duration in normal host

- Cardinal signs of inflammation include rubor (redness); calor (heat); tumor (swelling); dolor (pain); functio laesa (loss of function).

The important components of acute inflammation are hemodynamic changes, **neutrophils**, and chemical mediators.

Hemodynamic Changes

- Initial transient vasoconstriction

- Massive vasodilatation mediated by histamine, bradykinin, and prostaglandins

- Increased vascular permeability

  ○ Chemical mediators of increased permeability include vasoactive amines (histamine and serotonin), bradykinin (an end-product of the kinin cascade), leukotrienes (e.g., LTC4, LTD4, LTE4).

  ○ The mechanism of increased vascular permeability involves endothelial cell and pericyte contraction; direct endothelial cell injury; and leukocyte injury of endothelium.

- Blood flow slows (stasis) due to increased viscosity, allows neutrophils to marginate

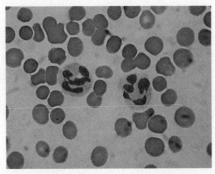

Source: commons.wikimedia.org (Mgiganteus)

Lobed nucleus, small granules

Neutrophil

Neutrophils

- Life span in tissue 1–2 days

- Synonyms: segmented neutrophils, polymorphonuclear leukocytes (PMN)

- Primary (azurophilic) granules contain myeloperoxidase, phospholipase A2, lysozyme (damages bacterial cell walls by catalyzing hydrolysis of 1,4-beta-linkages), and acid hydrolases. Also present are elastase, defensins (microbicidal peptides active against many gram-negative and gram-positive bacteria, fungi, and enveloped viruses), and bactericidal permeability increasing protein (BPI).

- Secondary (specific) granules contain phospholipase A2, lysozyme, leukocyte alkaline phosphatase (LAP), collagenase, lactoferrin (chelates iron), and vitamin B12-binding proteins.

- **Macrophages** (life span in tissue compartment is 60–120 days) have acid hydrolases, elastase, and collagenase.

Neutrophil margination and adhesion. Adhesion is mediated by complementary molecules on the surface of neutrophils and endothelium.

- In **step 1**, the endothelial cells at sites of inflammation have increased expression of *E-selectin* and *P-selectin*.

- In **step 2**, neutrophils weakly bind to the endothelial selectins and roll along the surface.

- In **step 3**, neutrophils are stimulated by chemokines to express their integrins.

- In **step 4**, binding of the integrins to cellular adhesion molecules (ICAM-1 and VCAM-1) allows the neutrophils to firmly adhere to the endothelial cell.

Clinical Correlate

- A normal mature neutrophil has a segmented nucleus (3–4 segments).
- Hypersegmented neutrophils (>5 segments) are thought to be pathognomonic of the class of anemias called megaloblastic anemias (vitamin B12 or folate deficiencies).

Note

Selectins: weak binding; initiate rolling

Integrins: stable binding and adhesion

Table 3-1. Selectin and Integrin Distribution in the Endothelium and Leukocyte

	Endothelium	Leukocyte
Selectins	P-Selectin	Sialyl-Lewis X & PSGL-1
	E-Selectin	Sialyl-Lewis X & PSGL-1
	GlyCam-1/CD34	L-Selectin
Integrins	ICAM-1	LFA-1 & MAC-1
	VCAM-1	VLA-4

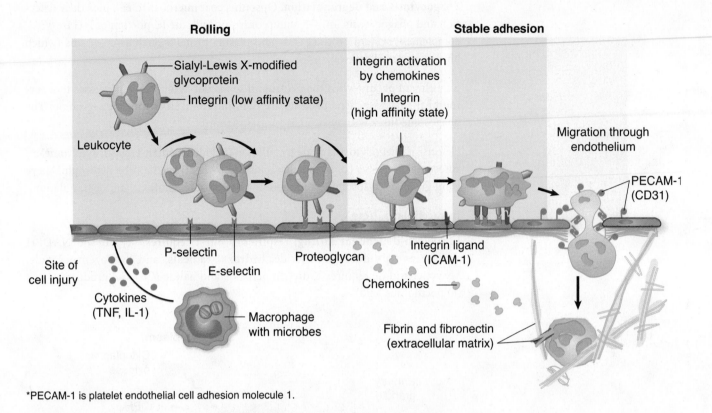

Figure 3-1. Adhesion and Migration

*PECAM-1 is platelet endothelial cell adhesion molecule 1.

Modulation of adhesion molecules in inflammation occurs as follows. The fastest step involves redistribution of adhesion molecules to the surface; for example, P-selectin is normally present in the Weibel-Palade bodies of endothelial cells and can be mobilized to the cell surface by exposure to inflammatory mediators such as histamine and thrombin.

- Additionally, synthesis of adhesion molecules occurs. For example, proinflammatory cytokines IL-1 and TNF induce production of E-selectin, ICAM-1, and VCAM-1 in endothelial cells.

- There can also be increased binding affinity, as when chemotactic agents cause a conformational change in the leukocyte integrin LFA-1, which is converted to a high-affinity binding state.

Defects in adhesion can be seen in diabetes mellitus, corticosteroid use, acute alcohol intoxication, and leukocyte adhesion deficiency (autosomal recessive condition with recurrent bacterial infections).

In **emigration (diapedesis),** leukocytes emigrate from the vasculature (postcapillary venule) by extending pseudopods between the endothelial cells. They then move between the endothelial cells, migrating through the basement membrane toward the inflammatory stimulus.

Chemotaxis is the attraction of cells toward a chemical mediator that is released in the area of inflammation. Important chemotactic factors for neutrophils include bacterial products such as *N*-formyl-methionine and host derived molecules such as leukotriene B4 (LTB4), complement system product C5a, and α-chemokines (IL-8).

Clinical Correlate

Leukocyte adhesion deficiency type I

- Autosomal recessive
- Deficiency of β2 integrin subunit (CD18)
- Recurrent bacterial infection
- Delay in umbilical cord sloughing

Phagocytosis and degranulation. Opsonins coat microbes to enhance their detection and phagocytosis. Important opsonins include the Fc portion of IgG isotypes, complement system product C3b, and plasma proteins such as collectins (which bind to bacterial cell walls).

Engulfment occurs when the neutrophil sends out cytoplasmic processes that surround the bacteria. The bacteria are then internalized within a phagosome. The phagosome fuses with lysosomes (degranulation).

Defects in phagocytosis and degranulation include Chédiak-Higashi syndrome, an autosomal recessive condition characterized by neutropenia. The neutrophils have giant granules (lysosomes) and there is a defect in chemotaxis and degranulation.

Intracellular killing.

In oxygen-dependent killing, respiratory burst requires oxygen and NADPH oxidase and produces superoxide, hydroxyl radicals, and hydrogen peroxide. Myeloperoxidase requires hydrogen peroxide and halide (Cl^-) and produces HOCl (hypochlorous acid).

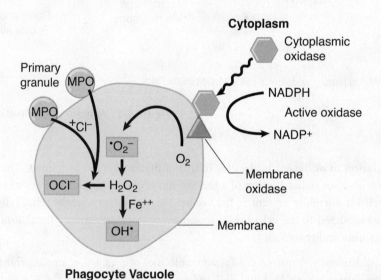

Figure 3-2. Oxygen-Dependent Killing

Oxygen-independent killing involves lysozyme, lactoferrin, acid hydrolases, bactericidal permeability increasing protein (BPI), and defensins.

Deficiencies of oxygen-dependent killing include:

- Chronic granulomatous disease of childhood can be X-linked or autosomal recessive. It is characterized by a deficiency of NADPH oxidase, lack of superoxide and hydrogen peroxide, and recurrent bacterial infections with catalase-positive organisms (*S. aureus*). The nitroblue tetrazolium test will be negative.

- Myeloperoxidase deficiency is an autosomal recessive condition characterized by infections with *Candida*. In contrast to chronic granulomatous disease, the nitroblue tetrazolium test will be positive.

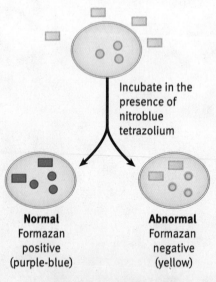

Normal
Formazan
positive
(purple-blue)

Abnormal
Formazan
negative
(yellow)

Incubate in the presence of nitroblue tetrazolium

Nitroblue Tetrazolium Reduction

Chemical Mediators of Inflammation

Vasoactive amines

- **Histamine** is produced by basophils, platelets, and mast cells. It causes vasodilation and increased vascular permeability. Triggers for release include IgE-mediated mast cell reactions, physical injury, anaphylatoxins (C3a and C5a), and cytokines (IL-1).

- **Serotonin** is produced by platelets and causes vasodilation and increased vascular permeability.

Kinin system

- Activated Hageman factor (factor XII) converts prekallikrein → kallikrein

- Kallikrein cleaves high molecular weight kininogen (HMWK) → bradykinin

- Effects of bradykinin include increased vascular permeability, pain, vasodilation, bronchoconstriction, and pain

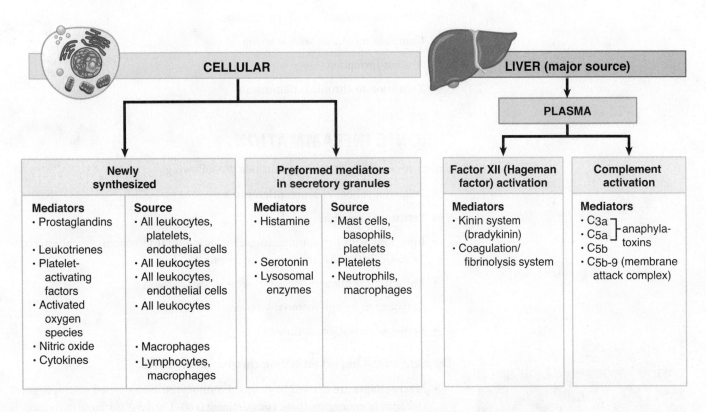

Figure 3-3. Sources of Chemical Mediators of Inflammation

Arachidonic acid products

- **Cyclooxygenase pathway**

  ○ Thromboxane A2 is produced by platelets and causes vasoconstriction and platelet aggregation.

  ○ Prostacyclin (PGI2) is produced by vascular endothelium and causes vasodilation and inhibition of platelet aggregation.

  ○ Prostaglandin E_2 causes pain.

  ○ Prostaglandins PGE2, PGD2, and PGF2 cause vasodilatation.

In a Nutshell
Mediators of Pain

- Bradykinin
- Prostaglandins (E_2)

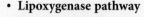

- **Lipoxygenase pathway**

  Leukotriene B4 (LTB4) causes neutrophil chemotaxis, while leukotriene C4, D4, E4 cause vasoconstriction. Lipoxins are antiinflammatory products which inhibit neutrophil chemotaxis.

Important products in the complement cascade include C5b-C9 (membrane attack complex), C3a,C5a (anaphylatoxins stimulate the release of histamine), C5a (leukocyte chemotactic factor), and C3b (opsonin for phagocytosis).

Cytokines

- IL-1 and TNF cause fever and induce acute phase reactants; enhance adhesion molecules; and stimulate and activate fibroblasts, endothelial cells, and neutrophils.

- IL-8 is a neutrophil chemoattractant produced by macrophages.

Four Outcomes of Acute Inflammation

- Complete resolution with regeneration

- Complete resolution with scarring

- Abscess formation

- Transition to chronic inflammation

CHRONIC INFLAMMATION

Causes of chronic inflammation include the following:

- Following a bout of acute inflammation

- Persistent infections

- Infections with certain organisms, including viral infections, mycobacteria, parasitic infections, and fungal infections

- Autoimmune diseases

- Response to foreign material

- Response to malignant tumors

There are several **important cells** in chronic inflammation.

- **Macrophages** are derived from blood monocytes. Tissue-based macrophages (life span in connective tissue compartment is 60–120 days) are found in connective tissue (histiocyte), lung (pulmonary alveolar macrophages), liver (Kupffer cells), bone (osteoclasts), and brain (microglia). During inflammation circulating monocytes emigrate from the blood to the periphery and differentiate into macrophages.

  ° Respond to chemotactic factors: C5a, MCP-1, MIP-1α, PDGF, TGF-β

  ° Secrete a wide variety of active products (monokines)

  ° May be modified into epithelioid cells in granulomatous processes

- **Lymphocytes** include B cells and plasma cells, as well as T cells. Lymphotaxin is the lymphocyte chemokine.

In a Nutshell
Mediators of Fever

- Cytokines IL-1, IL-6, and TNF-α
- Prostaglandins

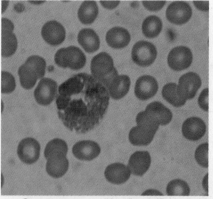

Source: commons.wikimedia.org (Bobjgalindo)

Bilobed nucleus, large granules (pink)

Eosinophil

- **Eosinophils** play an important role in parasitic infections and IgE-mediated allergic reactions. The eosinophilic chemokine is eotaxin. Eosinophil granules contain major basic protein, which is toxic to parasites.

- **Basophils** contain similar chemical mediators as mast cells in their granules. Mast cells are present in high numbers in the lung and skin. Both basophils and mast cells play an important role in IgE-mediated reactions (allergies and anaphylaxis) and can release histamine.

Chronic granulomatous inflammation is a specialized form of chronic inflammation characterized by small aggregates of modified macrophages (epithelioid cells and multinucleated giant cells) usually populated by CD4+ Th1 lymphocytes.

Composition of a granuloma is as follows:

- Epithelioid cells, located centrally, form when IFN-γ transforms macrophages to epithelioid cells. They are enlarged cells with abundant pink cytoplasm.

- Multinucleated giant cells, located centrally, are formed by the fusion of epithelioid cells. Types include Langhans-type giant cell (peripheral arrangement of nuclei) and foreign body type giant cell (haphazard arrangement of nuclei).

- Lymphocytes and plasma cells are present at the periphery.

- Central necrosis occurs in granulomata due to excessive enzymatic breakdown and is commonly seen in *Mycobacterium tuberculosis* infection as well as fungal infections and a few bacterial infections. Because of the public health risk of tuberculosis, necrotizing granulomas should be considered tuberculosis until proven otherwise.

Bilobed nucleus, large granules (blue)

Basophil

Clinical Correlate

Patients who are to be placed on tumor necrosis factor (TNF) inhibitors such as infliximab must undergo a PPD test before starting therapy. The PPD checks for latent tuberculosis infection, which can be reactivated by the TNF alpha inhibitor.

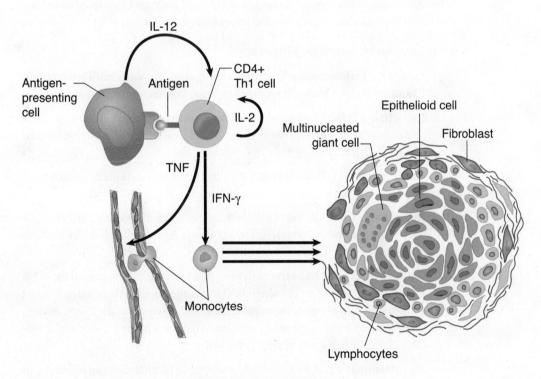

Figure 3-4. Granuloma Formation

Granulomatous diseases include tuberculosis (caseating granulomas), cat-scratch fever, syphilis, leprosy, fungal infections (e.g., coccidioidomycosis), parasitic infections (e.g., schistosomiasis), foreign bodies, beryllium, and sarcoidosis.

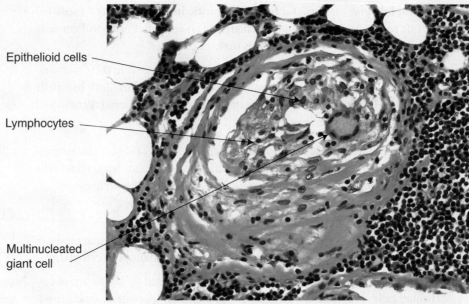

Epithelioid cells

Lymphocytes

Multinucleated
giant cell

© Henry Sanchez, M.D.
Used with permission.

Figure 3-5. A Granuloma Is Seen in the Large,
Poorly Circumscribed Nodule in the Center of the Field

TISSUE RESPONSES TO INFECTIOUS AGENTS

Infectious diseases are very prevalent worldwide and are a major cause of morbidity and mortality. Infectious agents tend to have **tropism** for specific tissues and organs.

There are **6 major histologic patterns:**

- **Exudative inflammation** is acute inflammatory response with neutrophils. Examples include bacterial meningitis, bronchopneumonia, and abscess.

- **Necrotizing inflammation** occurs when a virulent organism produces severe tissue damage and extensive cell death. Examples include necrotizing fasciitis and necrotizing pharyngitis.

- **Granulomatous inflammation.** Granulomatous response predominates with slow-growing organisms such as mycobacteria, fungi, and parasites.

- **Interstitial inflammation** is a diffuse mononuclear interstitial infiltrate that is a common response to viral infectious agents. Examples include myocarditis (Coxsackie virus) and viral hepatitis.

- **Cytopathic/cytoproliferative** inflammation refers to inflammation in which the infected/injured cell is altered. The changes may include intranuclear/cytoplasmic inclusions (cytomegalic inclusion disease, rabies [Negri body]); syncytia formation (respiratory syncytial virus and herpes virus); and apoptosis (Councilman body in viral hepatitis).

- **No inflammation.** An inflammatory response to microbes cannot occur in severely immunosuppressed individuals due to primary immunodeficiencies or acquired immunodeficient states (e.g., AIDS).

Chapter Summary

- Acute inflammation is an immediate response to injury or infection that can cause redness, heat, swelling, pain, and loss of function.

- Hemodynamic changes in acute inflammation are mediated by vasoactive chemicals and, after a transient initial vasoconstriction, produce massive dilation with increased vascular permeability.

- Neutrophils are important WBCs in acute inflammation; they contain granules with many degradative enzymes. Neutrophils leave the bloodstream in a highly regulated process involving margination (moving toward the vessel wall), adhesion (binding to the endothelium), and emigration (moving between endothelial cells to leave the postcapillary venule). Defects in adhesion can contribute to the immunosuppression seen in diabetes mellitus and corticosteroid use.

- Chemotaxis is the attraction of cells toward a chemical mediator, which is released in the area of inflammation.

- The phagocytosis of bacteria by neutrophils is improved if opsonins, such as the Fc portion of immunoglobulin (Ig) G isotypes or the complement product C3B, are bound to the surface of the microbe. Chediak-Higashi syndrome is an example of a genetic disease with defective neutrophil degranulation.

- Once a bacterium has been phagocytized, both oxygen-requiring and oxygen-independent enzymes can contribute to the killing of the bacteria. Chronic granulomatous disease of childhood and myeloperoxidase deficiency are genetic immunodeficiencies related to defects in of oxygen-dependent killing.

- Chemical mediators of inflammation include vasoactive amines, the kinin system, arachidonic acid products, the complement cascade, and cytokines.

- Acute inflammation may result in tissue regeneration, scarring, abscess formation, or chronic inflammation.

- Cells important in chronic inflammation include macrophages, lymphocytes, eosinophils, and basophils.

- Chronic granulomatous inflammation is a specialized form of chronic inflammation with modified macrophages (epithelioid cells and multinucleated giant cells) usually surrounded by a rim of lymphocytes. A wide variety of diseases can cause chronic granulomatous inflammation, most notably TB, syphilis, leprosy, and fungal infections.

- Patterns of tissue response to infectious agents can include exudative inflammation, necrotizing inflammation, granulomatous inflammation, interstitial inflammation, and cytopathic/cytoproliferative inflammation.

Learning Objectives

❑ Demonstrate understanding of regeneration and healing

❑ Answer questions about aberrations in wound healing

REGENERATION AND HEALING

Regeneration and healing of damaged cells and tissues starts almost as soon as the inflammatory process begins. Tissue repair involves 5 overlapping processes:

- Hemostasis (coagulation, platelets)

- Inflammation (neutrophils, macrophages, lymphocytes, mast cells)

- Regeneration (stem cells and differentiated cells)

- Fibrosis (macrophages, granulation tissue [fibroblasts, angiogenesis], type III collagen)

- Remodeling (macrophages, fibroblasts, converting collagen III to I)

The extracellular matrix (ECM) is an important tissue scaffold with 2 forms, the interstitial matrix and the basement membrane (type IV collagen and laminin). There are 3 ECM components:

- Collagens and elastins

- Gels (proteoglycans and hyaluronan)

- Glycoproteins and cell adhesion molecules

Different tissues have different **regenerative** capacities.

- **Labile cells** (primarily stem cells) regenerate throughout life. Examples include surface epithelial cells (skin and mucosal lining cells), hematopoietic cells, stem cells, etc.

- **Stable cells** (stem cells and differentiated cells) replicate at a low level throughout life and have the capacity to divide if stimulated by some initiating event. Examples include hepatocytes, proximal tubule cells, endothelium, etc.

- **Permanent cells** (few stem cells and/or differentiated cells with the capacity to replicate) have a very low level of replicative capacity. Examples include neurons and cardiac muscle.

Scar formation occurs in a series of steps when repair cannot be effected by regeneration.

- Angiogenesis is promoted by vascular endothelial growth factor (VEGF) and the fibroblast growth factor (FGF) family of growth factors

- Platelet-derived growth factor (PDGF), fibroblast growth factor 2 (FGF-2), and transforming growth factor β (TGF-β) drive fibroblast activation

- TGF-β, PDGF, and FGF drive ECM deposition. Cytokines IL-1 and IL-13 stimulate collagen production.

Types of Wound Healing

Primary union (healing by first intention) occurs when wounds are closed physically with sutures, metal staples, dermal adhesive, etc.

Secondary union (healing by secondary intention) occurs when wounds are allowed to heal by wound contraction and is mediated by myofibroblasts at the edge of the wound.

Repair in specific organs occurs as follows:

- **Liver:** Mild injury is repaired by regeneration of hepatocytes, sometimes with restoration to normal pathology. Severe or persistent injury causes formation of regenerative nodules that may be surrounded by fibrosis, leading to hepatic cirrhosis.

- In the **brain**, neurons do not regenerate, but microglia remove debris and astrocytes proliferate, causing gliosis.

- Damaged **heart muscle** cannot regenerate, so the heart heals by fibrosis.

- In the **lung**, type II pneumocytes replace type I pneumocytes after injury.

- In **peripheral nerves**, the distal part of the axon degenerates while the proximal part regrows slowly, using axonal sprouts to follow Schwann cells to the muscle.

ABERRATIONS IN WOUND HEALING

- **Delayed wound healing** may be seen in wounds complicated by foreign bodies, infection, ischemia, diabetes, malnutrition, scurvy, etc.

- **Hypertrophic scar** results in a prominent scar that is localized to the wound, due to excess production of granulation tissue and collagen. It is common in burn patients.

- **Keloid formation** is a genetic predisposition that is common in African Americans. It tends to affect the earlobes, face, neck, sternum, and forearms, and it may produce large tumor-like scars extending beyond the injury site. There is excess production of collagen that is predominantly type III.

Note

Clinicians make decisions about wound healing techniques based on clinical information and the size of the tissue defect.

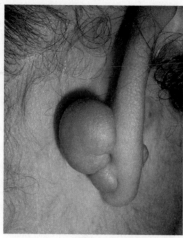

© Richard P. Usatine, M.D.
Used with permission.

Figure 4-1. Keloid on Posterior Surface of Ear (Auricle)

Chapter Summary

- Tissue repair involves regeneration of the damaged tissue by cells of the same type and healing with replacement by connective tissue.

- Tissue repair involves 5 overlapping processes: hemostasis, inflammation, regeneration, fibrosis, and remodeling.

- The extracellular matrix is an important tissue scaffold.

- Tissues vary in their regenerative capacities. Labile cell populations that regenerate throughout life include surface epithelial cells, hematopoietic cells, and stem cells. Stable cells that replicate at a low level through life, but can divide if stimulated, include hepatocytes, proximal tubule cells, and endothelial cells. Permanent cells that cannot replicate in adult life include neurons and cardiac muscle.

- Healing with replacement of a damaged area by a connective tissue scar is mediated by many growth factors and cytokines, primarily from macrophages. Initially granulation tissue forms, which later undergoes wound contraction mediated by myofibroblasts, eventually resulting in true scar formation.

- Wound healing by first intention (primary union) occurs after clean wounds have been physically closed, with sutures, for example. Wound healing by second intention (secondary union) relies on wound contraction by myofibroblasts.

- Problems that can occur with wound healing include delayed wound healing, hypertrophic scar formation, and keloid formation.

Circulatory Pathology

Learning Objectives

❏ Use knowledge of edema, hemostasis, and bleeding disorders to solve problems

❏ Answer questions about thrombosis, embolism, and infarction

❏ Solve problems concerning shock

Note
Edema can be localized or generalized, depending on the etiology and severity.

EDEMA

Edema is the presence of excess fluid in the intercellular space. It has many causes.

- **Increased hydrostatic pressure** causes edema in congestive heart failure (generalized edema), portal hypertension, renal retention of salt and water, and venous thrombosis (local edema).

- **Hypoalbuminemia and decreased colloid osmotic pressure** cause edema in liver disease, nephrotic syndrome, and protein deficiency (e.g., kwashiorkor).

- **Lymphatic obstruction** (lymphedema) causes edema in tumor, following surgical removal of lymph node drainage, and in parasitic infestation (filariasis → elephantiasis).

- **Increased endothelial permeability** causes edema in inflammation, type I hypersensitivity reactions, and with some drugs (e.g., bleomycin, heroin, etc.).

- **Increased interstitial sodium** causes edema when there is increased sodium intake, primary hyperaldosteronism, and renal failure.

- Specialized forms of tissue swelling due to **increased extracellular glycosaminoglycans** also occur, notably in pretibial myxedema and exophthalmos (Graves disease).

Anasarca is severe generalized edema. **Effusion** is fluid within the body cavities.

Types of Edema Fluid

- **Transudate** is edema fluid with low protein content.

- **Exudate** is edema fluid with high protein content and cells. Types of exudates include purulent (pus), fibrinous, eosinophilic, and hemorrhagic.

- **Lymphedema** related to lymphatic obstruction leads to accumulation of protein-rich fluid which produces a non-pitting edema.

- **Glycosaminoglycan-rich** edema fluid shows increased hyaluronic acid and chondroitin sulfate, and causes myxedema.

Active hyperemia versus congestion (passive hyperemia): an excessive amount of blood in a tissue or organ can accumulate secondary to vasodilatation (active, e.g., inflammation) or diminished venous outflow (passive, e.g., hepatic congestion).

HEMOSTASIS AND BLEEDING DISORDERS

Hemostasis is a sequence of events leading to the cessation of bleeding by the formation of a stable fibrin-platelet hemostatic plug. It involves interactions between the vascular wall, platelets, and the coagulation system.

Vascular Wall Injury

Transient vasoconstriction is mediated by endothelin-1. Thrombogenic factors include a variety of processes:

- Changes in blood flow cause turbulence and stasis favor clot formation.
- Release of tissue factor from injured cells activates factor VII (extrinsic pathway).
- Exposure of thrombogenic subendothelial collagen activates factor XII (intrinsic pathway).
- Release of von Willebrand factor (vWF) binds to exposed collagen and facilitates platelet adhesion.
- Decreased endothelial synthesis of antithrombogenic substances (prostacyclin, nitric oxide [NO_2], tissue plasminogin activator, and thrombomodulin)

Platelets

Platelets are derived from megakaryocytes in the bone marrow. They form a thrombus through a series of steps.

- **Step 1: Platelet adhesion** occurs when vWF adheres to subendothelial collagen and then platelets adhere to vWF by glycoprotein Ib.
- **Step 2: Platelet activation** occurs when platelets undergo a shape change and degranulation occurs. Platelets synthesize thromboxane A2. Platelets also show membrane expression of the phospholipid complex, which is an important substrate for the coagulation cascade.
- **Step 3: Platelet aggregation** occurs when additional platelets are recruited from the bloodstream. ADP and thromboxane A2 are potent mediators of aggregation. Platelets bind to each other by binding to fibrinogen using GPIIb-IIIa.

Laboratory tests for platelets include platelet count (normal 150,000–400,000 mm^3) and platelet aggregometry.

Bernard-Soulier syndrome and Glanzmann thrombasthenia present as mucocutaneous bleeding in childhood.

Table 5-1. Contents of Platelet Alpha Granules and Dense Bodies

Alpha Granules	Dense Bodies
• Fibrinogen	• ADP (potent platelet aggregator)
• Fibronectin	• Calcium
• Factor V and vWF	• Histamine and serotonin
• Platelet factor 4	• Epinephrine
• Platelet-derived growth factor (PDGF)	

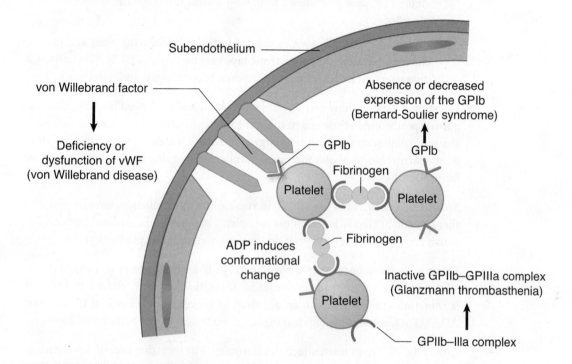

Figure 5-1. Platelet Aggregation

Table 5-2. Common Platelet Disorders

Thrombocytopenia	Qualitative Defects
Decreased production	• von Willebrand disease
• Aplastic anemia (drugs, virus, etc.)	• Bernard-Soulier syndrome
• Tumor	• Glanzmann thrombasthenia
	• Drugs (aspirin)
	• Uremia
Increased destruction	
• Immune thrombocytopenia (ITP)	
• Thrombotic thrombocytopenic purpura (TTP)	
• Disseminated intravascular coagulation (DIC)	
• Hypersplenism	

In a Nutshell

Glanzmann Thrombasthenia

- Autosomal recessive
- Defective GPIIb-IIIa receptor
- Defective platelet aggregation

Immune thrombocytopenia purpura (ITP) is an immune-mediated attack (usually IgG antiplatelet antibodies) against platelets leading to decreased platelets (thrombocytopenia) which result in petechiae, purpura (bruises), and a bleeding diathesis (e.g., hematomas).

The etiology involves antiplatelet antibodies against platelet antigens such as GPIIb-IIIa and GPIb-IX (type II hypersensitivity reaction). The antibodies are made in the spleen, and the platelets are destroyed peripherally in the spleen by macrophages, which have Fc receptors that bind IgG-coated platelets.

Forms of ITP include:

- Acute ITP, seen in children following a viral infection and is a self-limited disorder.
- Chronic ITP, usually seen in women in their childbearing years and may be the first manifestation of systemic lupus erythematosus (SLE). Clinically, it is characterized by petechiae, ecchymoses, menorrhagia, and nosebleeds.

Lab studies usually show decreased platelet count and prolonged bleeding time but normal prothrombin time and partial thromboplastin time. Peripheral blood smear shows thrombocytopenia with enlarged immature platelets (megathrombocytes). Bone marrow biopsy shows increased numbers of megakaryocytes with immature forms.

Treatment is corticosteroids, which decrease antibody production; immunoglobulin therapy, which floods Fc receptors on splenic macrophages; and/or splenectomy, which removes the site of platelet destruction and antibody production.

Thrombotic thrombocytopenic purpura (TTP) is a rare disorder of hemostasis in which there is widespread intravascular formation of fibrin-platelet thrombi. It is sometimes associated with an acquired or inherited deficiency of the enzyme ADAMTS13, responsible for cleaving large multimers of von Willebrand factor.

Clinically, TTP most often affects adult women. The inclusion criteria are microangiopathic hemolytic anemia and thrombocytopenia, with or without renal failure or neurologic abnormalities. Pathology includes widespread formation of platelet thrombi with fibrin (hyaline thrombi) leading to intravascular hemolysis (thrombotic microangiopathy).

Lab studies typically show decreased platelet count and prolonged bleeding time but normal prothrombin time and partial thromboplastin time. Peripheral blood smear shows thrombocytopenia, schistocytes, and reticulocytosis. Treatment is plasma exchange.

Hemolytic uremic syndrome (HUS) is a form of thrombotic microangiopathy due to endothelial cell damage. It occurs mostly in children, typically after a gastroenteritis (typically due to Shiga toxin-producing *E. coli* 0157:H7).

Typical HUS presents with abdominal pain, diarrhea (an atypical variant is diarrhea-negative), microangiopathic hemolytic anemia, thrombocytopenia, and renal failure. Renal involvement is seen more commonly than in TTP. The kidney shows fibrin thrombi in the glomeruli. Renal glomerular endothelial cells are targeted by the bacterial toxin. Glomerular scarring may ensue.

Treatment is supportive (fluid management, dialysis, erythrocyte transfusions); plasma exchange is only used for atypical cases.

Coagulation factors. The majority of the clotting factors are produced by the liver. The factors are proenzymes that must be converted to the active form. Some conversions occur on a phospholipid surface, and some conversions require calcium.

- The **intrinsic coagulation pathway** is activated by the contact factors, which include contact with subendothelial collagen, high molecular weight kininogen (HMWK), and kallikrein.

- The **extrinsic coagulation pathway** is activated by the release of tissue factor.

Note
- Patients on warfarin therapy should be monitored using prothrombin time (WEPT = warfarin, extrinsic PT).
- Patients on heparin therapy should be monitored using partial thromboplastin time (HIPTT = heparin, intrinsic PTT).

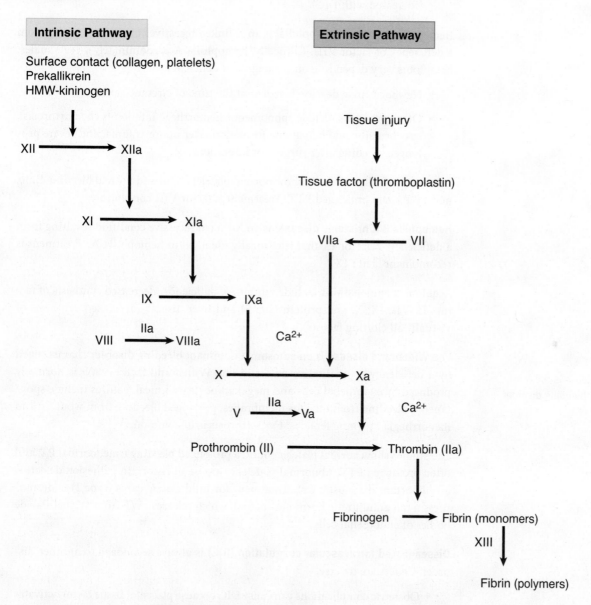

Figure 5-2. Coagulation Cascade

Lab tests for coagulation include the following:

- Prothrombin time (PT), which tests the extrinsic and common coagulation pathways (more specifically, it tests factors VII, X, V, prothrombin, and fibrinogen). The international normalized ratio (INR) standardizes the PT test so that results throughout the world can be compared. A longer time means blood takes longer to clot.

- Partial thromboplastin time (PTT), which tests the intrinsic and common coagulation pathways (more specifically, it tests factors XII, XI, IX, VIII, X, V, prothrombin, and fibrinogen).

- Thrombin time (TT), which tests for adequate fibrinogen levels.

- Fibrin degradation products (FDP), which tests the fibrinolytic system (increased with DIC).

Hemophilia A (classic hemophilia) is an X-linked recessive condition resulting from a deficiency of factor VIII. Clinically, hemophilia A predominately affects males. Symptoms vary depending on the degree of deficiency.

- Newborns may develop bleeding at the time of circumcision.

- Other problems include spontaneous hemorrhage into joints (hemarthrosis), easy bruising and hematoma formation after minor trauma, and severe prolonged bleeding after surgery or lacerations.

Laboratory studies typically show normal platelet count and normal bleeding time, normal PT and prolonged PTT. Treatment is factor VIII concentrate.

Hemophilia B (Christmas disease) is an X-linked recessive condition resulting from a deficiency of factor IX that is clinically identical to hemophilia A. Treatment is recombinant factor IX.

Acquired coagulopathies include vitamin K deficiency (decreased synthesis of factors II, VII, IX, X, and protein C & S) and liver disease (decreased synthesis of virtually all clotting factors).

Note

Von Willebrand disease is the most common inherited bleeding disorder.

Von Willebrand disease is an autosomal dominant bleeding disorder characterized by a deficiency or qualitative defect in von Willebrand factor. vWF is normally produced by endothelial cells and megakaryocytes. Clinical features include spontaneous bleeding from mucous membranes, prolonged bleeding from wounds, and menorrhagia in young females. Hemarthrosis is uncommon.

Lab studies show normal platelet count, a prolonged bleeding time, normal PT, and often prolonged PTT. Abnormal platelet response to ristocetin (adhesion defect) is an important diagnostic test. Treatment for mild classic cases (type I) is desmopressin (an antidiuretic hormone analog), which releases vWF from Weibel-Palade bodies of endothelial cells.

Disseminated intravascular coagulation (DIC) is always secondary to another disorder. Causes are diverse.

- Obstetric complications can cause DIC because placental tissue factor activates clotting.

- Gram-negative sepsis can cause DIC because tumor necrosis factor activates clotting.

- Microorganisms (especially meningococcus and rickettsiae)

- AML M3 (cytoplasmic granules in neoplastic promyelocytes activate clotting)

- Adenocarcinomas (mucin activates clotting)

DIC causes widespread microthrombi with consumption of platelets and clotting factors, causing hemorrhage. Laboratory studies show decreased platelet count, prolonged PT/PTT, decreased fibrinogen, and elevated fibrin split products (D dimers). Treat the underlying disorder.

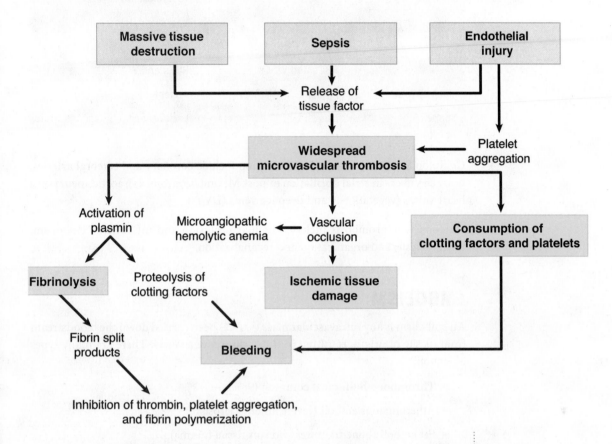

Figure 5-3. Disseminated Intravascular Coagulation

THROMBOSIS

Thrombosis is the pathologic formation of an intravascular fibrin-platelet thrombus during life. Factors involved in thrombus formation (**Virchow's triad**) include:

- Endothelial injury due to atherosclerosis, vasculitis, or many other causes

- Alterations in laminar blood flow predisposing for DIC occur with stasis of blood (e.g., immobilization); turbulence (e.g., aneurysms); and hyperviscosity of blood (e.g., polycythemia vera)

- Hypercoagulability of blood can be seen with clotting disorders (factor V Leiden; deficiency of antithrombin III, protein C, or protein S); tissue injury (postoperative and trauma); neoplasia; nephrotic syndrome; advanced age; pregnancy; and oral contraceptives (estrogen increases synthetic activity of the liver, including clotting factors)

Table 5-3. Comparison of a Thrombus with a Blood Clot

	Thrombus	Blood Clot
Location	Intravascular	Extravascular or intravascular (postmortem)
Composition	Platelets	Lacks platelets
	Fibrin	Fibrin
	RBCs and WBCs	RBCs and WBCs
Lines of Zahn	Present	Absent
Shape	Has shape	Lacks shape

Common locations of thrombus formation include coronary and cerebral arteries; heart chambers in atrial fibrillation or post-MI (mural thrombus); aortic aneurysms; heart valves (vegetations); and deep leg veins (DVTs).

Outcomes of thrombosis include vascular occlusion and infarctions; embolism; thrombolysis; and organization and recanalization.

EMBOLISM

An embolism is any intravascular mass that has been carried down the bloodstream from its site of origin, resulting in the occlusion of a vessel. There are many types of emboli:

- **Thromboemboli:** most common (98%)

- Atheromatous emboli (severe atherosclerosis)

- Fat emboli (bone fractures and soft tissue trauma)

- Bone marrow emboli (bone fractures and cardiopulmonary resuscitation [CPR])

- Gas emboli cause decompression sickness ("the bends" and caisson disease) when rapid ascent results in nitrogen gas bubbles in the blood vessels

- Amniotic fluid emboli are a complication of labor that may result in DIC; fetal squamous cells are seen in the maternal pulmonary vessels

- Tumor emboli (metastasis)

- Talc emboli (IV drug abuse)

- Bacterial/septic emboli (infectious endocarditis)

Bridge to Anatomy

The dual blood supply to the lungs is from the pulmonary artery and the bronchial arteries.

Clinical Correlate

The classic presentation of pulmonary embolism, which occurs in <20% of patients, includes hemoptysis, dyspnea, and chest pain.

Pulmonary emboli (PE) are often clinically silent and are the most commonly missed diagnosis in hospitalized patients. They are found in almost 50% of all hospital autopsies. Most PE (95%) arise from deep leg vein thrombosis (DVT) in the leg; other sources include the right side of the heart and the pelvic venous plexuses of the prostate and uterus.

Diagnosis of a PE can be established when V/Q lung shows a scan V/Q mismatch. Doppler ultrasound of the leg veins can be used to detect a DVT. Additionally, plasma D-dimer ELISA test is elevated.

Most cases are clinically silent and resolve.

Infarction is more common in patients with cardiopulmonary compromise. Symptoms include shortness of breath, hemoptysis, pleuritic chest pain, and pleural effusion. On gross examination there is typically a hemorrhagic wedge-shaped infarct. The infarction heals by regeneration or scar formation.

- Sudden death can occur when large emboli lodge in the bifurcation (saddle embolus) or large pulmonary artery branches.

- Chronic secondary pulmonary hypertension is caused by recurrent PEs, which increase pulmonary resistance and lead to secondary pulmonary hypertension.

INFARCTION

Infarction is a localized area of necrosis secondary to ischemia. Common sites of infarction include heart, brain, lungs, intestines, kidneys. Infarcts have multiple causes.

- Most infarcts (99%) result from thrombotic or embolic occlusion of an artery or vein.

- Less common causes include vasospasm and torsion of arteries and veins (e.g., volvulus, ovarian, and testicular torsion).

On gross examination infarctions typically have a wedge shape, with the apex of the wedge tending to point to the occlusion.

- **Anemic infarcts (pale or white color)** occur in solid organs with a single blood supply such as the spleen, kidney, and heart.

- **Hemorrhagic infarcts (red color)** occur in organs with a dual blood supply or collateral circulation, such as the lung and intestines, and can also occur with venous occlusion (e.g., testicular torsion).

Microscopic pathology of infarction can show either coagulative necrosis (most organs) or liquifactive necrosis (brain). The general sequence of tissue changes after infarction is as follows:

ischemia → coagulative necrosis → inflammation → granulation tissue → fibrous scar

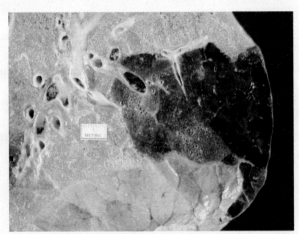

© Katsumi M. Miyai, M.D., Ph.D.; Regents of the University of California.
Used with permission.

Figure 5-4. Wedge-Shaped Pulmonary Infarction

SHOCK

Shock is characterized by vascular collapse and widespread hypoperfusion of cells and tissue due to reduced blood volume, cardiac output, or vascular tone. The cellular injury is initially reversible; if the hypoxia persists, the cellular injury becomes irreversible, leading to the death of cells and the patient.

Major Causes of Shock

- **Cardiogenic shock** (pump failure) can be due to myocardial infarction, cardiac arrhythmias, pulmonary embolism, and cardiac tamponade.

- **Hypovolemic shock** (reduced blood volume) can be due to hemorrhage, fluid loss secondary to severe burns, and severe dehydration.

- **Septic shock** (viral or bacterial infection) causes cytokines to trigger vasodilatation and hypotension, acute respiratory distress syndrome (ARDS), DIC, and multiple organ dysfunction syndrome. Mortality rate is 20%.

- **Neurogenic shock** (generalized vasodilatation) can be seen with anesthesia and brain or spinal cord injury.

- **Anaphylactic shock** (generalized vasodilatation) is a type I hypersensitivity reaction.

Stages of Shock

The stages of shock are arbitrarily defined as follows.

- **Stage I: compensation**

  Perfusion to vital organs is maintained by reflex mechanisms. Compensation is characterized by increased sympathetic tone, release of catecholamines, and activation of the renin-angiotensin system.

- **Stage II: decompensation**

  There is a progressive decrease in tissue perfusion, leading to potentially reversible tissue injury with development of a metabolic (lactic) acidosis, electrolyte imbalances, and renal insufficiency.

- **Stage III: irreversible tissue injury and organ failure**

  This ultimately results in death.

The organs show various manifestations of shock:

- Kidneys show fibrin thrombi in glomeruli and ultimately, acute tubular failure ensues, which causes oliguria and electrolyte imbalances.

- Lungs undergo diffuse alveolar damage ("shock lung").

- Intestines show superficial mucosal ischemic necrosis and hemorrhages, and with prolonged injury, bacteremia may ensue.

Chapter Summary

- Edema is the presence of excess fluid in the intercellular space. Causes include increased hydrostatic pressure, increased interstitial sodium, hypoalbuminemia and decreased colloid pressure, lymphatic obstruction, and increased endothelial permeability.

- Transudates have low protein content while exudates have high protein content.

- Hyperemia is an excessive amount of blood in a tissue or organ and can caused by vasodilation or diminished venous outflow.

- Hemostasis is the sequence of events leading to cessation of bleeding by the formation of a stable fibrin-platelet hemostatic plug. Vascular wall injury triggers transient vasoconstriction, facilitation of platelet adhesion, and activation of both the extrinsic and intrinsic clotting pathways. Formation of a platelet thrombus occurs when platelets adhere to von Willebrand factor attached to subendothelial collagen, undergo shape change and degranulation, and then aggregate with additional platelets.

- Causes of thrombocytopenia due to decreased platelet production include aplastic anemia and tumor. Causes of thrombocytopenia due to increased platelet destruction include ITP, TTP, DIC, and hypersplenism. Causes of qualitative platelet defects include von Willebrand disease, Bernard-Soulier syndrome, Glanzmann thrombasthenia, aspirin, and uremia.

- In ITP, antiplatelet antibodies destroy platelets, primarily in the spleen. In TTP, there is widespread formation of platelet thrombi with fibrin but without activation of the coagulation system. Hemolytic uremic syndrome can clinically resemble TTP and is triggered by E. coli strain 0157:H7.

- The intrinsic coagulation pathway is activated by contact factors and is clinically tested with the partial thromboplastin time (PTT). The extrinsic coagulation pathway is activated by the release of tissue factor, and is tested with the prothrombin time (PT), which also tests the common coagulation pathway.

- Hemophilia A is an X-linked recessive deficiency of factor VIII. Clinically, hemophilia B closely resembles hemophilia A but is due to deficiency of factor IX. Acquired coagulopathies can be due to vitamin K deficiency and liver disease. Von Willebrand is an inherited bleeding disorder characterized by a deficiency or qualitative defect in von Willebrand factor, which facilitates formation of platelet clots.

- DIC can be triggered by a variety of severe medical conditions and results in formation of many microthrombi that consume platelets and clotting factors, leading, in turn, to a superimposed bleeding tendency.

- Factors involved in thrombus formation include endothelial injury, alterations in laminar blood flow, and hypercoagulability of blood. Thrombi can lead to a spectrum of outcomes, including vascular occlusion and infarction, embolism, thrombolysis, and organization and recanalization. Embolism is used for any intravascular mass (solid, liquid, or gas) that has been carried downstream from its site of origin, resulting in occlusion of a vessel. Most emboli are thromboemboli, but many other materials have also formed emboli. Pulmonary emboli are a common form of emboli that are often clinically silent but can cause infarction or sudden death. Most pulmonary emboli arise from deep vein thromboses. Systemic arterial emboli usually arise in the heart and may cause infarction in a variety of sites, depending upon where they lodge.

(continued)

Chapter Summary *(cont'd)*

- Infarction is a localized area of necrosis secondary to ischemia. Most infarcts result from thrombotic occlusion of an artery. Anemic infarcts occur in organs with a single blood supply, whereas hemorrhagic infarcts occur in organs with a dual blood supply or secondary to venous occlusion. After infarction, ischemia leads to coagulative necrosis, which leads to inflammation, which leads to granulation tissue, which leads to fibrous scar.

- Shock is characterized by vascular collapse and widespread hypoperfusion of cells and tissues due to reduced blood volume, cardiac output, or vascular tone. Major forms of shock include cardiogenic shock, hypovolemic shock, septic shock, neurogenic shock, and anaphylactic shock.

Learning Objectives

❏ Answer questions about disorders involving an extra autosome and chromosomal deletions

❏ Demonstrate understanding of Mendelian disorders, autosomal recessive/dominant, and x-linked recessive/dominant conditions

❏ Solve problems concerning triplet repeat mutations

❏ Explain information related to mitochondrial DNA disorders and multifactorial inheritance

DISORDERS INVOLVING AN EXTRA AUTOSOME

Down syndrome (trisomy 21).

The most common **karyotype** is 47, XX, +21. Down syndrome is the **most common of the chromosomal disorders**. The risk increases with maternal age to an incidence of 1 in 25 live births in women age ≥45. The pathogenesis involves meiotic nondisjunction (95%), Robertsonian translocation (4%), or mosaicism due to mitotic nondisjunction during embryogenesis (1%).

Clinical findings can include intellectual disability; mongoloid facial features (flat face, low-bridged nose, and epicanthal folds); Brushfield spots (speckled appearance of the iris); muscular hypotonia; broad short neck; palmar (simian) crease; and congenital heart defects. Endocardial cushion defect, if present, leads to the formation of an atrioventricular canal (a common connection between all 4 chambers of the heart). Additional clinical problems that can develop include duodenal atresia ("double-bubble" sign); Hirschsprung disease; increased risk (15–20 fold) of acute lymphoblastic leukemia (ALL); and Alzheimer disease (by age 40 virtually all will develop Alzheimer disease).

Prenatal tests include maternal serum tests, ultrasonography, amniocentesis, and chorionic villus sampling.

Median life expectancy is 47 years.

Note

Robertsonian Translocation

Defined as a translocation involving 2 acrocentric chromosomes with the break points occurring close to the centromeres. This results in an extremely large chromosome and a tiny one, which is typically lost.

Note

Mosaicism is defined as the presence of ≥2 populations of cells within an individual.

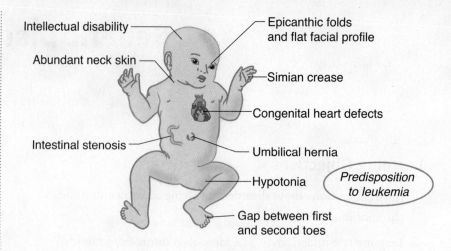

Figure 6-1. Down Syndrome

Edwards syndrome (trisomy 18) is caused by nondisjunction. The risk increases with maternal age.

Clinical findings can include intellectual disability; low-set ears and micrognathia; congenital heart defects; overlapping flexed fingers; and rocker-bottom feet. There is a very poor prognosis due to severe congenital malformations.

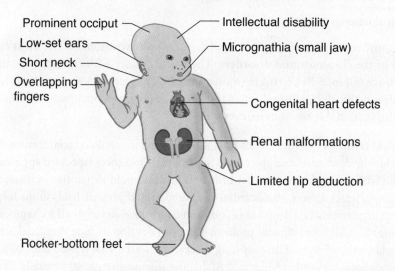

Figure 6-2. Edwards Syndrome

Patau syndrome (trisomy 13) is caused by nondisjunction. The risk increases with maternal age.

Clinical findings can include intellectual disability; cleft lip and/or palate; cardiac defects; renal abnormalities; microcephaly; holoprosencephaly; and polydactyly. The very poor prognosis is due to severe congenital malformations.

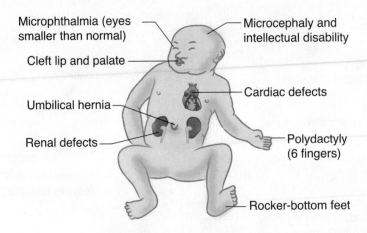

Microphthalmia (eyes smaller than normal)

Microcephaly and intellectual disability

Cleft lip and palate

Cardiac defects

Umbilical hernia

Renal defects

Polydactyly (6 fingers)

Rocker-bottom feet

Figure 6-3. Patau Syndrome

DISORDERS INVOLVING CHROMOSOMAL DELETIONS

Cri du chat syndrome is due to deletion of the short arm of chromosome 5. Clinical findings include a characteristic high-pitched catlike cry; intellectual disability; congenital heart disease; and microcephaly. **Microdeletions** include 13q14 (retinoblastoma gene) and 11p13 (WAGR complex [Wilms tumor, aniridia, genitourinary anomalies, and intellectual disability [previously known as mental retardation]). Microdeletions are too small to be detected by karyotyping and require molecular techniques for detection.

DISORDERS INVOLVING SEX CHROMOSOMES

Klinefelter syndrome is caused by meiotic nondisjunction and is a common cause of male hypogonadism. The most common karyotype is 47,XXY. Lab studies show elevated FSH and LH with low levels of testosterone. Clinical findings include testicular atrophy, infertility due to azoospermia, eunuchoid body habitus, high-pitched voice; female distribution of hair; and gynecomastia.

Turner syndrome is a common cause of female hypogonadism. The most common karyotype is 45,X. The second X chromosome is necessary for oogenesis and normal development of the ovary. Clinically, patients fail to develop secondary sex characteristics and have short stature with widely spaced nipples. Other features include gonadal dysgenesis with atrophic streak ovaries; primary amenorrhea; and infertility.

Clinical features involving other organ systems include cystic hygroma and webbing of the neck; hypothyroidism; congenital heart disease (preductal coarctation of the aorta and bicuspid aortic valve); and hydrops fetalis. Females with 45,X/46,XY mosaicism are at risk for gonadoblastoma.

Note

The presence of a Y chromosome determines male phenotype due to the presence of the testes-determining factor gene (also called the sex-determining region Y [SRY]) on the Y chromosome.

In a Nutshell

Lyon's Hypothesis of X-Inactivation

- Only one X is genetically active.
- Most, but not all, of the genes on the other X chromosome are inactivated.
- Females are mosaics.
- Either the maternal or paternal X chromosome is inactivated at random.

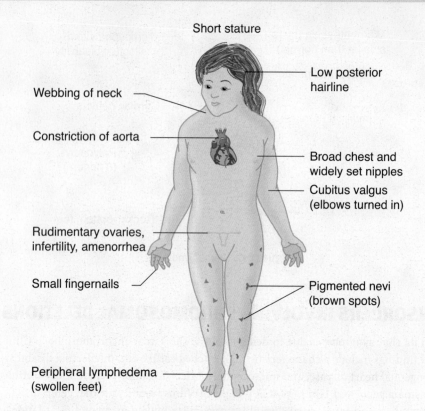

Figure 6-4. Turner Syndrome

DISORDERS OF SEXUAL DEVELOPMENT (DSD)

Determination of sex can be established by a variety of methods that do not necessarily completely agree.

- **Karyotypic** (genetic) sex refers to which sex chromosomes an individual has; the presence of a Y chromosome results in testicular development.

- **Gonadal** sex refers to the presence of ovarian or testicular tissue.

- **Ductal sex** refers to the presence of Müllerian (female – Fallopian tube, uterus, cervix, and upper portion of vagina) or Wolffian (male – epididymis, vas deferens, seminal vesicles, and ejaculatory ducts) duct adult derivatives.

- **Phenotypic** (genital) sex refers to the external appearance of the genitalia.

Individuals with **ovotesticular disorder** have both ovarian and testicular tissue, which is an extremely rare condition. The most common karyotype of ovotesticular disorder is 46,XX. The gonadal sex can be either an ovary on one side and testis on the other, or ovotestes, in which there is a gonad with both testicular and ovarian tissue. The ductal sex is often mixed, and the phenotypic sex shows ambiguous genitalia.

The **46,XX DSD category** includes individuals (formerly characterized as female pseudohermaphrodites) with disorders of ovarian development, androgen excess, vaginal atresia, and cloacal exstrophy. The **46,XY category** includes individuals (formerly characterized as male pseudohermaphrodites) with disorders of testicular development, disorders of androgen synthesis, severe hypospadias and cloacal exstrophy.

MENDELIAN DISORDERS

Mendelian disorders are characterized by single gene mutations. Common types of mutations include point mutations and frameshift mutations.

- **Point mutations** occur with a single nucleotide base substitution, which may produce a variety of effects. The form of point mutation called synonymous mutation (silent mutation) occurs when a base substitution results in a codon that codes for the same amino acid. The form of point mutation called missense mutation occurs when a base substitution results in a new codon and a change in amino acids. The form of point mutation called a nonsense mutation occurs when a base substitution produces a stop codon and therefore produces a truncated protein.

- **Frameshift mutations** occur when insertion or deletion of bases leads to a shift in the reading frame of the gene.

The location of a mutation will alter its potential effects. Mutations involving coding regions of DNA may result in abnormal amino acid sequences; decreased production of the protein; truncated or abnormally folded protein; or altered or lost function of the protein. Mutations of promoter or enhancer regions may interfere with transcription factors, resulting in decreased transcription of the gene.

Patterns of inheritance for genetic diseases show wide variation, and the genetic pattern of a disease may be classified as autosomal dominant; autosomal recessive; X-linked recessive; X-linked dominant; triplet repeat mutations; genomic imprinting; mitochondrial; or multifactorial.

Table 6-1. Autosomal Dominant and Recessive Diseases

	Autosomal Recessive	Autosomal Dominant
Onset	Early uniform onset (infancy/childhood)	Variable onset (may be delayed into adulthood)
Penetrance	Complete penetrance	Incomplete penetrance with variable expression
Mutation	Usually an enzyme protein	Usually a structural protein or receptor
Requires	Mutation of both alleles	Mutation of one allele

AUTOSOMAL RECESSIVE DISORDERS

(This material is included here for reinforcement. It is also covered in the Physiology Lecture Notes.)

Cystic fibrosis (CF) is the most common lethal genetic disorder in Caucasians. It is due to mutation of the chloride channel protein, cystic fibrosis transmembrane conductance regulator (CFTR), whose *CFTR* gene is located on chromosome 7 and most commonly has been damaged by a deletion of the amino acid phenylalanine at position 508 (ΔF508). The defective chloride channel protein leads to abnormally thick viscous mucus, which obstructs the ducts of exocrine organs.

Note

CF seems to break 2 rules of genetics:

- Inheritance is autosomal recessive, even though the affected protein is a receptor protein.
- The clinical manifestations vary widely, which is more characteristic of autosomal dominant disorders.

The **distribution of disease** reflects the distribution of eccrine sweat glands and exocrine glands.

- In the lungs, CF may cause recurrent pulmonary infections; chronic bronchitis; and bronchiectasis.

- In the pancreas, CF may cause plugging of pancreatic ducts resulting in atrophy and fibrosis; and pancreatic insufficiency leading to fat malabsorption, malodorous steatorrhea, and deficiency of fat-soluble vitamins.

- In the male reproductive system, CF may be associated with absence or obstruction of the vas deferens and epididymis, which often leads to male infertility.

- In the liver, plugging of the biliary canaliculi may result in biliary cirrhosis.

- In the GI tract, the thick secretions may cause small intestinal obstruction (meconium ileus).

Diagnosis can be established with a sweat test (elevated NaCl) or DNA probes. Due to improved therapies, some patients live into their forties, but with this increase in longevity there has been an increase in liver disease. Patients succumb to pulmonary disease. The 3 most common pulmonary infections are *S. aureus*, *H. influenzae*, and *P. aeruginosa*. Lung transplantation is a treatment option. Patients infected with *Burkholderia cepacia* complex who undergo transplant have a worse prognosis.

Bridge to Biochemistry

Most CF cases result from deletion of phenylalanine at position 508 (ΔF508), which interferes with proper protein folding and the post-translational processing of oligosaccharide side chains. The abnormal chloride channel protein is degraded by the cytosolic proteasome complex rather than translocated to the cell membrane.

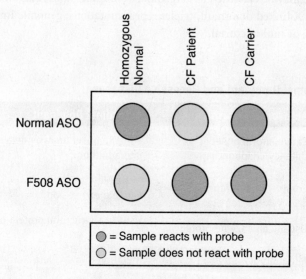

Figure 6-5. The Use of Allele-Specific Oligonucleotide (ASO) Probes for Cystic Fibrosis

Bridge to Biochemistry

Phenylalanine hydroxylase converts phenylalanine into tyrosine.

Phenylketonuria (PKU) is due to deficiency of phenylalanine hydroxylase, resulting in toxic levels of phenylalanine and a lack of tyrosine.

Clinically, affected children are normal at birth but, if undiagnosed and untreated, develop intellectual development disorder by age 6 months. The lack of tyrosine causes light-colored skin and hair, since melanin is a tyrosine derivative. Affected children may have a mousy or musty odor to the sweat and urine (secondary to metabolite [phenylacetate] accumulation).

Screening for PKU is done at birth. Treatment is dietary restriction of phenylalanine, including avoidance of the artificial sweetener aspartame.

A genetic variant, **benign hyperphenylalaninemia**, has partial enzyme deficiency with mildly increased levels of phenylalanine which are insufficient to cause intellectual disability.

In a minority of cases, an abnormality of the cofactor tetrahydrobiopterin causes a variant that does not respond to dietary restriction.

Transplacental accumulation of phenylalanine can cause problems with fetal development in cases of maternal PKU. Prevention requires maternal dietary restriction.

Alkaptonuria (ochronosis) occurs when deficiency of homogentisic acid oxidase results in the accumulation of homogentisic acid. The homogentisic acid has an affinity for connective tissues (especially cartilage), resulting in a black discoloration (as a consequence of oxidation of homogentisic acid).

Clinical features include urine that is initially pale yellow but turns black upon standing, and black-stained cartilage, which causes discoloration of the nose and ears. Alkaptonuria also predisposes for early onset of degenerative arthritis.

Albinism is caused by a lack of the enzyme tyrosinase needed for melanin production. Affected individuals show deficiency of melanin pigmentation in the skin, hair follicles, and eyes (oculocutaneous albinism), with resulting increased risk of basal cell and squamous cell carcinomas.

The **glycogen storage diseases** are a group of rare diseases that have in common a deficiency of one of the enzymes necessary for the metabolism of glycogen, which results in the accumulation of glycogen in the liver, heart, and skeletal muscle.

- **Type I (von Gierke disease)** is due to a deficiency of *glucose-6-phosphatase*, and is characterized clinically by hepatomegaly and hypoglycemia.

- **Type II (Pompe disease)** is due to a deficiency of *lysosomal α-1,4-glucosidase (acid maltase)*, and is characterized clinically by hepatomegaly, skeletal muscle hypotonia, cardiomegaly, and death from cardiac failure by age 2 years.

- **Type V (McArdle syndrome)** is due to a deficiency of *muscle glycogen phosphorylase*, and is characterized clinically by exercise-induced muscle cramps.

Tay-Sachs disease is due to a deficiency of hexosaminidase A (due to mutation of *HEXA* gene on chromosome 15), which leads to the accumulation of GM2 ganglioside in the lysosomes of the CNS and retina. Tay-Sachs is common in Ashkenazi Jews (1 in 30 carrier rate).

The distribution of disease involves the retina (cherry-red spot due to accentuation of the macula) and central nervous system (dilated neurons with cytoplasmic vacuoles). Affected children are normal at birth, but by 6 months show onset of symptoms (progressive mental deterioration and motor incoordination) that progress to death by age 2–3 years. **Electron microscopy** shows distended lysosomes with whorled membranes; the diagnosis can also be established with enzyme assays and DNA probes.

Note

Lysosomal Storage Diseases

Defined as a deficiency of a lysosomal enzyme (acid hydrolase), which leads to the accumulation of a complex substrate within the lysosome leading to enlarged cells that become dysfunctional

- Tay-Sachs
- Niemann-Pick
- Gaucher
- Mucopolysaccharidosis
- Fabry
- Metachromatic leukodystrophy

Table 6-2. Lysosomal Storage Diseases

Disease	Enzyme Deficiency	Accumulating Substance
Tay-Sachs disease	Hexosaminidase A	GM$_2$ ganglioside
Niemann-Pick disease types A and B	Sphingomyelinase	Sphingomyelin
Gaucher disease	Glucocerebrosidase	Glucocerebroside
Fabry disease	α -galactosidase A	Ceramide trihexoside
Metachromatic leukodystrophy	Arylsulfatase A	Sulfatide
Hurler syndrome	α -L-iduronidase	Dermatan sulfate Heparan sulfate
Hunter syndrome	L-iduronate sulfatase	Dermatan sulfate Heparan sulfate

Note

"Zebra bodies" are concentric lamellated inclusions seen in the cytoplasm on electron microscopy. Although they are present in Neimann-Pick disease, they are also present in other diseases including Fabry disease and Hurler syndrome.

Niemann-Pick disease is caused by a deficiency of sphingomyelinase, which leads to the accumulation of sphingomyelin within the lysosomes of the CNS and reticuloendothelial system (monocytes and macrophages located in reticular connective tissue). Niemann-Pick is common in Ashkenazi Jews (note similarity to Tay-Sachs disease).

The distribution of disease depends on the form of disease, but can involve the retina (cherry-red spot, note similarity to Tay-Sachs disease); central nervous system (distended neurons with a foamy cytoplasmic vacuolization, note similarity to Tay-Sachs disease); and reticuloendothelial system (hepatosplenomegaly, lymphadenopathy, and bone marrow involvement; note difference from Tay-Sachs disease).

In Neimann-Pick **types A and B**, there is a mutation affecting an enzyme that metabolizes lipids; organomegaly occurs, and with type A, there is severe neurologic damage. In **type C**—the most common form—a defect in cholesterol transport causes ataxia, dysarthria, and learning difficulties. All forms are lethal, usually before adulthood.

Gaucher disease is the most common lysosomal storage disorder. Deficiency of glucocerebrosidase leads to the accumulation of glucocerebroside, predominately in the lysosomes of the reticuloendothelial system (monocytes and macrophages located in reticular connective tissue).

Type I represents 99% of cases and presents in adulthood with hepatosplenomegaly; thrombocytopenia/pancytopenia secondary to hypersplenism; lymphadenopathy; and bone marrow involvement that may lead to bone pain, deformities, and fractures. Central nervous system manifestations occur in **types II and III**.

The characteristic **Gaucher cells** are enlarged macrophages with a fibrillary (tissue paper–like) cytoplasm. Diagnosis can be established with biochemical enzyme assay of glucocerebrosidase activity.

Mucopolysaccharidosis (MPS) is a group of lysosomal storage disorders characterized by deficiencies in the lysosomal enzymes required for the degradation of mucopolysaccharides (glycosaminoglycans).

Clinical features include intellectual disability; cloudy cornea; hepatosplenomegaly; skeletal deformities and coarse facial features; joint abnormalities; and cardiac lesions. MPS I (Hurler syndrome) is the severe form and is due to deficiency of α-L-iduronidase. MPS II (Hunter syndrome) is a milder form; it shows X-linked recessive inheritance and is due to a deficiency of L-iduronate sulfatase.

AUTOSOMAL DOMINANT DISORDERS

Familial hypercholesterolemia is the most common inherited disorder (incidence 1 in 500) and is due to a mutation in the low density lipoprotein (LDL) receptor gene (LDLR) on chromosome 19. The mutations in the LDL receptor cause increased levels of circulating cholesterol, loss of feedback inhibition of HMG-coenzyme A (HMG-CoA) reductase, and increased phagocytosis of LDL by macrophages.

There are 5 major **classes of mutation**.

- **Class I:** no LDL receptor synthesis
- **Class II:** defect in transport out of the endoplasmic reticulum
- **Class III:** defect in LDL receptor binding
- **Class IV:** defect in ability to internalize bound LDL
- **Class V:** defect in the recycling of the LDL receptor

Clinical features include elevated serum cholesterol (heterozygotes have elevations of 2–3 times the normal level and homozygotes have elevations of 5–6 times the normal level), skin xanthomas (collections of lipid-laden macrophages), xanthelasma around the eyes, and premature atherosclerosis (homozygotes often develop myocardial infarctions in late teens and twenties).

Marfan syndrome is due to a mutation of the **fibrillin** gene (*FBN1*) on chromosome 15q21. Fibrillin is a glycoprotein that functions as a scaffold for the alignment of elastic fibers.

Clinical features include skeletal changes (tall, thin build with long extremities, hyperextensible joints, pectus excavatum [inwardly depressed sternum], and pectus carinatum [pigeon breast]) and abnormal eyes (ectopia lentis, characterized by bilateral subluxation of the lens). The cardiovascular system is also particularly vulnerable; it may show cystic medial degeneration of the media of elastic arteries with a loss of elastic fibers and smooth muscle cells with increased risk of dissecting aortic aneurysm (a major cause of death), dilatation of the aortic ring potentially leading to aortic valve insufficiency, and/or mitral valve prolapse.

Ehlers-Danlos syndrome (EDS) is a group of inherited connective tissue diseases that have in common a defect in collagen structure or synthesis. Clinically, the disease causes hyperextensible skin that is easily traumatized and hyperextensible joints secondary to effects on the joints and adjacent ligaments.

There are a number of variants with different modes of inheritance.

- **Kyphoscoliotic EDS**: autosomal recessive form
- **Vascular variant EDS**: autosomal dominant form that causes rupture of vessels and bowel wall
- **Classical EDS**: autosomal dominant form that causes a type V collagen defect; patients have a normal lifespan

Bridge to Biochemistry

HMG-CoA reductase is the rate-limiting enzyme in the synthesis of cholesterol. Normally, cholesterol represses the expression of the HMG-CoA reductase gene (negative feedback).

Note

Disorders of collagen biosynthesis include scurvy, osteogenesis imperfecta, Ehlers-Danlos syndrome, Alport syndrome, and Menkes disease.

Neurofibromatosis

Type 1 (**von Recklinghausen disease**) neurofibromatosis (90% of cases) has an incidence of 1 in 3,000. The condition is due to a mutation of the tumor suppressor gene *NF1* located on chromosome 17 (17q11.2). The normal gene product (neurofibromin) inhibits p21 ras oncoprotein.

- Affected individuals characteristically have multiple neurofibromas and benign tumors of peripheral nerves that are often numerous and may be disfiguring. The plexiform variant of the neurofibromas are diagnostic.

- Rarely (3%), malignant transformation of a neurofibroma may occur.

- Other clinical features include pigmented skin lesions (6 or more "cafe-au-lait spots" that are light brown macules usually located over nerves); pigmented iris hamartomas (Lisch nodules); and increased risk of meningiomas and pheochromocytoma, an adrenal tumor that also occurs with von Hippel-Lindau disease and MEN 2.

Type 2 (**bilateral acoustic**) neurofibromatosis (10% of cases) has an incidence of 1 in 45,000.

- There is a mutated tumor suppressor gene *NF-2* (22q12.2) on chromosome 22.

- The normal gene product (merlin) is a critical regulator of contact-dependent inhibition of proliferation.

- Clinical features include vestibular schwannomas (acoustic neuromas), and increased risk of meningioma and ependymomas.

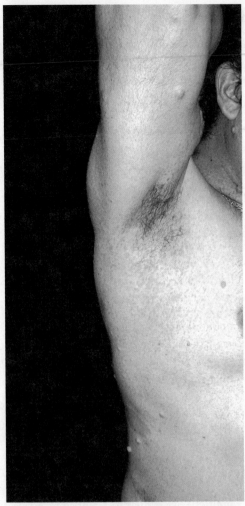

© Richard P. Usatine, M.D.
Used with permission.

Figure 6-6. Multiple Subcutaneous Neural Tumors of Neurofibromatosis

von Hippel-Lindau disease is due to a mutation of the tumor suppressor gene *VHL* on chromosome 3p (3p26-p25). The normal gene product's main action is to tag proteins (e.g., hypoxia inducible factor 1a [a transcription factor that induces the expression of angiogenesis factors]) with ubiquitin for degradation.

Clinical manifestations can include retinal hemangioblastoma (von Hippel tumor); hemangioblastomas of the cerebellum, brain stem, and spinal cord (Lindau tumor); cysts of the liver, pancreas, and kidneys; and multiple bilateral renal cell carcinomas.

X-LINKED RECESSIVE CONDITIONS

In **X-linked recessive conditions**, males with a mutant recessive gene on the X chromosome have the condition, while daughters of affected males are obligate carriers, who in many situations are asymptomatic.

- Sons of affected males do not carry the mutation.
- Daughters of carrier females may be either normal or carriers.
- Sons of carrier females may be affected or normal (because males are hemizygous for the X chromosome).

Lesch-Nyhan syndrome results from deficiency of hypoxanthine-guanine phophoribosyltransferase (HGPRT), which impairs salvaging of the purines hypoxanthine and guanine. Clinical features include intellectual disability, hyperuricemia, and self-mutilation.

Testicular feminization is an androgen insensitivity that causes failure of normal masculinization of external genitalia of XY males.

In **Bruton agammaglobulinemia**, defective Bruton tyrosine kinase (*Btk*) at band Xq21.3 causes complete failure of immunoglobulin production characterized clinically by complete absence of antibodies in serum and recurrent bacterial infections. (*See* the Immunopathology chapter 7.)

In **Menkes disease**, a mutation of the *ATP7A* gene impairs copper distribution. Infants show failure to thrive, and death occurs in the first decade.

X-LINKED DOMINANT CONDITIONS

X-linked dominant conditions are similar to X-linked recessive, but both males and females show disease. An example is Alport syndrome, which is a hereditary glomerulonephritis with nerve deafness. Alport syndrome can also be inherited in other patterns.

TRIPLET REPEAT MUTATIONS

Fragile X syndrome is due to triplet nucleotide repeat mutations, so that the nucleotide sequence CGG repeats typically hundreds to thousands of times. The mutation occurs in the *FMR-1* gene (fragile X mental retardation-1) on the X chromosome (Xq27.3), and the disease behaves as an X-linked dominant disease that causes intellectual disability in all affected males and 50% of female carriers. The characteristic phenotype includes elongated face with a large jaw, large everted ears, and macroorchidism. The condition can be diagnosed with DNA probe analysis.

Huntington disease is due to a triplet repeat mutation (CAG) of the *HTT* gene that produces an abnormal protein (huntingtin), which is neurotoxic and causes atrophy of the caudate nucleus. Huntington disease has an early onset (age range: 20–50 years) of progressive dementia with choreiform movements.

Note

Most common genetic causes of intellectual developmental disorder:

- Down syndrome
- Fragile X syndrome

Note

Triplet repeat expansion can occur in a coding region (Huntington and spinobulbar muscular atrophy) or in an untranslated region of the gene (fragile X and myotonic dystrophy).

GENOMIC IMPRINTING

Genomic imprinting refers to differential expression of genes based on chromosomal inheritance from maternal versus paternal origin.

- In **Prader-Willi syndrome**, microdeletion on paternal chromosome 15 {del(15) (q11;q13)} causes intellectual disability, obesity, hypogonadism, and hypotonia.

- In **Angelman syndrome**, microdeletion on maternal chromosome 15 {del(15) (q11;q13)} causes intellectual disability, seizures, ataxia, and inappropriate laughter.

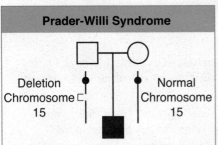
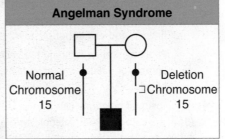

Figure 6-7. Genomic Imprinting

> The inheritance of a deletion on chromosome 15 from a male produces Prader-Willi syndrome, whereas inheritance of the same deletion from a female produces Angelman syndrome.

MITOCHONDRIAL DNA DISORDERS

Mitochondrial DNA codes for mitochondrial oxidative phosphorylation enzymes; inheritance is only from mother to child, because only the ovum contributes mitochondria to the zygote. Examples include:

- **Leber hereditary optic neuropathy** causes loss of retinal cells, which leads to central vision loss.

- **Myoclonic epilepsy with ragged red fibers (MERRF)** is a mitochondrial disorder characterized by epilepsy, ataxia, peripheral neuropathy and deterioration in cognitive ability. Sensorineural hearing loss and ocular dysfunction can also develop. Patients have short stature and cardiomyopathy. On muscle biopsy, ragged red fibers are seen on Gomori trichrome staining due to the accumulation of mitochondria.

MULTIFACTORIAL INHERITANCE

Multifactorial inheritance refers to disease caused by a combination of multiple minor gene mutations and environmental factors. Examples include open neural tube defects and type 2 diabetes mellitus.

Chapter Summary

- Disorders involving an extra autosomal chromosome include Down, Edwards, and Patau syndromes.

  - Down syndrome (trisomy 21) is the most common of the chromosomal disorders and is characterized by intellectual disability, mongoloid facial features, hypotonia, and palmar creases. Serious complications include congenital heart disease (endocardial cushion defects), duodenal atresia, Hirschsprung disease, acute lymphoblastic leukemia, and early onset of Alzheimer disease.

  - Edwards syndrome (trisomy 18) is characterized by intellectual disability, low-set ears, micrognathia, congenital heart defects, overlapping flexed fingers, and rocker-bottom feet.

  - Patau syndrome (trisomy 13) is characterized by intellectual disability, cleft lip and/or palate, cardiac defects, renal abnormalities, microcephaly, and polydactyly.

- Chromosomal deletions can also cause genetic disease. Cri du chat syndrome (5p-) is a chromosomal deletion syndrome characterized by a high-pitched, catlike cry; intellectual disability; congenital heart disease; and microcephaly. Microdeletions are associated with retinoblastoma and Wilms tumor.

- Klinefelter and Turner syndromes are important disorders of sex chromosomes.

  - Klinefelter (47 XXY) is a common cause of male hypogonadism.
  - Turner (45 XO) is a common cause of female hypogonadism.

- Individuals with ovotesticular disorder have both ovarian and testicular tissue and are exceptionally rare. Individuals with 46,XX DSD were previously characterized as female pseudohermaphrodites. Individuals with 46,XY DSD were previously characterized as male pseudohermaphrodites.

- Mendelian disorders are characterized by single gene mutations, which may be either point mutations or frameshift mutations. These mutations may produce autosomal dominant, autosomal recessive, or X-linked diseases.

- Cystic fibrosis is a common autosomal recessive disorder due to a defect in the chloride channel protein, the cystic fibrosis transmembrane conductance regulator (CFTR), and can be diagnosed when elevated NaCl is identified in sweat.

- Phenylketonuria is an autosomal recessive disease due to deficiency of phenylalanine hydroxylase; it can cause severe intellectual developmental disability if not identified by biochemical screening at birth.

- Alkaptonuria is an autosomal recessive disease due to deficiency of homogentisic acid.

- Albinism is an autosomal recessive deficiency of melanin pigmentation in the skin, hair follicles, and eyes, which occurs secondary to tyrosinase deficiency.

- Glycogen storage diseases are rare diseases due to abnormalities of glycogen metabolism; they result in accumulation of glycogen in liver, heart, and skeletal muscle. Important subtypes include von Gierke disease, Pompe disease, and McArdle syndrome.

(continued)

Chapter Summary *(cont'd)*

- Tay-Sachs is an autosomal recessive disease seen in Ashkenazi Jews, which is due to deficiency of hexosaminidase A, leading to GM2 ganglioside deposition.

- Niemann-Pick is an autosomal recessive disorder with 3 forms; all are lethal before adulthood. Lipid metabolism is impaired.

- Gaucher is an autosomal recessive deficiency of glucocerebrosidase, leading to accumulation of glucocerebroside, with hepatosplenomegaly and bone marrow involvement. Most cases present in adulthood.

- The mucopolysaccharidoses (MPS) are lysosomal storage disorders characterized by deficiencies in the lysosomal enzymes required for the degradation of mucopolysaccharides (glycosaminoglycans). Hunter syndrome (MPS II) is less severe than Hurler syndrome (MPS I).

- Familial hypercholesterolemia is a common autosomal dominant disorder with atherosclerotic manifestations (worse in homozygotes) due to genetic defects of several forms involving the LDL receptor gene.

- Marfan syndrome is an autosomal dominant disorder due to mutation of the fibrillin gene (*FBN1*) characterized by skeletal abnormalities (tall build with hyperextensible joints and chest abnormalities), subluxation of the lens, and cardiovascular system problems (cystic medial necrosis, dissecting aortic aneurysm, valvular insufficiency).

- Ehlers-Danlos is a group of inherited connective tissue diseases that have in common a defect in collagen structure or synthesis.

- Von Recklinghausen (neurofibromatosis type 1) is an autosomal dominant defect in the tumor suppressor gene *NF-1*. Bilateral acoustic neurofibromatosis (neurofibromatosis type 2) is less common and caused by a defect in tumor suppressor gene *NF-2*.

- Von Hippel-Lindau is caused by an abnormality of a tumor suppressor gene on chromosome 3p.

- Fragile X syndrome is an important cause of familial mental retardation and is due to a triple nucleotide repeat mutation in the *FMR-1* gene on the X chromosome.

- Huntington disease is due to a triple repeat mutation of the *HTT*, which clinically produces atrophy of the caudate nucleus with choreiform movements and progressive dementia.

- Genomic imprinting refers to differential expression of genes based on chromosomal inheritance from maternal versus paternal origin. The classic examples are Prader-Willi and Angelman syndromes.

- Most X-linked disorders are recessive, with males expressing the disease and producing daughter carriers; examples include Lesch-Nyhan syndrome (hyperuricemia, intellectual disability, and self-mutilation due to impaired purine salvage), testicular feminization (androgen insensitivity leads to failure of normal masculinization), and Bruton agammaglobulinemia (lack of immunoglobulin production causes recurrent bacterial infections).

(continued)

Chapter Summary (cont'd)

- Rare X-linked disorders are dominant, causing disease in both daughters and sons. Alport disease (hereditary glomerulonephritis with nerve deafness) is an example.

- Mitochondrial DNA disorders are transmitted from the mother, but not the father, to the offspring. These include Leber hereditary optic neuropathy and myoclonic epilepsy with ragged red fibers.

- Multifactorial inheritance occurs when disease is caused by multiple gene mutations and environmental factors; examples include open neural tube defects and type 2 DM.

Immunopathology 7

Learning Objectives

❏ Explain information related to hypersensitivity reactions and autoimmune diseases

❏ Answer questions about primary/secondary immune deficiency syndromes

❏ Demonstrate understanding of AIDS

❏ Answer questions about immunology of transplant rejection

HYPERSENSITIVITY REACTIONS

(This material is included here for reinforcement. It is also covered in the Immunology Lecture Notes.)

Type I (immediate) hypersensitivity reactions (**anaphylactic type**) are characterized by IgE-dependent release of chemical mediators from mast cells and basophils. Cross-linking of IgE bound to antigen to IgE Fc receptors on the surface of mast cells and basophils causes degranulation. This binding triggers release of chemical mediators that include histamine and heparin; eosinophil chemotactic factor; leukotriene B4 and neutrophil chemotactic factor; and prostaglandin D4, platelet-activating factor (PAF), and leukotrienes C4 and D4. Influx of eosinophils amplifies and perpetuates the reaction. Effects may be systemic (anaphylaxis, as for example due to bee stings or drugs) or localized (food allergies, atopy, and asthma).

Type II hypersensitivity reactions (antibody-mediated) are mediated by IgG or IgM antibodies directed against a specific target cell or tissue. Reactions can take several forms.

- In complement-dependent cytotoxicity, fixation of complement results in osmotic lysis or opsonization of antibody-coated cells; examples include autoimmune hemolytic anemia, transfusion reactions, and erythroblastosis fetalis.

- In antibody-dependent cell-mediated cytoxicity (ADCC), cytotoxic killing of an antibody-coated cell occurs; an example is pernicious anemia. Antireceptor antibodies can activate or interfere with receptors; examples include Graves disease and myasthenia gravis.

Type III hypersensitivity reactions (**immune complex disease**) are characterized by the formation of in situ or circulating antibody-antigen immune complexes, which deposit in tissue resulting in inflammation and tissue injury. Examples include serum sickness, systemic lupus erythematosus (SLE), and glomerulonephritis.

Type IV hypersensitivity reactions (**cell-mediated type**) are mediated by sensitized T lymphocytes. In delayed type hypersensitivity, CD4+ TH1 lymphocytes mediate granuloma formation; examples include the PPD skin test and tuberculosis.

In cytotoxic T-cell–mediated hypersensitivity, CD8+ T-cell lymphocytes destroy antigen-containing cells; examples include type 1 diabetes, virus-infected cells, immune reaction to tumor-associated antigens, and graft rejection.

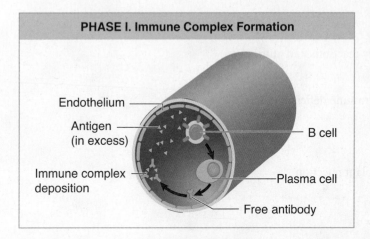

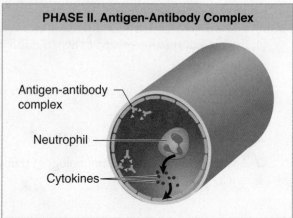

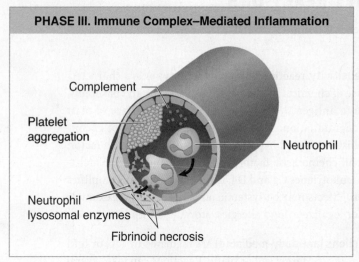

Figure 7-1. Type III Hypersensitivity

AUTOIMMUNE DISEASES

Note

Multiple autoantibodies may be produced and are commonly directed against nuclear antigens (DNA, histones, nonhistone nuclear RNA proteins) and blood cells.

Systemic lupus erythematosus (SLE) is a chronic systemic autoimmune disease characterized by loss of self-tolerance and production of autoantibodies. Females are affected much more often than males (M:F = 1:9); peak incidence is age 20–45; and African Americans are affected more often than Caucasians. The mechanism of injury in lupus is a mix of type II and III hypersensitivity reactions.

- Important **autoantibodies** that may be detected in the sera from lupus patients include antinuclear antibody (ANA) (>95%); anti-dsDNA (40–60%); anti-Sm (20–30%); antihistone antibodies; nonhistone nuclear RNA proteins; and blood cells.

- SLE affects **many organ systems**.

  ○ Hematologic (type II hypersensitivity reaction) manifestations can include hemolytic anemia, thrombocytopenia, neutropenia, and lymphopenia.

  ○ Skeletal manifestations include an arthritis characterized by polyarthralgia and synovitis without joint deformity (type III hypersensitivity reaction).

  ○ Skin (type III hypersensitivity reaction) manifestations can include a malar "butterfly" rash; maculopapular rash; and ulcerations and bullae formation.

  ○ Serosal surfaces may also be affected, with resulting pericarditis, pleuritis, or pleural effusions (type III hypersensitivity reaction).

  ○ Central nervous system manifestations include focal neurologic symptoms, seizures, and psychosis (type III hypersensitivity reaction).

  ○ Cardiac manifestations include Libman-Sacks endocarditis (nonbacterial verrucous endocarditis) (type III hypersensitivity reaction).

- Of particular importance are the renal manifestations (type III hypersensitivity) classified by the Society of Nephrology/Renal Pathology Society as follows.

  ○ **Class I**: minimal mesangial lupus nephritis

  ○ **Class II**: mesangial proliferative lupus nephritis

  ○ **Class III**: focal (< 50%) lupus nephritis

  ○ **Class IV**: diffuse (> 50%) lupus nephritis

  ○ **Class V**: membranous lupus nephritis

  ○ **Class VI**: advanced sclerosing lupus nephritis

- Lupus is treated with **steroids** and **immunosuppressive agents**. It tends to have a chronic, unpredictable course with remissions and relapses. The 10-year survival is 85%, with death frequently being due to renal failure or infections.

Sjögren syndrome (sicca syndrome) is an autoimmune disease characterized by destruction of the lacrimal and salivary glands, resulting in the inability to produce saliva and tears. Females are affected more often than males, with typical age 30–50.

Clinical manifestations include keratoconjunctivitis sicca (dry eyes) and corneal ulcers; xerostomia (dry mouth); and Mikulicz syndrome (enlargement of the salivary and lacrimal glands). Sjögren syndrome is often associated with rheumatoid arthritis and other autoimmune diseases. The characteristic autoantibodies are the anti-ribonucleoprotein antibodies SS-A (Ro) and SS-B (La). There is an increased risk of developing non-Hodgkin lymphoma.

Scleroderma (progressive systemic sclerosis) is an autoimmune disease characterized by fibroblast stimulation and deposition of collagen in the skin and internal organs. It affects females more than males, with typical age range of 20 to 55 years. The pathogenesis involves activation of fibroblasts by cytokines interleukin 1 (IL-1), platelet-derived growth factor (PDGF), and/or fibroblast growth factor (FGF) with the resulting activated fibroblasts causing fibrosis.

- **Diffuse scleroderma** has anti-DNA topoisomerase I antibodies (Scl-70) (70%), widespread skin involvement, and early involvement of the visceral organs. Organs that can be affected include the esophagus (dysphagia), GI tract (malabsorption), lungs (pulmonary fibrosis which causes dyspnea on exertion), heart (cardiac fibrosis which may manifest as arrhythmias), and kidney (fibrosis that may manifest as renal insufficiency).

Clinical Correlate

Antihistone antibodies: Hydralazine, isonizide, and procainamide can cause a lupus-like syndrome with antihistone antibodies.

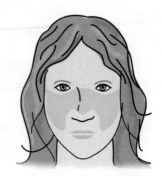

Butterfly Rash

Clinical Correlate

Maternal **anti-Ro (SS-A) antibodies** have been implicated in the pathogenesis of congenital complete heart block.

In a Nutshell
CREST Syndrome
- Calcinosis
- Raynaud phenomenon
- Esophageal dysmotility
- Sclerodactyly
- Telangiectasia

- **Localized scleroderma** (CREST syndrome) has anti-centromere antibodies, skin involvement of the face and hands, late involvement of visceral organs, and a relatively benign clinical course.

Dermatomyositis and polymyositis. See Skeletal Muscle chapter.

Mixed connective tissue disease is an overlap condition with features of systemic lupus erythematosus, systemic sclerosis, and polymyositis. Antiribonucleoprotein antibodies are nearly always positive.

PRIMARY IMMUNE DEFICIENCY SYNDROMES

X-linked agammaglobulinemia of Bruton is an immunodeficiency characterized by a developmental failure to produce mature B cells and plasma cells, resulting in agammablobulinemia. The condition occurs because of loss of function mutations of B-cell Bruton tyrosine kinase (BTK). Clinically, the disease affects male infants who have recurrent infections beginning at 6 months of life due to the loss of passive maternal immunity. Common infections include pharyngitis, otitis media, bronchitis, and pneumonia; common infecting organisms include *H. influenza, S. pneumococcus,* and *S. aureus.*

Common variable immunodeficiency is a group of disorders characterized by defects in B-cell maturation that can lead to defective IgA or IgG production. Clinically, both sexes are affected with onset in childhood of recurrent bacterial infections and with increased susceptibility to *Giardia lamblia*. Complications include increased frequency of developing autoimmune disease, non-Hodgkin lymphoma, and gastric cancer.

DiGeorge syndrome is an embryologic failure to develop the 3rd and 4th pharyngeal pouches, resulting in the absence of the parathyroid glands and thymus. Clinical findings can include neonatal hypocalcemia and tetany, T-cell deficiency, and recurrent infections with viral and fungal organisms.

Severe combined immunodeficiency (SCID) is a combined deficiency of cell-mediated and humoral immunity that is often caused by a progenitor-cell defect. The modes of inheritance are variable and can include X-linked (mutation of the common [gamma] chain of the interleukin receptors IL-2, IL-4, IL-7, IL-9, IL-15, and IL-21) and autosomal recessive (deficiency of adenosine deaminase). Clinical features include recurrent infections with bacteria, fungi, viruses, and protozoa; susceptibility to *Candida*, cytomegalovirus (CMV), and *Pneumocystis jirovecii* infections, and adverse reactions to live virus immunizations. SCID is treated with hematopoietic stem cell transplantation since the prognosis without treatment is death of most infants within a year.

Wiskott-Aldrich syndrome is an X-linked recessive disease with mutation in the gene for Wiskott-Aldrich syndrome protein (WASP). The disease has a clinical triad of recurrent infections, severe thrombocytopenia, and eczema (chronic spongiform dermatitis). Treatment is hematopoietic stem cell transplantation. Complications include increased risk of non-Hodgkin lymphoma and death due to infection or hemorrhage.

Complement system disorders can involve a variety of factors, with deficiencies of different factors producing different clinical patterns.

Note

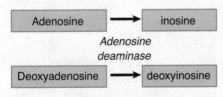

Adenosine deaminase is an important enzyme in purine metabolism; a deficiency of it results in accumulation of deoxyadenosine within lymphoid progenitor cells.

In both the classical and alternate pathways, C3 deficiency causes both recurrent bacterial infections and immune complex disease, while C5, C6, C7, and C8 deficiencies cause recurrent meningococcal and gonococcal infections.

- In the classical pathway only, C1q, C1r, C1s, C2, and C4 deficiencies cause marked increases in immune complex diseases, including infections with pyogenic bacteria.

- In the alternate pathway, Factor B and properdin deficiencies cause increased neisserial infections. Deficiencies in complement regulatory proteins can cause C1-INH deficiency (hereditary angioedema), which is characterized clinically by edema at mucosal surfaces with low C2 and C4 levels.

MHC class II deficiency can be caused by defects in positive selection of thymocytes. Few CD4+ lymphocytes develop and as a result, patients suffer from severe immunodeficiency. Mutations in genes (i.e., *CIITA*) that encode proteins that regulate MHC class II gene expression are the cause. CD8+ T cells are unaffected.

Hyper IgM syndrome is characterized by normal B and T lymphocyte numbers and normal to elevated IgM levels but significantly decreased IgA, IgG and IgE levels. Mutations in the gene for CD40 ligand result in the most common form of X-linked hyper IgM syndrome.

Selective IgA deficiency has unknown genetic etiology. Many affected individuals appear healthy while others have significant illness. Sinopulmonary infections, diarrhea and adverse reactions to transfusions can occur. Levels of IgA are undetectable whereas levels of other isotypes are normal. There is an association with autoimmune disease.

Phagocyte deficiencies (*See* chronic granulomatous disease in Inflammation chapter.)

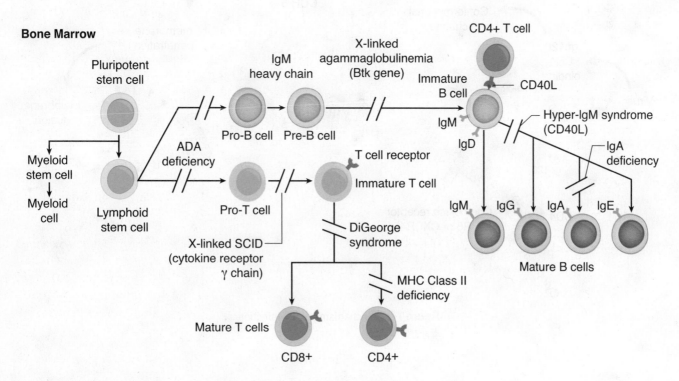

Figure 7-2. Primary Immune Deficiency Syndromes

SECONDARY IMMUNE DEFICIENCY SYNDROMES

Systemic diseases that can cause secondary immunodeficiency include diabetes mellitus, collagen vascular disease (e.g., systemic lupus erythematosus), and chronic alcoholism. Secondary immunodeficiency is more common.

ACQUIRED IMMUNODEFICIENCY SYNDROME (AIDS)

AIDS can be diagnosed when a person is HIV-positive and has CD4 count <200 cells/mL, **or** when a person is HIV-positive and has an AIDS-defining disease. Males are affected more frequently than females.

The *human immunodeficiency virus* (HIV) is an enveloped RNA retrovirus that contains reverse transcriptase. HIV infects CD4-positive cells, including CD4+ T lymphocytes, all macrophages, lymph node follicular dendritic cells, and Langerhans cells. The mechanism of infection is by binding of CD4 by the viral gp120, followed by entry into cell by fusion, which requires gp41 and coreceptors CCR5 (β-chemokine receptor 5) and CXCR4 (α-chemokine receptor).

Transmission of HIV can occur by many mechanisms, including sexual contact (most common mode, including both homosexual transmission and an increasing rate of heterosexual transmission, with important cofactors including herpes and syphilis infection); parenteral transmission; IV drug use; blood transfusions (including those done in hemophiliacs); accidental needle sticks in hospital workers; and vertical transmission.

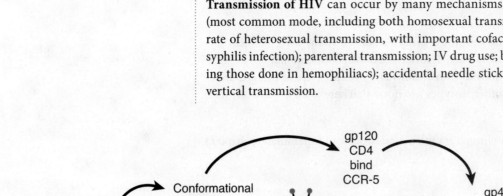

Retrovirus

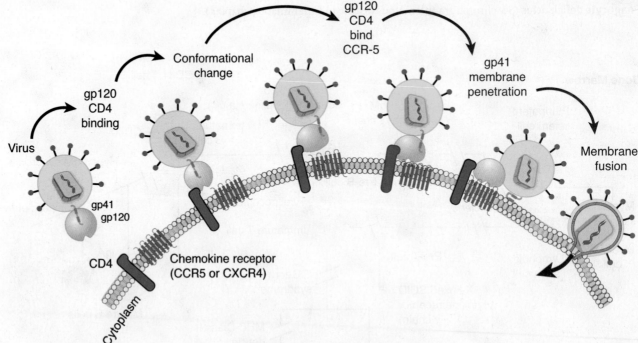

Figure 7-3. Mechanisms of HIV Infection

Diagnosis. The CDC recommends initial testing with an antigen/antibody combination immunoassay, followed by a confirmatory HIV-1/HIV-2 antibody differentiation immunoassay. If the confirmatory test is negative, testing with an HIV-1 nucleic acid test is done. Treatment varies, and can include combination antiretroviral treatment, reverse transcriptase inhibitors, protease inhibitors, and prophylaxis for opportunistic infections based on CD4 count.

The clinical manifestations of HIV infection vary over time.

- The **acute phase** is characterized by viremia with a reduction in CD4 count, mononucleosis-like viral symptoms and lymphadenopathy, and seroconversion.

- The **latent phase** is characterized by asymptomatic or persistent generalized lymphadenopathy with continued viral replication in the lymph nodes and spleen, low level of virus in the blood, and minor opportunistic infections including oral thrush (candidiasis) and herpes zoster. The average duration of latent phase is 10 years.

- **Progression to AIDS** (third phase) occurs with reduction of CD4 count to <200 cells/mL, which is accompanied by reemergence of viremia and development of AIDS-defining diseases, possibly to eventual death.

Table 7-1.
Opportunistic Infection and Common Sites of Infection in AIDS Patients

Opportunistic Infection	Common Sites of Infection
Pneumocystis jiroveci	Lung (pneumonia), bone marrow
Mycobacterium tuberculosis	Lung, disseminated
Mycobacterium avium-intracellulare	Lung, GI tract, disseminated
Coccidioidomycosis	Lung, disseminated
Histoplasmosis	Lung, disseminated
Cytomegalovirus	Lung, retina, adrenals, and GI tract
Giardia lamblia	GI tract
Cryptosporidium	GI tract
Herpes simplex virus	Esophagus and CNS (encephalitis)
Candida	Oral pharynx and esophagus
Aspergillus	CNS, lungs, blood vessels
Toxoplasmosis	CNS
Cryptococcus	CNS (meningitis)
JC virus	CNS (progressive multifocal leukoencephalopathy)
Bartonella spp.	Skin, mucosa, bone (bacillary angiomatosis)

Note

Macrophages and follicular dendritic cells are reservoirs for the virus.

Note

The CD4+ cell count is used to determine the health of the immune system and for recommendations on instituting prophylaxis for opportunistic diseases. Viral load is followed to assess treatment efficacy.

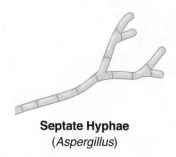

Septate Hyphae
(*Aspergillus*)

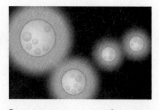

Cryptococcus neoformans

AIDS-Defining Diseases

Hairy leukoplakia is an Epstein-Barr virus (EBV)–associated condition due to infection of squamous cells. White plaques are present on the tongue.

Kaposi sarcoma is the most common neoplasm in AIDS patients. (*See* Vascular Pathology chapter.)

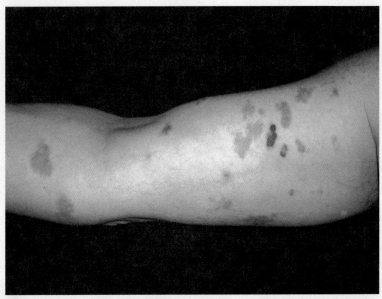

© Richard P. Usatine, M.D.
Used with permission.

Figure 7-4. Kaposi Sarcoma in an AIDS Patient

Non-Hodgkin lymphomas tend to be high-grade B-cell lymphomas; extranodal CNS lymphomas are common.

Other AIDS-defining diseases include cervical cancer, HIV-wasting syndrome, AIDS nephropathy, and AIDS dementia complex.

IMMUNOLOGY OF TRANSPLANT REJECTION

Rejection is caused largely by differences in HLA alleles between donor and recipient. Immunosuppressive agents are used to prevent and mitigate rejection.

- **Hyperacute rejection** occurs within minutes to hours due to preformed antibodies in the recipient. Lymphocyte cross-matching has almost eliminated this problem.

- **Acute rejection** occurs in the first 6 months and may be cellular (CD8+ T lymphocytes kill graft cells) or antibody-mediated.

- **Chronic rejection** occurs after months or years and may be cell-mediated or antibody-mediated. The vasculature components are targeted, and the histopathologic changes depend on the organ involved.

Chapter Summary

- **Type I hypersensitivity** (anaphylactic type) reactions are characterized by IgE-dependent release of chemical mediators from mast cells and basophils following exposure to an antigen. Examples include systemic anaphylaxis following bee stings and drugs. Localized forms of anaphylactic reaction include food allergies, atopy, and asthma.

- **Type II hypersensitivity** (cytotoxic type) reactions are characterized by production of IgG or IgM antibody directed against a specific target cell or tissue. Examples include the complement-dependent cytotoxicity of autoimmune hemolytic anemia, the antibody-dependent cell-mediated cytotoxicity of pernicious anemia, and the antireceptor antibodies of Graves disease.

- **Type III hypersensitivity** (immune complex disease) reactions are characterized by the formation of in situ or circulating antibody-antigen complexes that deposit in tissue, resulting in inflammation and tissue injury. Examples include serum sickness, systemic lupus erythematosus, and glomerulonephritis.

- **Type IV hypersensitivity** (cell-mediated type) reactions are mediated by sensitized T lymphocytes. Examples include the delayed hypersensitivity of PPD skin tests and TB and the cytotoxic T-cell–mediated destruction of antigen-containing cells in viral infections, immune reaction to tumor-associated antigens, type 1 diabetes, and graft rejection.

- Systemic lupus erythematosus is a chronic systemic autoimmune disease characterized by a loss of self-tolerance and production of autoantibodies.

- Sjögren syndrome (sicca syndrome) is an autoimmune disease characterized by destruction of the lacrimal and salivary glands resulting in the inability to produce saliva and tears.

- Scleroderma (progressive systemic sclerosis) is an autoimmune disease characterized by fibroblast stimulation and deposition of collagen in the skin and internal organs. Scleroderma can have anti-DNA topoisomerase I antibodies (Scl-70), widespread skin involvement, and early involvement of the esophagus, GI tract, lung, heart, and kidney.

- X-linked agammaglobulinemia of Bruton is an inherited immunodeficiency characterized by a developmental failure to produce mature B cells and plasma cells.

- Common variable immunodeficiency is a group of disorders characterized by a B-cell maturation defect leading to defects in IgA and IgG production.

- DiGeorge is an embryologic failure to develop the third and fourth pharyngeal pouches, resulting in the absence of the parathyroid glands and thymus.

- Severe combined immunodeficiency (SCID) is a combined deficiency of cell-mediated and humoral immunity often caused by a progenitor cell defect that, without treatment, causes death by infection within 1 year.

- Wiskott-Aldrich is an X-linked condition characterized by recurrent infections, severe thrombocytopenia, and eczema.

(continued)

Chapter Summary *(cont'd)*

- Secondary immune deficiency syndromes can be caused by systemic diseases such as DM, collagen vascular disease (i.e., SLE), and chronic alcoholism.

- AIDS is said to be present when a patient is HIV positive with CD4 count ‹200 cells/mL or HIV positive with an AIDS-defining disease. HIV can be spread by sexual contact, parenteral transmission, or vertical transmission. The virus is an RNA retrovirus with reverse transcriptase and a predilection for infecting CD4+ cells.

- HIV infection produces a mononucleosis-like acute phase, an asymptomatic latent phase, and then progression to AIDS. Clinical AIDS is characterized by susceptibility to a wide variety of opportunistic infections.

- Rejection following tissue transplantation can occur in 3 patterns:

  - **Hyperacute** rejection, due to preformed antibodies
  - **Acute** rejection, mediated by T cells and antibodies
  - **Chronic** rejection, mediated by T cells and antibodies targeting the vasculature

Learning Objectives

❑ Answer questions about composition of amyloid

❑ Explain information related to systemic types of amyloid

❑ Demonstrate understanding of localized types of amyloid

COMPOSITION OF AMYLOID

Amyloidosis is a group of diseases characterized by the deposition of an extracellular protein that has specific properties.

- Individual molecular subunits form β-pleated sheets. Amorphous eosinophilic extracellular deposits of amyloid are seen on the H&E stain. These deposits stain red with the Congo red stain, and apple green birefringence of the amyloid is seen on the Congo red stain under polarized light.

- The fibrillary protein of amyloid varies with each disease. Also present in amyloid are serum amyloid P (SAP) and glycosaminoglycans (heparan sulfate).

SYSTEMIC TYPES OF AMYLOID

Primary amyloidosis has amyloid light chain (AL) amyloid, whose fibrillary protein is made of kappa or lambda light chains. Primary amyloidosis may be seen in plasma cell disorders (multiple myeloma, B-cell lymphomas, etc.) but most cases occur independent of other diseases.

Reactive systemic amyloidosis (secondary amyloidosis) has amyloid-associated (AA) protein, whose precursor is serum amyloid A (SAA), an acute phase reactant produced by the liver which is elevated with ongoing chronic inflammation and neoplasia. Reactive systemic amyloidosis can be seen with a wide variety of chronic diseases, including rheumatoid arthritis, systemic lupus erythematosus, tuberculosis, bronchiectasis, osteomyelitis, inflammatory bowel disease, and cancer.

Familial Mediterranean fever has AA type amyloid with fibrillary protein composed of serum amyloid A (SAA). This autosomal recessive disease is characterized by recurrent inflammation, fever, and neutrophil dysfunction. Gain of function mutations of *pyrin* are present.

Hemodialysis-associated amyloidosis has Aβ2M type amyloid with precursor protein β2-microglobulin. This form of amyloidosis may cause carpal tunnel syndrome and joint disease.

Clinical Correlate

Carpal tunnel syndrome is caused when fibrosis, edema, or another pathologic process compresses and damages the median nerve within the tunnel formed by the carpal bones and flexor retinaculum.

LOCALIZED TYPES OF AMYLOID

Senile cerebral amyloidosis (Alzheimer disease) has Aβ type amyloid with fibrillary protein composed of β-amyloid precursor protein (βAPP). It is found in Alzheimer plaques and in cerebral vessels. The gene for βAPP is located on chromosome 21.

TTR = transporter of thyroxine and retinol

Senile cardiac/systemic amyloidosis has ATTR type amyloid with fibrillary protein composed of transthyretin. This type of amyloidosis is seen in men older than 70 years and may cause heart failure as a result of restrictive/infiltrative cardiomyopathy. Four percent of African Americans have a transthyretin (TTR) V1221 mutation with 1% being homozygous, serving as a risk for cardiac disease.

Endocrine type amyloidosis is seen in medullary carcinoma of the thyroid (procalcitonin), adult-onset diabetes (amylin), and pancreatic islet cell tumors (amylin).

CLINICAL FEATURES

In **systemic forms** of amyloidosis, the kidney is the most commonly involved organ, and patients may experience nephrotic syndrome and/or progressive renal failure. Cardiac involvement may cause restrictive cardiomyopathy and conduction disturbances. Other clinical features include hepatosplenomegaly and involvement of the gastrointestinal tract, which may produce tongue enlargement (macroglossia, primarily in AL type) and malabsorption.

Diagnosis in systemic forms of amyloidosis can be established with biopsy of the rectal mucosa, gingiva, or the abdominal fat pad; Congo red stain shows apple green birefringence under polarized light of amyloid deposits. The prognosis of systemic amyloidosis is poor. AL amyloidosis is diagnosed by serum and urinary protein electrophoresis and immunoelectrophoresis. Proteomic analysis is another diagnostic tool.

Chapter Summary

- Amyloidosis is a group of diseases characterized by the deposition of an extracellular protein that tends to form β-pleated sheets and stain red with apple green birefringence with Congo red stain.

- Amyloid is composed of a fibrillary protein, amyloid P component, and glycosaminoglycans. The specific composition of the protein varies with each disease producing amyloidosis.

- In primary amyloidosis, the amyloid protein is AL, and the fibrillary protein is kappa or lambda light chains.

- Reactive systemic amyloidosis (secondary amyloidosis) can complicate neoplasia and ongoing inflammation due to chronic disease. The amyloid protein in reactive systemic amyloidosis is AA, and the fibrillary protein is serum amyloid A (SAA), which is an acute phase reactant produced by the liver.

- Familial Mediterranean fever is an autosomal recessive inflammatory disease with amyloid protein AA and fibrillary protein SAA.

- Hemodialysis-associated amyloidosis is associated with amyloid protein Aβ2M and fibrillary protein β2-microglobulin.

- Localized forms of amyloidosis are seen in senile cerebral amyloidosis (amyloid protein Aβ and fibrillary protein β-amyloid precursor protein); senile cardiac/systemic amyloidosis (amyloid protein ATTR and fibrillary protein transthyretin); and some endocrine diseases.

Principles of Neoplasia 9

Learning Objectives

❏ Use knowledge of epidemiology of neoplasias

❏ Answer questions about carcinogenic agents

❏ Solve problems concerning carcinogenesis

❏ Answer questions about diagnosis of cancer

DEFINITION

In **neoplasia**, an abnormal cell or tissue grows more rapidly than normal cells or tissue; it does so by acquiring multiple genetic changes over time and by continuing to grow after the stimuli that initiated the new growth have been removed.

EPIDEMIOLOGY

Cancer is the **second leading cause of death** in the United States. In 2015, the estimated number of new cancers diagnosed was 1,658,370, and the estimated number of deaths from cancer was 589,430.

In men, the sites with the highest new cancer rates are (in order of decreasing frequency):

- Prostate
- Lung and bronchus
- Colon and rectum

These same sites have the highest mortality rate, although lung and bronchus cancers more commonly cause death than prostate cancer.

In women, the sites with the highest new cancer rates are (in order of decreasing frequency):

- Breast
- Lung and bronchus
- Colon and rectum

These same sites have the highest mortality rate, although lung and bronchus cancers more commonly cause death than breast cancer.

In children, the most common cancers are acute lymphocytic leukemia, CNS malignancy, neuroblastoma, and non-Hodgkin lymphoma.

Predisposition to cancer involves many factors. Geographic and racial factors can be important:

- Stomach cancer is **much more prevalent** in Japan than in the United States.
- Breast cancer is **much more prevalent** in the United States than in Japan.
- Liver hepatoma is **much more prevalent** in Asia than in the United States.
- Prostate cancer is **more prevalent** in African Americans than in Caucasians.

Heredity predisposition can be seen in many cancers, including familial retinoblastoma, multiple endocrine neoplasia, and familial polyposis coli.

Acquired preneoplastic disorders also affect cancer incidence, with examples including cervical dysplasia (characterized by changes in cell size and shape), endometrial hyperplasia, cirrhosis, inflammatory bowel disease, and chronic atrophic gastritis.

CARCINOGENIC AGENTS

Chemical carcinogens. Carcinogenesis is a multistep process involving a sequence of initiation (mutation) followed by promotion (proliferation). Initiators can be either direct-acting chemical carcinogens (mutagens which cause cancer directly by modifying DNA) or indirect-acting chemical carcinogens (procarcinogens which require metabolic conversion to form active carcinogens). Promotors cause cellular proliferation of mutated (initiated) cells, which may lead to accumulation of additional mutations.

- **Clinically important chemical carcinogens** are numerous, and include nitrosamines (gastric cancer), cigarette smoke (multiple malignancies), polycyclic aromatic hydrocarbons (bronchogenic carcinoma), asbestos (bronchogenic carcinoma, mesothelioma), chromium and nickel (bronchogenic carcinoma), arsenic (squamous cell carcinomas of skin and lung, angiosarcoma of liver), vinyl chloride (angiosarcoma of liver), aromatic amines and azo dyes (hepatocellular carcinoma), alkylating agents (leukemia, lymphoma, other cancers), benzene (leukemia), and naphthylamine (bladder cancer). Potential carcinogens are screened by the Ames test, which detects any mutagenic effects of potential carcinogens on bacterial cells in culture; mutagenicity *in vitro* correlates well with carcinogenicity in vivo.

Bridge to Biochemistry

Diseases associated with DNA repair include xeroderma pigmentosum and hereditary nonpolyposis colorectal cancer.

Radiation. Ultraviolet B sunlight is the most carcinogenic because it produces pyrimidine dimers in DNA, leading to transcriptional errors and mutations of oncogenes and tumor suppressor genes, thereby increasing the risk of skin cancer. Xeroderma pigmentosum is an autosomal recessive inherited defect in DNA repair, in which the pyrimidine dimers formed with ultraviolet B sunlight cannot be repaired; this defect predisposes to skin cancer. Ionizing radiation includes x-rays and gamma rays, alpha and beta particles, protons, and neutrons. Cells in mitosis or the G2 phase of the cell cycle are most sensitive to radiation. Radiation causes cross-linking and chain breaks in nucleic acids. Atomic bomb survivors experienced an increased incidence of leukemias, thyroid cancer, and other cancers. Uranium miners historically had increased lung cancer, related to inhalation of radioactive radon, which is a decay product of uranium.

Oncogenic viruses.

RNA oncogenic viruses. Human T-cell leukemia virus (HTLV-1) causes adult T-cell leukemia/lymphoma.

DNA oncogenic viruses include the following:

- Hepatitis B virus (hepatocellular carcinoma)
- Epstein-Barr virus (EBV), which has been implicated in Burkitt lymphoma, B-cell lymphomas in immunosuppressed patients, nasopharyngeal carcinoma
- Human papilloma virus (HPV), which causes benign squamous papillomas (warts-condyloma acuminatum) and a variety of carcinomas (cervical, vulvar, vaginal, penile, and anal)
- Kaposi-sarcoma-associated herpesvirus (HHV8) which causes Kaposi sarcoma

Loss of immune regulation. Immunosurveillance normally destroys neoplastic cells via recognition of "non-self" antigens, and both humoral and cell-mediated immune responses play a role. Patients with immune system dysfunction have an increased number of neoplasms, especially malignant lymphomas.

CARCINOGENESIS

Carcinogenesis is a multistep process, and development of all human cancers appears to require the accumulation of multiple genetic changes. These changes can involve either inherited germline mutations or acquired mutations. Once a single severely mutated cell forms, monoclonal expansion of the cell's line can cause a tumor. Most important mutations in tumorogenesis involve growth promoting genes (proto-oncogenes), growth inhibiting tumor suppressor genes, or the genes regulating apoptosis and senescence.

Activation of growth promoting oncogenes. Proto-oncogenes are normal cellular genes involved with growth and cellular differentiation. Oncogenes are derived from proto-oncogenes by either a change in the gene sequence, resulting in a new gene product (oncoprotein), or a loss of gene regulation resulting in overexpression of the normal gene product. Mechanisms of oncogene activation include point mutations, chromosomal translocations, gene amplification, and insertional mutagenesis. Activated oncogenes lack regulatory control and are overexpressed, resulting in unregulated cellular proliferation.

Table 9-1. Clinically Important Oncogenes

Oncogene	Tumor	Gene Product	Mechanism of Activation
FGF3 & FGF4	Cancer of the stomach, breast, bladder, and Kaposi sarcoma	**Growth factors** Fibroblast growth factor	Overexpression
PDGFRA	Astrocytoma	Platelet-derived growth factor	Overexpression
ERBB1	Squamous cell carcinoma of lung	**Growth factor receptors** Epidermal growth factor receptor	Overexpression
ERBB2	Breast, ovary, lung	Epidermal growth factor receptor	Amplification
ERBB3	Breast	Epidermal growth factor receptor	Overexpression
RET	MEN 2A & 2B, familial thyroid (medullary) cancer	Glial neurotrophic factor receptor	Point mutation
ABL	CML, ALL	**Signal transduction proteins** bcr-abl fusion protein with tyrosine kinase activity	Translocation t(9;22)
KRAS	Lung, pancreas, and colon	GTP binding protein	Point mutation
MYC	Burkitt lymphoma	Nuclear regulatory protein	Translocation t(8;14)
MYCL	Small cell lung carcinoma	Nuclear regulatory protein	Amplification
MYCN	Neuroblastoma	Nuclear regulatory protein	Amplification
CCND1	Mantle cell lymphoma	**Cell cycle regulatory proteins** Cyclin D protein	Translocation t(11;14)
CDK4	Melanoma, GBM	Cyclin dependent kinase	Amplification

Inactivation of tumor suppressor genes. Tumor suppressor genes encode proteins that regulate and suppress cell proliferation by inhibiting progression of the cell through the cell cycle. The mechanism of action of tumor suppressor genes may vary. As examples, p53 prevents a cell with damaged DNA from entering S-phase, while Rb prevents the cell from entering S-phase until the appropriate growth signals are present.

- **Knudson's "two hit hypothesis"** states that at least 2 tumor suppressor genes must be inactivated for oncogenesis. In cancers arising in individuals with inherited germline mutations, the "first hit" is the inherited germline mutation and the "second hit" is an acquired somatic mutation. Examples of inherited germline mutations include familial retinoblastoma (in which germline mutation of *RB1* on chromosome 13 is associated with a high rate of retinoblastoma and osteosarcoma) and Li-Fraumini syndrome (in which germline mutation of *TP53* on chromosome 17 is associated with a high rate of many types of tumors).

Table 9-2. Clinically Important Tumor Suppressor Genes

Chromosome	Gene	Tumors
3p25.3	VHL	von Hippel-Lindau disease, renal cell carcinoma
11p13	WT1	Wilms tumor
11p15.5	WT2	Wilms tumor
13q14.2	RB1	Retinoblastoma, osteosarcoma
17p13.1	TP53	Lung, breast, colon, and others
17q21.31	BRCA1	Hereditary breast and ovary cancer
13q13.1	BRCA2	Hereditary breast cancer
5q22.2	APC	Adenomatous polyps and colon cancer
18q21.2	DCC	Colon cancer
17q11.2	NF1	Neurofibromas
22q12.2	NF2	Acoustic neuromas, meningiomas

Regulation of apoptosis. Tumor genesis related to changes in regulation of apotosis occurs in the follicular lymphomas that have the translocation t(14;18). Normally, Bcl-2 prevents apoptosis (programmed cell death). In the follicular lymphomas with this translocation, the Bcl-2 regulator of apoptosis is overexpressed, because the translocation connects the immunoglobulin heavy chain gene on chromosome 14 (which turns on easily in B lymphocytes) to the *BCL2* gene on chromosome 18, thereby leading to a situation in which lymphocytes fail to die as expected and instead produce a tumor.

Other examples of apoptosis regulators include Bax, Bad, bcl-xS, and Bid; p53 promotes apoptosis in mutated cells by stimulating bax synthesis. The protein c-myc promotes cellular proliferation and when associated with p53 leads to apoptosis and when associated with Bcl-2 inhibits apoptosis.

Limitless replication is possible due in part to upregulation of telomerase.

Sustained angiogenesis is possible due in part to activation of the Notch signaling pathway.

Invasiveness/metastasis. Malignant cells must dissociate from tumors (loss of E-cadherin function) and degrade the extracellular matrix before spreading to distant sites. Cancer-associated glycans are being investigated for their role in cancer spread and as targets for therapy.

DIAGNOSIS OF CANCER

Table 9-3. General Features of Benign versus Malignant Neoplasms

	Benign	Malignant
Gross	• Small size • Slow growing • Encapsulated or well-demarcated borders	• Larger in size • Rapid growth • Necrosis and hemorrhage are commonly seen • Poorly demarcated
Micro	• Expansile growth with well-circumscribed borders • Tend to be well differentiated • Resemble the normal tissue counterpart from which they arise • Noninvasive and never metastasize	• Vary from well to poorly (anaplastic) differentiated • Tumor cells vary in size and shape (pleomorphism) • Increased nuclear to cytoplasmic ratios • Nuclear hyperchromasia and prominent nucleoli • High mitotic activity with abnormal mitotic figures • *Invasive growth pattern* • *Has potential to metastasize*

Histologic diagnosis of cancer. Microscopic examination of tissue or cells is required to make the diagnosis of cancer. Material suitable for diagnosis of a tumor may be obtained by complete excision, biopsy, fine needle aspiration, or cytologic smears (Pap test).

- **Immunohistochemistry** may be helpful in confirming the tissue of origin of metastatic or poorly differentiated tumors. The technique uses monoclonal antibodies that are specific for a cellular component. Among the many antibodies that are clinically useful are:

  - All of the serum tumor markers
  - Thyroglobulin (thyroid cancers)
  - S100 (melanoma and neural tumors)
  - Actin (smooth and skeletal muscle)
  - CD markers (lymphomas/leukemias)
  - Estrogen receptors (breast cancer)
  - Intermediate filaments

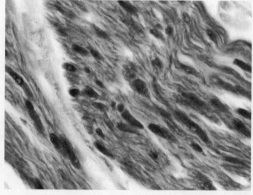

© Gregg Barré, M.D.
Used with permission.

Figure 9-1. S100 Staining of a Neurofibroma

- **Ancillary tests** for the diagnosis of cancer include electron microscopy, flow cytometry, cytogenetics, and PCR/DNA probes.

Table 9-4.
Expression of Intermediate Filaments by Normal and Malignant Cells

Intermediate Filament	Normal Tissue Expression	Tumor
Keratin	All epithelial cells	Carcinomas
Vimentin	Mesenchymal cells	Sarcomas
Desmin	Muscle cells	Uterine leiomyoma Rhabdomyosarcoma
Neurofilament	CNS and PNS neurons Neural crest derivatives	Pheochromocytoma Neuroblastoma
Glial fibrillary acidic protein (GFAP)	Glial cells	Astrocytomas Ependymomas

Serum tumor markers. Tumor markers are usually normal cellular components that are increased in neoplasms but may also be elevated in nonneoplastic conditions. Serum tumor markers are used for screening (e.g., prostate specific antigen [PSA]) for cancer, monitoring treatment efficacy, and detecting recurrence of cancers.

- **Clinically useful tumor markers** include alpha-fetoprotein (AFP, used for hepatoma, nonseminomatous testicular germ cell tumors); beta human chorionic gonadotropin (hCG, used for trophoblastic tumors, choriocarcinoma); calcitonin (used for medullary carcinoma of the thyroid); carcinoembryonic antigen (CEA, used for carcinomas of the lung, pancreas, stomach, breast, and colon); CA-125 (used for malignant ovarian epithelial tumors); CA19-9 (used for malignant pancreatic adenocarcinoma); placental alkaline phosphatase (used for seminoma); and prostate specific antigen (PSA, used for prostate cancer).

Grading and staging. Tumor grade is a histologic estimate of the malignancy of a tumor, and typically uses criteria such as the degree of differentiation from low grade (well-differentiated) to high grade (poorly differentiated/anaplastic) and the number of mitoses.

Tumor stage is a clinical estimate of the extent of tumor spread. TNM staging system criteria is used for most tumor types:

- **T** indicates the size of the primary tumor.
- **N** indicates extent of regional lymph node spread.
- **M** indicates the presence or absence of metastatic disease.

In general, staging is a better predictor of prognosis than tumor grade.

Note

Most neoplasms (90%) arise from epithelium, with the remainder from mesenchymal cells.

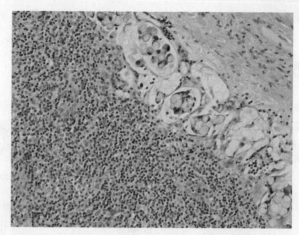

Figure 9-2. Involvement of Lymph Node by Signet Ring Cell Carcinoma

Tumor progression refers to the tendency of a tumor to become more malignant over time. This progression can be related to both natural selection (evolution of a more malignant clone over time due to a selective growth advantage) and genetic instability (malignant cells are more prone to mutate and accumulate additional genetic defects).

Metastasis. Lymphatic spread is the most common initial route of spread for epithelial carcinomas. Early hematogenous spread is typically seen with most sarcomas (e.g., osteogenic sarcoma), renal cell carcinoma (because of the proximity of the large renal vein), hepatocellular carcinoma (because of the presence of the hepatic sinusoids), follicular carcinoma of the thyroid, and choriocarcinoma (because of its propensity to seek vessels). Seeding of body cavities and surfaces occurs in ovarian carcinoma. Transplantation via mechanical manipulation (e.g., surgical incision, needle tracts) may occur but is relatively rare.

Chapter Summary

- Cancer is the second leading cause of death in the United States in both adults and children.

  - In men, the sites with the highest new cancer rates are (in order of decreasing frequency): prostate, lung and bronchus, and colon and rectum.
    - These same sites have the highest mortality rate, although lung and bronchus cancers more commonly cause death than prostate cancer.
  - In women, the sites with the highest new cancer rate are (in order of decreasing frequency): breast, lung and bronchus, and colon and rectum.
    - These same sites have the highest mortality rate, although lung and bronchus cancers more commonly cause death than breast cancer.

- The incidence of different cancers can vary with geographic site, racial factors, occupational exposures, age, hereditary predisposition, and acquired preneoplastic disorders.

- A variety of chemical carcinogens have been identified that can act as initiators or promoters of specific cancers. Ultraviolet light and ionizing radiation are also carcinogenic. A relatively small number of cancers have been linked to infection with specific viruses. Patients with immune system dysfunction also have an increased number of neoplasms.

- Carcinogenesis is a multistep process requiring the accumulation of multiple genetic changes as the result of either inherited germline mutations or acquired mutations, leading to the monoclonal expansion of a mutated cell.

- Cancer growth can involve either activation of growth promoting oncogenes or inactivation of tumor suppressor genes.

- Activated oncogenes lack regulatory control and are overexpressed, resulting in unregulated cellular proliferation. Examples of clinically important oncogenes include *ERBB2*, *RAS*, and *MYC*.

- Tumor suppressor genes encode proteins that regulate and suppress cell proliferation by inhibiting progression of the cell through the cell cycle. Inactivation of these genes leads to uncontrolled cellular proliferation with tumor formation. Examples of clinically important tumor suppressor genes include *VHL*, *TP53*, *RB1*, *APC*, *DCC*, and *NF1*.

- Cancers can also develop if apoptosis (programmed cell death) is prevented by mutations in genes such as *BCL2*, *BAX*, *BAD*, and *BCLXS*.

- Malignant neoplasms tend to be more rapidly growing than similar benign lesions due to a greater portion of cells that are in mitosis; tend to have areas of necrosis and hemorrhage; tend to have invasive growth pattern; tend to have the potential to metastasize; tend to have high mitotic activity with abnormal mitotic figures; and tend to have pleomorphic cells with increased nuclear to cytoplasmic ratio, nuclear hyperchromasia, and prominent nucleoli.

- Serum tumor markers are usually normal cellular components that are increased in neoplasms but may also be elevated in non-neoplastic conditions. They can be used for screening, monitoring of treatment efficacy, and detecting recurrence.

- Tumor grade is a histologic estimate of the malignancy of a tumor. Tumor stage is a clinical estimate of the extent of tumor spread.

(continued)

Chapter Summary (cont'd)

- Many tumors tend to become more malignant over time as a result of natural selection of more malignant clones and genetic instability of malignant cells.

- Lymphatic spread is the most common route of spread for epithelial carcinomas. Hematogenous spread is most likely to be seen with sarcomas, renal cell carcinoma, hepatocellular carcinoma, follicular carcinoma of the thyroid, and choriocarcinoma. Tumors are also less commonly spread by seeding of body cavities and surfaces and via mechanical manipulations such as surgical incisions and needle tracts.

Skin Pathology 10

Learning Objectives

❏ Solve problems concerning disorders of pigmentation

❏ Answer questions about melanocytic tumors

❏ Explain information related to epidermal and dermal lesions

❏ Explain information related to malignant tumors

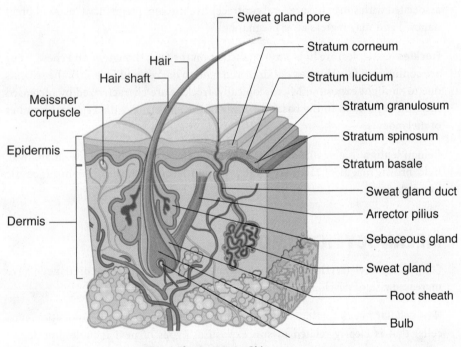

Figure 10-1. Skin

DISORDERS OF PIGMENTATION

Vitiligo causes irregular, completely depigmented skin patches. It is common and can affect any race; there may also be a familial predisposition. The disease has an unknown etiology that is possibly autoimmune. Microscopically, affected areas are devoid of epidermal melanocytes.

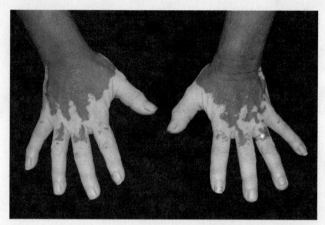

© Richard P. Usatine, M.D.
Used with permission.

Figure 10-2. Vitiligo

Melasma causes irregular blotchy patches of hyperpigmentation on the face; it is associated with sun exposure, oral contraceptive use, and pregnancy ("mask of pregnancy") and may regress after pregnancy.

Freckles (ephelides) are light brown macules on the face, shoulders, and chest. They are common in fair-skinned children and tend to darken and fade with the seasons due to sunlight exposure. Microscopically, freckles are characterized by increased melanin deposition in the basal cell layer of the epidermis with a normal number of melanocytes.

Benign **lentigo** is a localized proliferation of melanocytes which cause small, oval, light brown macules. Microscopically, benign lentigos show linear melanocytic hyperplasia.

MELANOCYTIC TUMORS

Congenital nevi (birthmarks) are present at birth; giant congenital nevi have increased risk of developing melanoma.

Nevocellular nevus (mole) is a benign tumor of melanocytes (melanocytic nevus cells) that is clearly related to sun exposure. Types of nevi include junctional, compound, and intradermal. Nevi have uniform tan to brown color with sharp, well-circumscribed borders and tend to be stable in shape and size. Malignant transformation is uncommon.

Dysplastic nevi (BK moles) are larger and more irregular than common nevi, and they may have pigment variation. Microscopically, the nevus exhibits cytological and architectural atypia. Dysplastic nevus syndrome is autosomal dominant (*CMM1* locus on chromosome 1); patients often have multiple dysplastic nevi; and there is increased risk of developing melanoma.

Malignant melanoma is a malignancy of melanocytes whose incidence is increasing at a rapid rate, with peak in ages 40–70. Risk factors include chronic sun exposure, sunburn, fair skin, dysplastic nevus syndrome, and familial melanoma (associated with loss of function mutation of the p16 tumor suppressor gene, *CDKN2A*, on chromosome 9; somatic mutations of *NRAS* and *BRAF* also occur). Melanomas characteristically form skin lesions of large diameter with asymmetric and irregular borders and variegated color; the lesions may be macules, papules, or nodules. Melanomas on males have increased frequency on the upper back; females have increased frequency on the back and legs.

Several **types of melanomas** occur:

- Lentigo maligna melanoma is usually located on the face or neck of older individuals and has the best prognosis.

- Superficial spreading melanoma is the most common type of melanoma and has a primarily horizontal growth pattern.

- Acral lentiginous melanoma is the most common melanoma in dark-skinned individuals; it affects palms, soles, and subungual area.

- Nodular melanoma is a nodular tumor with a vertical growth pattern that has the worst prognosis of the melanomas.

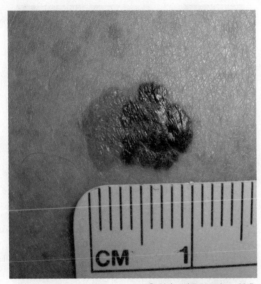

© Richard P. Usatine, M.D.
Used with permission.

Figure 10-3. Melanoma

Note the size, irregular borders, and variegated color.

The **prognosis** of melanomas is determined by TNM staging; T status is based on the depth of invasion (Breslow thickness measured histologically in millimeters).

Local disease is treated with wide surgical excision and sometimes sentinel node biopsy. Systemic disease is treated with chemotherapy or immunotherapy. Metastases may occur after years of dormancy.

EPIDERMAL AND DERMAL LESIONS

Acanthosis nigricans causes thickened, hyperpigmented skin of the posterior neck, axillae, and groin; it is often associated with obesity and hyperinsulinism. On rare occasions it is associated with internal malignancy (stomach and other gastrointestinal malignancies).

Seborrheic keratoses are benign squamoproliferative neoplasms that are very common in middle-aged and elderly individuals; they may occur on the trunk, head, neck, and the extremities. The lesions are tan to brown coin-shaped plaques that have a granular surface with a "stuck on" appearance, characterized microscopically by basaloid epidermal hyperplasia and "horn cysts" (keratin-filled epidermal pseudocysts). They are usually left untreated, but may be removed if they become irritated or for cosmetic purposes. The sign of Leser-Trélat (paraneoplastic syndrome) is the sudden development of multiple lesions which may accompany an internal malignancy.

Psoriasis is an autoimmune disorder with a clear genetic component that causes increased proliferation and turnover of epidermal keratinocytes; it affects 1% of the U.S. population. The most common form is psoriasis vulgaris. Common sites of involvement include the knees, elbows, and scalp; the classic skin lesion is a well-demarcated erythematous plaque with a silvery scale. Removal of scale results in pinpoint bleeding (Auspitz sign). Nail beds show pitting and discoloration. Psoriasis may be associated with arthritis, enteropathy, and myopathy.

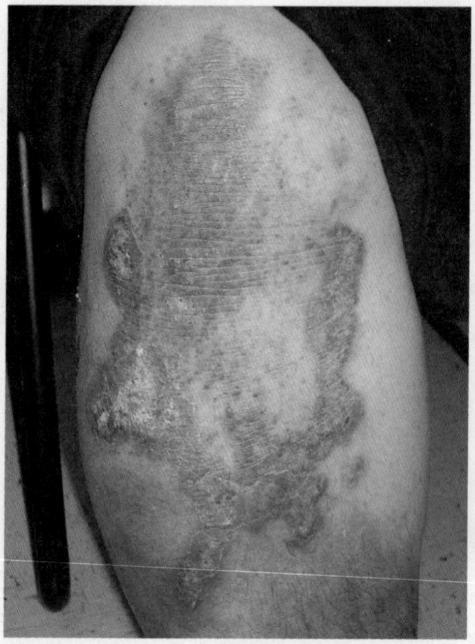

© Richard P. Usatine, M.D.
Used with permission.

Figure 10-4. The Silvery Plaques of Psoriasis

- **Microscopically**, the lesions show epidermal hyperplasia (acanthosis), patchy hyperkeratinization with parakeratosis, uniform elongation and thickening of the rete ridges, thinning of the epidermis over the dermal papillae, and Munro microabscesses.
- Treatment is topical steroids and ultraviolet irradiation; severe systemic disease may be treated with methotrexate.

Pemphigus is a rare, potentially fatal autoimmune disorder that is characterized by intraepidermal blister formation. Pemphigus vulgaris is the most common form. The pathogenesis involves the production of autoantibodies directed against a part of the keratinocyte desmosome called desmoglein 3, with resulting loss of intercellular adhesion (acantholysis) and blister formation. Pemphigus causes mucosal lesions and easily ruptured, flaccid blisters. Oral involvement is common.

- Microscopic examination shows intraepidermal acantholysis; the acantholysis leaves behind a basal layer of keratinocytes, which has a tombstone-like arrangement. Immunofluorescence shows a net-like pattern of IgG staining between the epidermal keratinocytes that create bullae.

- Treatment is with immunosuppression.

Bullous pemphigoid is a relatively common autoimmune disorder of older individuals characterized by subepidermal blister formation with tense bullae that do not rupture easily. The condition results from production of autoantibodies directed against a part of the keratinocyte hemidesmosome called *bullous pemphigoid antigens 1 and 2*. Immunofluorescence shows linear deposits of IgG at the dermal-epidermal junction.

Dermatitis herpetiformis is a rare immune disorder that is often associated with celiac sprue; it is characterized by subepidermal blister formation with itchy, grouped vesicles and occasional bullae on the extensor surfaces. Production of IgA antibodies directed against gliadin and other antigens deposit in the tips of the dermal papillae and result in subepidermal blister formation. Routine microscopy shows microabscesses at the tips of the dermal papillae that can lead to eventual subepidermal separation results in blister formation; immunofluorescence shows granular IgA deposits at the tips of the dermal papillae. Dermatitis herpetiformis often responds to a gluten-free diet.

Porphyria cutanea tarda is an acquired and familial disorder of heme synthesis. Patients experience upper extremity blistering secondary to sun exposure and minor trauma. Microscopically, there are subepidermal blisters with minimal inflammation. Dermal vessels are thickened. Direct immunofluorescence shows deposition of immunoglobulins and complement at the epidermal basement membrane and around dermal vessels.

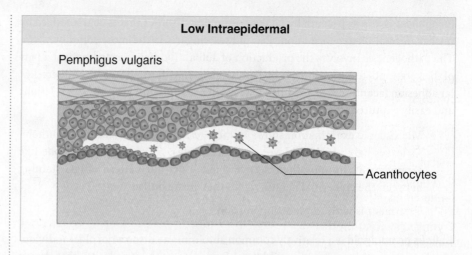

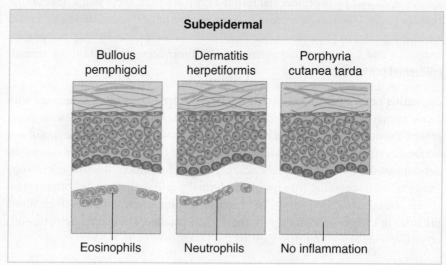

Figure 10-5. Intraepidermal and Subepidermal Blisters

Ichthyosis vulgaris is a common inherited (autosomal dominant) skin disorder characterized by a thickened stratum corneum with absent stratum granulosum. Onset is in childhood. Patients have hyperkeratotic, dry skin on the trunk and extensor surfaces of limb areas.

Xerosis is a common cause of pruritus and dry skin in the elderly that is due to decreased skin lipids. Cancer patients receiving epidermal growth factor receptor inhibitor are susceptible. Treatment is with emollients.

Eczema is a group of related inflammatory skin diseases characterized by pruritus and epidermal spongiosis (edema).

- Acute eczema causes a vesicular, erythematous rash.

- Chronic eczema develops following repetitive scratching, and is characterized by dry, thickened, hyperkeratotic skin.

- Atopic dermatitis is often inherited. Defects in the keratinocyte barrier are due to mutations in the filaggrin gene (*FLG*).

- Contact dermatitis can be either allergic type (poison ivy, nickel in jewelry) or photodermatitis type (such as photosensitivity reaction after tetracycline).

Polymorphous light eruption is the most common idiopathic form of photodermatosis and causes pruritic erythematous macules, papules, plaques, or vesicles on exposure to sunlight. There is dermal edema and inflammation.

Verrucae (warts) are caused by human papillomavirus. Verruca vulgaris is the most common type.

Cutaneous lupus erythematosus may be acute (facial butterfly rash), subacute (photosensitive rash on anterior chest, upper back and upper extremities), or chronic (discoid plaques, usually above the neck). Direct immunofluorescence shows deposition of immunoglobulin and complement at the dermal-epidermal junction. Serologies for autoantibodies and clinical correlation help establish the diagnosis.

Erythema multiforme is a hypersensitivity skin reaction to infections (*Mycoplasma pneumoniae*, herpes simplex) or drugs (sulfonamides, penicillin, barbiturates, phenytoin) characterized by vesicles, bullae, and "targetoid" erythematous lesions. The most severe form is Stevens-Johnson syndrome, which has extensive involvement of skin and mucous membranes.

Pityriasis rosea causes a pruritic rash that starts with an oval-shaped "herald patch" and progresses to a papular eruption of the trunk to produce a "Christmas tree" distribution. It is clinically diagnosed, self-limiting and possibly a viral exanthem.

Granuloma annulare is a chronic inflammatory disorder that causes papules and plaques. Palisaded granulomas are present microscopically. The pathogenesis is immunologic, but most cases occur in healthy patients.

Erythema nodosum causes raised, erythematous, painful nodules of subcutaneous adipose tissue, typically on the anterior shins, which can be associated with granulomatous diseases and streptococcal infection.

Epidermoid cyst is a common benign skin cyst lined with stratified squamous epithelium and filled with keratin debris.

MALIGNANT TUMORS

Squamous cell carcinoma (SCC) has peak incidence at age 60. Risk factors include chronic sun exposure (ultraviolet UVB); fair complexion; chronic skin ulcers or sinus tracts; long-term exposure to hydrocarbons, arsenic, burns, and radiation; immunosuppression; and xeroderma pigmentosum. Common mutations include *TP53* and *HRAS*.

- Precursors include actinic keratosis (a sun-induced dysplasia of the keratinocytes that causes rough, red papules on the face, arms, and hands) and Bowen disease (squamous cell carcinoma *in situ*).

- Squamous cell carcinoma occurs on sun-exposed areas (face and hands) and causes a tan nodular mass which commonly ulcerates. Microscopic examination shows nests of atypical keratinocytes that invade the dermis, (oftentimes) formation of keratin pearls, and intercellular bridges (desmosomes) between tumor cells. Squamous cell carcinoma of the skin rarely metastasizes and complete excision is usually curative.

- A variant is **keratoacanthoma** (well differentiated Squamous cell carcinoma), which causes rapidly growing, dome-shaped nodules with a central keratin-filled crater; these are often self-limited and may regress spontaneously.

Basal cell carcinoma (BCC) is the most common tumor in adults in the Western world; it is most common in middle-aged or elderly individuals and arises from the basal cells of hair follicles. Risk factors include chronic sun exposure, fair complexion, immunosuppression, and xeroderma pigmentosum.

BCC occurs on sun-exposed, hair-bearing areas (face), and may form pearly papules; nodules with heaped-up, translucent borders, telangiectasia, or ulcers (rodent ulcer). Microscopically, BCCs show invasive nests of basaloid cells with a palisading growth pattern.

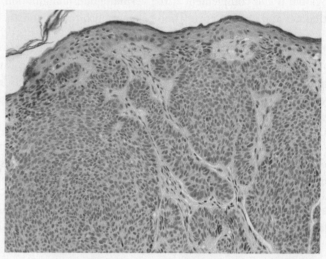

© Gregg Barré, M.D.
Used with permission.

Figure 10-6. Basal Cell Carcinoma

BCC grows slowly and rarely metastasizes, but it may be locally aggressive. Shave biopsies have a 50% recurrence rate, but complete excision is usually curative. Mutations affecting the Hedgehog pathway are seen in sporadic and familial cases.

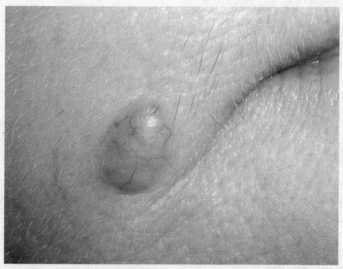

© Richard P. Usatine, M.D.
Used with permission.

Figure 10-7. Pearly Papule Characteristic of a Basal Cell Carcinoma

Chapter Summary

- Disorders of skin pigmentation include vitiligo (irregular depigmented patches due to lack of melanocytes of possibly autoimmune etiology), melasma ("mask of pregnancy"), ephelides (freckles), and benign lentigos.

- Melanocytic tumors include congenital nevi (birthmarks, giant ones have increased risk of melanoma), nevocellular nevi (common moles with proliferating nevus cells; subclassified as junctional, compound, and intradermal), dysplastic nevi (larger, more irregular, and with more pigment variation than common moles, cytological and architectural atypia, may be part of autosomal dominant nevus syndrome with increased risk of melanoma if multiple), and malignant melanoma.

- Malignant melanoma has a rapidly increasing incidence (peak middle age and older) and prognosis ranging from excellent (thin lesions that can be completely excised) to poor (metastatic lesions, often arising in primary sites with tumor thickness >1 mm). In general melanomas cause asymmetric, irregular, large-diameter macules, papules, or nodules with variegated color, found most often on the upper back of men and the back and legs of women.

  - Subtypes include lentigo maligna (best prognosis, face or neck of older individuals), superficial spreading (most common type, horizontal growth pattern), acral-lentiginous (palms, soles, and subungual area of dark-skinned individuals), and nodular melanoma (vertical growth pattern with worst prognosis).

- Benign epidermal and dermal lesions include acanthosis nigricans (thickened, hyperpigmented skin in axillae and groin that may be associated with internal malignancy), seborrheic keratoses (very common benign squamoproliferative tan to brown coin-shaped plaques that appear "stuck on" the trunk, head, neck, and extremities of middle-aged and elderly people), and psoriasis (well-demarcated erythematous plaques with silvery scale and pinpoint bleeding after scale removal commonly involving knees, elbows, and scalp; micro shows epidermal hyperplasia, parakeratosis, and Munro abscesses; genetic component and associations with arthritis, enteropathy, and myopathy).

- Pemphigus and bullous pemphigoid are autoimmune disorders; dermatitis herpetiformis is associated with celiac sprue, and porphyria cutanea tarda is a heme synthesis disorder.

- Other skin lesions include icthyosis vulgaris, xerosis, eczema, polymorphous light eruption, cutaneous lupus erythematosus, erythema multiforme, pityriasis rosea, granuloma annulare, erythema nodosum, and epidermoid cysts.

- In addition to melanoma, malignant tumors of the skin include squamous cell carcinoma and basal cell carcinoma.

Red Blood Cell Pathology: Anemias

Learning Objectives

❑ Explain information related to red blood cell morphology

❑ Solve problems using knowledge of microcytic, normocytic, and macrocytic anemias

❑ Demonstrate understanding of polycythemia vera

RED BLOOD CELL MORPHOLOGY

Red Cell Shapes

Abnormal size is called anisocytosis (*aniso* means unequal). Abnormal shape is called poikilocytosis (*poikilo* means various). **Elliptocytes** may be seen in hereditary elliptocytosis. **Spherocytes** result from decreased erythrocyte membrane, and they may be seen in hereditary spherocytosis and in autoimmune hemolytic anemia. **Target cells** result from increased erythrocyte membrane, and they may be seen in hemoglobinopathies, thalassemia, and liver disease. **Acanthocytes** have irregular spicules on their surfaces; numerous acanthocytes can be seen in abetalipoproteinemia. **Echinocytes** (burr cells) have smooth undulations on their surface; they may be seen in uremia or more commonly as an artifact.

Schistocytes are erythrocyte fragments (helmet cells are a type of schistocyte); they can be seen in microangiopathic hemolytic anemias or traumatic hemolysis. **Bite cells** are erythrocytes with "bites" of cytoplasm being removed by splenic macrophages; they may be seen in G6PD deficiency. **Teardrop cells** (dacrocytes) may be seen in thalassemia and myelofibrosis. **Sickle cells** (drepanocytes) are seen in sickle cell anemia. **Rouleaux** ("stack of coins") refers to erythrocytes lining up in a row. Rouleaux are characteristic of multiple myeloma.

Red Cell Inclusions

Basophilic stippling results from cytoplasmic remnants of RNA; it may indicate reticulocytosis or lead poisoning. **Howell-Jolly bodies** are remnants of nuclear chromatin that may occur in severe anemias or patients without spleens. **Pappenheimer bodies** are composed of iron, and they may be found in the peripheral blood following splenectomy. **Ring sideroblasts** have iron trapped abnormally in mitochondria, forming a ring around nucleus; they can be seen in sideroblastic anemia. **Heinz bodies** result from denatured hemoglobin; they can be seen with glucose-6-phosphate dehydrogenase deficiency.

ANEMIAS

Bridge to Physiology

Patients with anemia have normal SaO_2 and PaO_2, but they have reduced oxygen content due to the low level of hemoglobin.

Anemia is a reduction below normal limits of the total circulating red cell mass. Signs of anemia include palpitations, dizziness, angina, pallor of skin and nails, weakness, claudication, fatigue, and lethargy.

- **Reticulocytes** are immature, larger red cells (macrocytic cells) that are spherical and have a bluish color (polychromasia) due to free ribosomal RNA. Reticulocytes do not have a nucleus; note that any erythrocyte with a nucleus (nRBC) in peripheral blood is abnormal. Reticulocyte maturation to a mature erythrocyte takes about 1 day. The reticulocyte count is the percentage of red immature cells present in peripheral blood (normal 0.5–1.5%).

  The corrected reticulocyte count takes into consideration the degree of anemia and is calculated as (patient's hct/45) × (reticulocyte count); the idea behind the calculation is to scale the reticulocyte count by multiplying by the ratio of the patient's hematocrit to "normal" hematocrit of 45%. When interpreting the corrected reticulocyte count, <2% indicates poor bone marrow response and >3% indicates good bone marrow response.

- The reticulocyte production index is the corrected reticulocyte count/2; use this measure if bone marrow reticulocytes (shift cells) are present (polychromasia). The division by 2 is because shift cells take twice as long as reticulocytes to mature (2 days versus 1 day).

Laboratory terms used with respect to the population of erythrocytes:

- **Mean corpuscular volume** (MCV): average volume of a red blood cell

- **Mean corpuscular hemoglobin** (MCH): average content (mass) of hemoglobin per cell

- **Mean corpuscular hemoglobin concentration** (MCHC): average concentration of hemoglobin in a given volume of packed erythrocytes

- **Red cell distribution width** (RDW): coefficient of variation of red blood cell volume and a measure of anisocytosis

Classification of anemia can be based on color: normochromic anemias have normal red cell color (central pallor of about a third the diameter of the erythrocyte); hypochromic anemias have decreased color (seen as an increased central pallor of erythrocyte); and hyperchromic anemias, while theoretically possible, are usually instead called spherocytosis and have increased color (loss of central pallor of erythrocyte). Classification of anemia can also be based on size (MCV).

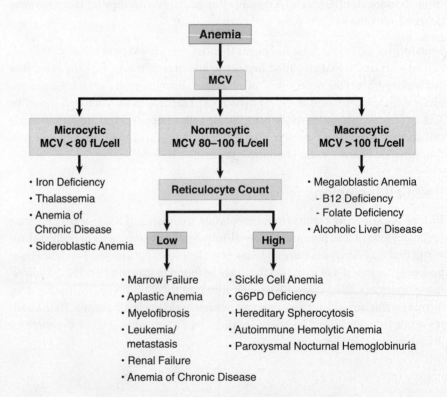

Figure 11-1. Classification of Anemias Based on MCV

The pathogenesis of anemia varies with the underlying disease. Blood loss can cause anemia. **Hemolytic anemias** are also important, and include hereditary spherocytosis, glucose-6-phosphate dehydrogenase deficiency, sickle cell disease, hemoglobin C disease, thalassemia, and paroxysmal nocturnal hemoglobinuria. **Immunohemolytic anemias**, which are hemolytic anemias with an immune component to the pathology, include autoimmune hemolytic anemia (AIHA), cold AIHA, incompatible blood transfusions, and hemolytic disease of the newborn. **Anemias of diminished erythropoiesis** include megaloblastic anemia (B12 and folate deficiencies), iron deficiency anemia, anemia of chronic disease, aplastic anemia, myelophthisic anemia, and sideroblastic anemia.

MICROCYTIC ANEMIAS

Iron Deficiency Anemia

Iron physiology. Functionally available iron is normally found in hemoglobin, myoglobin, and enzymes (catalase and cytochromes). Additionally, ferritin is the physiological storage form (plasma ferritin is normally close to the total body Fe), and hemosiderin (Prussian blue positive) is iron precipitated in tissues in the form of degraded ferritin mixed with lysosomal debris.

Iron is transported in the blood stream by transferrin. Transferrin saturation is reported as a percentage; it represents the ratio of the serum iron to the total iron-binding capacity, multiplied by 100.

Dietary deficiency of iron is seen in elderly populations, children, and the poor. Increased demand for iron is seen in children and pregnant women. Additionally, iron deficiency can develop because of decreased absorption, either due to generalized malabsorption or more specifically after gastrectomy (due to decreased acid, which is needed for ferrous absorption) or when there is decreased small intestinal transit time (causing "dumping syndrome"). Iron deficiency can also be due to chronic blood loss due to gynecologic (menstrual bleeding) or gastrointestinal causes (in the United States, think carcinoma; in the rest of the world, think hookworm).

The sequence of events during iron deficiency is as follows:

- **Initially**, decreased storage iron results in decreased serum ferritin and decreased bone marrow iron on Prussian blue stains.

- The **next stage** is decreased circulating iron, which causes decreased serum iron, increased total iron binding capacity, and decreased % saturation.

- The **last stage** is formation of microcytic/hypochromic anemia, with decreased MCV, decreased MCHC, and high RDW.

Other clinical features of iron deficiency include increased free erythrocyte protoporphyrin (FEP), oral epithelial atrophy if Plummer-Vinson syndrome is present, koilonychia (concave or spoon nails with abnormal ridging and splitting), and pica (eating nonfood substances, e.g. dirt).

Table 11-1. Iron Panel for Microcytic Anemias

	Iron Deficiency	AOCD	Thalassemia Minor
Serum iron	↓	↓	Normal
TIBC	↑	↓	Normal
% saturation	↓	↓	Normal
Serum ferritin	↓	↑	Normal

Anemia of chronic disease (AOCD) (or anemia of inflammation) is characterized by iron being trapped in bone marrow macrophages, leading to decreased utilization of endogenous iron stores. Laboratory studies show increased serum ferritin with decreased total iron binding capacity. Increased IL-6 increases plasma hepcidin, which is a negative regulator of iron uptake in the small intestine and of iron release from macrophages.

Thalassemia syndromes are quantitative, not qualitative, abnormalities of hemoglobin. α-thalassemia has decreased α-globin chains with relative excess β chains, while β-thalassemia has decreased β-globin chains with relative excess α chains. It is hypothesized that the thalassemia genes have been selectively preserved in the human genome because the thalassemias provide a protective advantage to carriers exposed to diseases such as malaria.

α-thalassemia. There are a total of 4 α-globin chain genes, 2 from each parent. α-thalassemia is due to gene deletions in the α-globin chain genes, and the clinical manifestations depend upon the number of genes that are affected. α chains are normally expressed prenatally and postnatally; therefore, there is prenatal and postnatal disease. In normal individuals, 4 α genes (αα/αα) are present and 100% of the α chains are normal.

- In the **silent carrier state**, one deletion is present, and the total number of α genes available is 3 (– α/αα), which produce 75% of the needed α chains. Individuals with the silent carrier state are completely asymptomatic and all lab tests are normal.

- In **α-thalassemia trait**, 2 deletions are present, and the total number of available α genes is 2, which produce 50% of the needed α chains. The genotype cis (– –/αα) is seen in Asians, while the genotype trans (–α/–α) is seen in African Americans (offspring don't develop hemoglobin H disease or hydrops fetalis).

- **Hemoglobin H disease** is characterized by 3 deletions, with the number of α genes being 1 (– –/– α), which produces 25% of the normal α chains. There is increased Hb H (β4,) which forms Heinz bodies that can be seen with crystal blue stain.

- **Hydrops fetalis** has 4 deletions and is lethal in utero, because the number of α genes is 0 (– –/– –), producing 0% α chains.

β-thalassemia. There are a total of 2 β-globin chain genes. In contrast to the α-globin chain genes, the 2 β-globin chain genes are expressed postnatally only, and therefore there is only postnatal disease and not prenatal disease. The damage to the genes is mainly by point mutations, which form either some β chains (β+) or none (β0).

Note

Composition of hemoglobins:

- HbA (2 alpha, 2 beta)
- HbA2 (2 alpha, 2 delta)
- HbF (2 alpha, 2 gamma)
- Hb Barts (4 gamma)
- Hb H (4 beta)

- **β-thalassemia minor** is seen when one of the β-globin chain genes has been damaged. The condition is asymptomatic, and characterized on laboratory studies by increased hemoglobin A2 (8%) and increased hemoglobin F (5%).

- **β-thalassemia intermedia** causes varying degrees of anemia, but no transfusions are needed.

- **β-thalassemia major** (Cooley anemia). Patients are normal at birth, and symptoms develop at about 6 months as hemoglobin F levels decline. Severe hemolytic anemia results from decreased erythrocyte life span. This severe anemia causes multiple problems:

  ° Intramedullary destruction results in "ineffective erythropoiesis."

  ° Hemolysis causes jaundice and an increased risk of pigment (bilirubin) gallstones.

  ° Lifelong transfusions are required, which result in secondary hemochromatosis.

  ° Congestive heart failure (CHF) is the most common cause of death.

Erythroid hyperplasia in the bone marrow causes "crewcut" skull x-ray and increased size of maxilla ("chipmunk face"). The peripheral blood shows microcytic/hypochromic anemia with numerous target cells and increased reticulocytes. Hemoglobin electrophoresis shows increased hemoglobin F (90%), normal or increased hemoglobin A2, and decreased hemoglobin A. Treatment is hematopoietic stem cell transplantation.

Sideroblastic anemia is a disorder in which the body has adequate iron stores, but is unable to incorporate the iron into hemoglobin. It is associated with ring sideroblasts (accumulated iron in mitochondria of erythroblasts) in bone marrow. Sideroblastic anemia may be either pyridoxine (vitamin B6) responsive or pyridoxine unresponsive; the latter is a form of myelodysplastic syndrome (refractory anemia with ring sideroblasts). The peripheral blood may show a dimorphic erythrocyte population. Laboratory studies show increased serum iron, ferritin, FEP, and % saturation of TIBC, with decreased TIBC.

NORMOCYTIC ANEMIAS

Anemias of blood loss. Acute blood loss may cause shock or death. If the patient survives, the resulting hemodilution caused by shift of water from the interstitium will lower the hematocrit. There will be a marked reticulocytosis in 5–7 days. Chronic blood loss, such as from the gastrointestinal tract or from the gynecologic system, may result in iron deficiency anemia.

Hemolytic anemias.

- In **intravascular (IV) hemolysis**, release of hemoglobin into the blood causes hemoglobinemia and hemoglobinuria; increased bilirubin from erythrocytes causes jaundice and an increased risk of pigment (bilirubin) gallstones. The hemoglobin may be oxidized to methemoglobin, which causes methemoglobinemia and methemoglobinuria. Markedly decreased (because they have been used up) hemoglobin-binding proteins in the blood, such as haptoglobin and hemopexin, are characteristic. No splenomegaly is seen.

• In **extravascular (EV) hemolysis**, splenomegaly results if the EV hemolysis occurs in the spleen and hepatomegaly results if the EV hemolysis occurs in the liver. EV hemolyis causes increased bilirubin and decreased haptoglobin, but not to the degree seen with intravascular hemolysis. In EV hemolysis, there is an absence of hemoglobinemia, hemoglobinuria, and methemoglobin formation.

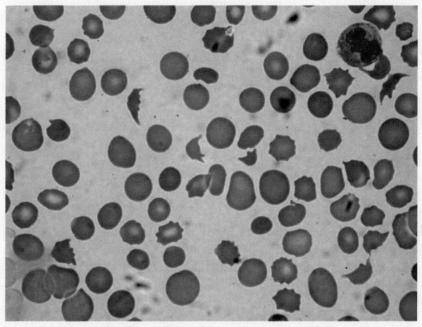

© commons.wikimedia.org.

Figure 11-2. DIC with Microangiopathic Hemolytic Anemia as Evidenced by Helmet Cells/Schistocytes

Sickle cell disease is an inherited blood disorder leading to the formation of hemoglobin S and increased propensity for the affected red blood cells to become sickle-shaped and occlude small vessels. The genetic abnormality is a single nucleotide change that causes valine (neutral) to replace normal glutamic acid (acidic) at the sixth position of the β-globin chain. This biochemical change then makes a critical point on the surface of the hemoglobin molecule become hydrophobic, making it feel "sticky" to an adjacent hemoglobin molecule, thereby favoring hemoglobin precipitation in crystalline form.

Heterozygous (AS) genome causes sickle cell trait. About 8% of African Americans are heterozygous for hemoglobin S. Patients with sickle trait have fewer symptoms than those with sickle disease, and also have resistance to *Plasmodium falciparum* infection (malaria), which may be why the disease has remained in the human genetic pool. Homozygous (SS) genome causes clinical disease (sickle cell anemia).

There are several factors affecting formation of irreversibly sickled red blood cells.

• **Increased concentration** (dehydration) makes symptoms worse; decreased concentration of sickled hemoglobin (as is seen if a sickle cell patient also has a thalassemia) makes symptoms better.

• **Decreased pH** decreases oxygen affinity and makes symptoms worse.

Note

Hemoglobin electrophoresis takes advantage of the differences in pH values between HbA and HbS (Glu6Val; glutamate at position 6 has been replaced by valine).

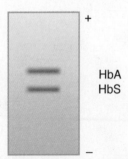

Hemoglobin electrophoresis at pH 8.4

- **Increased hemoglobin F** makes symptoms better (rationale for therapy with hydroxyurea, which increases blood hemoglobin F levels).

- The **presence of hemoglobin C** (SC: double-heterozygote individual) makes symptoms better.

Clinical features include increased erythrocyte destruction which causes a severe hemolytic anemia, accompanied by erythroid hyperplasia in the bone marrow and increased bilirubin leading to jaundice and gallstone (pigment) formation. Capillary thrombi result from sickle cells blocking small vessels and may cause vaso-occlusive (painful) crises; hand-foot syndrome (swelling) in children; and autosplenectomy, which is seen in older children and adults. Howell-Jolly bodies will appear in peripheral blood after autosplenectomy, and the lack of a functional spleen predisposes to increased incidence of infections (encapsulated organisms), increased incidence of *Salmonella* osteomyelitis (leg pain), leg ulcers, and risk of aplastic crisis (especially with *parvovirus B19* infection). Emergencies that may occur include priapism and acute chest syndrome.

For testing, hemoglobin electrophoresis is used to diagnose the disease, though genetic testing can be performed on amniotic fluid for prenatal diagnosis. Newborn screening is now mandatory in the United States and is commonly performed via high performance liquid chromatography. Treatment is hydroxyurea (to increase hemoglobin F) and hematopoietic stem cell transplantation.

Hemoglobin C disease occurs when a single nucleotide change in a codon causes lysine (basic) to replace normal glutamic acid (acidic) at the beta 6 position. Hemoglobin C disease is characterized by mild normochromic-normocytic anemia, splenomegaly, target cells, and rod-shaped crystals in erythrocytes (the latter being characteristic).

Glucose-6-phosphate dehydrogenase deficiency (G6PD) is a genetic disorder affecting the hexose monophosphate shunt pathway. It results in decreased levels of the antioxidant glutathione (GSH), leaving erythrocytes sensitive to injury by oxidant stresses leading to hemolysis. In some variants, G6PD is not due to decreased synthesis but rather to defective protein folding, resulting in a protein having a decreased half-life. The condition has X-linked inheritance.

- In **African Americans (A⁻ type)** with G6PD, the hemolysis is secondary to acute oxidative stress, such as oxidative drugs (primaquine, sulfonamides, anti-tuberculosis drugs), and more typically by viral or bacterial infections. The hemolysis is intermittent (even if the offending drug is continued) because only older erythrocytes have decreased levels of glucose-6-phosphate dehydrogenase.

- In individuals with G6PD of **Mediterranean type**, the disease is associated with favism due to ingestion of fava beans; more severe hemolysis occurs because all erythrocytes have decreased glucose-6-phosphate dehydrogenase activity in that there is both decreased synthesis and decreased stability.

- In **both forms**, the oxidation of hemoglobin forms **Heinz bodies**; these cannot be seen with normal peripheral blood stains (Wright-Giemsa) but can be visualized with supravital stains (methylene blue and crystal violet). The Heinz bodies are "eaten" by splenic macrophages (extravascular hemolysis), which may form "bite cell" erythrocytes that are visible on routine peripheral blood smears.

Bridge to Biochemistry

G6PD is the rate-limiting enzyme in the hexose-monophosphate shunt (HMP).

G6PD normally produces NADPH, which keeps glutathione reduced.

Glutathione protects RBCs by breaking down hydrogen peroxide.

Hereditary spherocytosis (HS) is an autosomal dominant disorder caused by a defect involving ankyrin and spectrin in the erythrocyte membrane; this causes a decrease in the erythrocyte surface membrane (spherocytosis). Spherocytes are not flexible and are removed in the spleen by macrophages (i.e., extravascular hemolysis). This causes multiple problems, including splenomegaly with a mild to moderate hemolytic anemia, increased bilirubin and increased risk for jaundice and pigment gallstones secondary to chronic hemolysis, and increased risk for acute red-cell aplasia due to parvovirus B19 infection. Laboratory testing shows increased osmotic fragility and normal MCH with increased MCHC. Treatment is splenectomy and folic acid.

Clinical Correlate

The differential diagnosis of spherocytes in the peripheral blood includes warm AIHA and hereditary spherocytosis. Use the osmotic fragility test (HS) and direct Coombs test (AIHA) to tell them apart. The Coombs test is negative in hereditary spherocytosis.

Autoimmune hemolytic anemia (AIHA) is most commonly warm AIHA, in which the antibodies are IgG that are usually against Rh antigens and are active at 37°C. Erythrocytes to which the antibodies attach are removed by splenic macrophages, which tends to induce splenomegaly as the spleen responds to the perceived need for increased phagocytosis.

The etiology varies; most cases are idiopathic, but some cases are related to auto-immune diseases such as systemic lupus erythematosus, chronic lymphocytic leukemia (CLL), small lymphocytic lymphoma (WDLL), or medications (penicillin). The peripheral blood smear typically shows microspherocytes, and laboratory confirmation can be obtained by demonstrating a positive direct Coombs test (direct antiglobulin test [DAT]).

Paroxysmal nocturnal hemoglobinuria (PNH) is a hemolytic anemia caused by an acquired somatic mutation of a gene (*PIGA*) that encodes an anchor for proteins (CD55 and CD59) in the cell membrane, causing complement-mediated lysis in red cells, white cells, and platelets. The condition causes episodes (paroxysms) of hemolysis at night.

Clinical Correlate

Increased levels of 2,3-bisphosphoglycerate (2,3 BPG) in cells can be seen in pyruvate kinase deficiency, which may affect tissue oxygenation. This will cause a "right shift" in the oxygen-hemoglobin dissociation curve, implying hemoglobin has a decreased affinity for oxygen.

Acidosis *in vivo* occurs during sleep (breathing slowly retains CO_2) and exercise (lactic acidosis), and the acidosis in turn causes activation of complement. PNH is a clonal stem cell disorder that affects all blood cell lines, leading to pancytopenia (anemia, leukopenia, and thrombocytopenia) that is apparent in the peripheral blood. Venous thrombosis may ensue.

Most PNH patients have mild disease and don't require treatment, but a monoclonal antibody against complement protein C5 can be therapeutic.

Pyruvate kinase deficiency is the most common enzyme deficiency in the glycolytic pathway and involves the enzyme that normally converts phosphoenolpyruvate to pyruvate. Deficiency leads to decreased ATP with resulting damage to the erythrocyte membrane. Clinically, there is a hemolytic anemia with jaundice from birth.

Hereditary elliptocytosis is a mild, hereditary, hemolytic anemia caused by a defect in spectrin. It is characterized by osmotically fragile ovoid erythrocytes ("elliptocytes").

Aplastic anemia is the term used when marrow failure causes a pancytopenia of the blood. Idiopathic causes for aplastic anemia are most commonly seen; when the etiology is known, the aplastic anemia may be due to medications (alkylating agents, chloramphenicol), chemical agents (benzene, insecticides), infection (EBV, CMV, parvovirus, hepatitis), or whole body radiation (therapeutic or nuclear exposure).

MACROCYTIC ANEMIAS

The basic cause of **megaloblastic anemias** is impaired DNA synthesis (delayed mitoses) without impairment of RNA synthesis; this produces a nuclear-cytoplasmic asynchrony that affects all rapidly proliferating cell lines, including cells of the bone marrow, gastrointestinal tract, and gynecologic system. The erythrocytes are the most obvious rapidly proliferating cells that exhibit these changes, and specifically show megaloblastic maturation, with megaloblasts in bone marrow forming macroovalocytes in peripheral blood. Autohemolysis of the affected megaloblasts in bone marrow (ineffective erythropoiesis) will cause increased bilirubin and increased lactate dehydrogenase (LDH). White blood cell changes include giant metamyelocytes in bone marrow and hypersegmented neutrophils (>5 lobes) in peripheral blood. Note that platelets are not increased in size.

Megaloblastic anemia due to vitamin B$_{12}$ (cobalamin) deficiency

- Dietary deficiency is rare because B$_{12}$ is stored in the liver and it takes years to develop dietary deficiency; it is usually seen only in strict vegetarians (diet with no animal protein, milk, or eggs).

- Decreased absorption of vitamin B$_{12}$ is more common and may be caused by decreased intrinsic factor associated with gastrectomy or pernicious anemia (an autoimmune gastritis); pancreatic insufficiency (pancreatic proteases normally break down B$_{12}$-R complexes in duodenum); or intestinal malabsorption due to parasites (fish tapeworm [*Diphyllobothrium latum*]), bacteria (blind-loop syndrome), or Crohn's disease of the ileum.

- Clinically, B$_{12}$ deficiency causes weakness due to anemia (megaloblastic anemia) and sore ("beefy") tongue due to generalized epithelial atrophy. Unlike folate deficiency, vitamin B$_{12}$ deficiency can also cause the central nervous system effects of subacute combined degeneration of the spinal cord, characterized by demyelination of the posterior and lateral columns of the spinal cord; the posterior (sensory) tract damage causes loss of vibratory and position sense, while the lateral cord damage involves dorsal spinocerebellar tracts (arm and leg dystaxia) and corticospinal tracts (spastic paralysis).

- Lab tests show low serum B$_{12}$, increased serum homocysteine, and increased methylmalonic acid in urine. Treatment is intramuscular vitamin B$_{12}$, which will cause increased reticulocytes in about 5 days.

Megaloblastic anemia due to folate deficiency can be caused by multiple processes:

- **Decreased intake** in chronic alcoholics and the elderly

- **Decreased absorption** in the upper small intestine

- **Increased requirement for folate** during pregnancy and infancy

- Folate antagonists, e.g., methotrexate

Clinically, folate deficiency produces megaloblastic anemia without neurologic disease symptoms. Lab tests show low serum folate levels and increased serum homocysteine. Treatment is folate replacement.

Note

Normal Sequence of B$_{12}$ Absorption

1. Dietary B12 binds to salivary haptocorrin.

2. Haptocorrin B$_{12}$ complex is broken down by pancreatic proteases.

3. Free B$_{12}$ binds to IF, which is secreted by gastric parietal cells.

4. B$_{12}$-IF complex is absorbed by ileal mucosal epithelial cells.

5. B$_{12}$ is transported in blood bound to transcobalamin.

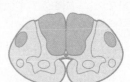

Subacute combined degeneration

POLYCYTHEMIA VERA

Polycythemia vera is caused by a clonal expansion of a multipotent myeloid stem cell that primarily produces extra erythrocytes. See discussion of myeloproliferative disorders in chapter 21.

Secondary polycythemia refers to increased red cell mass due to compromised ability of blood to supply oxygen to tissues. Causes include chronic obstructive pulmonary disease and cyanotic congenital heart disease. Erythropoietin levels can be appropriately high. Secondary polycythemia may also be caused by inappropriately high erythropoietin levels, with renal cell carcinoma excreting erythropoietin being the typical cause.

Relative polycythemia refers to an increased red cell count secondary to decreased plasma volume (typically due to dehydration). Red cell mass, erythropoietin, and blood oxygen content are normal.

Chapter Summary

- RBCs can have a variety of abnormal shapes or contain inclusions, either of which may suggest particular diagnoses.

- Anemia is the reduction below normal limits of the total circulating red cell mass, which may lead to palpitations, dizziness, angina, skin pallor, weakness, or other symptoms. Anemias can be classified based on size and red cell color. They can also be classified based on pathogenesis.

- Iron deficiency anemia is a microcytic anemia seen most often in the elderly and poor populations, children, pregnant women, and patients with chronic blood loss.

- Anemia of chronic disease can be seen in patients with a chronic systemic disease.

- Thalassemias are anemias due to quantitative abnormalities of synthesis of hemoglobin chains, and are subclassified as alpha thalassemias and beta thalassemias.

- Alpha-thalassemia has 4 clinical forms depending upon the number of alpha-globin genes affected: silent carrier, alpha-thalassemia trait, Hb H disease, and hydrops fetalis.

- Beta-thalassemia has 3 clinical presentations: minor, intermedia, and major.

- Sideroblastic anemias characteristically have ring sideroblasts in the bone marrow; some cases are a form of myelodysplastic syndrome.

- Anemia of blood loss occurs when a patient survives acute blood loss and undergoes hemodilution that lowers the hematocrit. Chronic cases may develop superimposed iron deficiency anemia.

- Hemolytic anemias can be due to either intravascular or extravascular hemolysis.

- Sickle cell anemia is due to a single nucleotide change in the beta-globin chain and is an important disease of African Americans. Hemoglobin C disease is also related to a single nucleotide change in a globin gene but produces milder disease than sickle cell anemia.

- Glucose-6-phosphate dehydrogenase deficiency is an enzyme deficiency that causes red cells to lyse under oxidant stresses.

- Hereditary spherocytosis is an autosomal dominant disorder due to an abnormal membrane-associated protein, spectrin, which leads to spherical erythrocyte morphology with mild to moderate hemolytic anemia.

- Autoimmune hemolytic anemias can be idiopathic or related to other autoimmune diseases, leukemias and lymphomas, or medications.

- Paroxysmal nocturnal hemoglobinuria produces episodic hemolysis as a result of increased erythrocyte sensitivity to the lytic actions of complement.

- Pyruvate kinase deficiency is a hereditary cause of hemolytic anemia due a deficiency of a glycolytic pathway enzyme, leading to decreased ATP and resulting in erythrocyte membrane damage. Hereditary elliptocytosis causes mild anemia. Aplastic anemia is a common end pathway of many different disease processes that destroy the marrow's ability to produce blood cells.

(continued)

Chapter Summary *(cont'd)*

- Megaloblastic anemias occur when there is impaired DNA synthesis, which leads to delayed mitoses. Important causes include vitamin B12 deficiency and folate deficiency.

- Polycythemia vera is a clonal disease leading to increased red cells (dominant process) accompanied by lesser degrees of increased granulocytes and platelets. Secondary polycythemia is polycythemia due to increased erythropoietin, which can be "appropriate" if it helps for a tissue oxygenation problem, or "inappropriate" if the erythropoietin is high because it is secreted by a tumor. Relative polycythemia is the term used for increased hematocrit in the absence of increased red cell mass and is usually due to decreased plasma volume (as in dehydration).

Learning Objectives

❏ Demonstrate understanding of the vasculitides

❏ Differentiate Raynaud disease from phenomenon

❏ Answer questions about arteriosclerosis, hypertension, aneurysms, and arteriovenous fistulas

❏ Explain information related to venous disease

❏ Demonstrate understanding of vascular neoplasms

THE VASCULITIDES

The vasculitides are a group of systemic disorders with vessel inflammation and myriad clinical presentations. There are many systems used to categorize them. The system below is based largely on the size of the vessels involved.

Large Vessel Vasculitides

Takayasu arteritis occurs in older adults (age >50). Initial symptoms may be nonspecific (fatigue) with a variable course to more severe symptoms (blindness) and involvement of the aortic arch. Microscopically, there is vessel wall thickening and variable inflammation (from a mononuclear adventitial infiltrate to medial necrosis with granulomas).

Giant cell arteritis was formerly called temporal arteritis, but the temporal arteries are not always involved. The vertebral and ophthalmic arteries and aorta are often involved. The typical presentation evolves from nonspecific symptoms (headache) to more severe symptoms (blindness). Microscopically, there are inner media granulomas in classic cases. Treatment is steroids and anti-TNF therapy.

Medium Vessel Vasculitides

Kawasaki disease presents with mucocutaneous symptoms and cervical lymph node enlargement in children. Involvement of the coronary arteries leads to cardiovascular sequelae, which can be circumvented with immunoglobulin therapy. Microscopically, there is transmural vascular inflammation.

Polyarteritis nodosa is a systemic necrotizing vasculitis occurring most often in young adults (M > F). It has an association with hepatitis B virus. The clinical course is one of episodic nonspecific symptoms (low-grade fever). Pulmonary involvement is rare; renal artery involvement can be fatal. Immunosuppressive therapy can achieve remission in most cases.

In a Nutshell

Thromboangiitis obliterans (Buerger's disease) is often categorized with the vasculitides, but the main lesion is thrombosis; inflammation may extend from vessels into adjacent soft tissue and nerves. The disease, which presents with severe distal extremity pain and ulceration, is seen most often in young male cigarette smokers. Pharmacologic therapies have not been successful.

Small Vessel Vasculitides

Small vessel vasculitides include those that are ANCA (antineutrophil cytoplasmic antibody)-associated (**granulomatosis with polyangiitis**, formerly known as Wegener's granulomatosis; and **eosinophilic granulomatosis with polyangiitis**, formerly known as Churg-Strauss syndrome) and those that are mediated by immune complexes (e.g., anti-glomerular basement membrane disease and IgA vasculitis, also known as Henoch-Schönlein purpura).

Granulomatosis with polyangiitis typically occurs in middle-aged men; it is characterized by granulomas of the lung and upper respiratory tract, glomerulonephritis, and a necrotizing granulomatous vasculitis. PR3-ANCAs are present in most cases.

Eosinophilic granulomatosis with polyangiitis is associated with asthma, extravascular granulomas (respiratory tract), and a systemic vasculitis that features eosinophils; eosinophil counts may be extremely high in peripheral blood. T lymphocytes and antibodies to MPO (P-ANCA) play a role in the etiology. There may be increased IgG4 levels. ANCA is present in cases with glomerulonephritis. The sequential phases are allergic, followed by eosinophilic and vasculitic. Cardiac involvement may be fatal. Steroids are therapeutic. Microscopic findings depend upon the organ biopsied: Purpuric leg lesions show a leukocytoclastic vasculitis; the glomerulonephritis tends not to show eosinophilic infiltrates; the extravascular pulmonary granulomas contain eosinophils.

Other small vessel vasculitides include **variable vessel vasculitides**, e.g., Behcet's disease; **single organ vasculitides**, e.g., CNS vasculitides; and **vasculitis associated with systemic disease**, e.g., rheumatoid vasculitis.

RAYNAUD DISEASE VERSUS PHENOMENON

Primary Raynaud phenomenon (Raynaud disease) typically occurs in young women as episodic small artery vasospasm in the extremities, nose, or ears; it results in blanching and cyanosis of the fingers or toes upon stress or (more commonly) exposure to cold. The pathogenesis may involve CNS and intravascular factors.

Secondary Raynaud phenomenon is caused by arterial insufficiency secondary to an underlying disease such as scleroderma (CREST).

ARTERIOSCLEROSIS

Mönckeberg medial calcific sclerosis is a medial calcification of medium-sized (muscular) arteries, such as femoral, tibial, radial, and ulnar arteries. It is asymptomatic, but may be detected by x-ray.

Arteriolosclerosis refers to sclerosis of arterioles; it affects small arteries and arterioles. Microscopically, either hyaline arteriolosclerosis (pink, glassy arterial wall thickening with luminal narrowing seen in benign hypertension, diabetes, and aging) or hyperplastic arteriolosclerosis (smooth-muscle proliferation resulting in concentric ["onion skin"] wall thickening and luminal narrowing seen in malignant hypertension) may occur.

Atherosclerosis is a common vascular disorder characterized by lipid deposition and intimal thickening of large and medium-sized (elastic and muscular) arteries,

In a Nutshell

Arteriosclerosis is a group of diseases that results in arterial wall thickening ("hardening of the arteries")

- Mönckeberg medial calcific sclerosis
- Arteriolosclerosis
- Atherosclerosis

resulting in fatty streaks and atheromatous plaques over a period of decades (a type of chronic inflammatory condition). Particularly likely to be affected are the aorta and a number of important muscular arteries (coronary, carotid, cerebral, renal, iliac, and popliteal arteries).

Risk factors for atherosclerosis are as follows:

Hyperlipidemia	Sedentary lifestyle
Hypertension	Stress (type A personality)
Smoking	Elevated homocysteine
Diabetes	Oral contraceptive use
Obesity	Increasing age
Male gender	Familial/genetic factors

- The earliest (clinically reversible) stage in atherosclerosis is the **fatty streak**, which is seen grossly as a flat, yellow intimal streak and is characterized microscopically by lipid-laden macrophages (foam cells).

- **Stable atheromatous plaques** have a dense fibrous cap, a small lipid core and less inflammation than their vulnerable counterparts. They cause chronic ischemia.

Vulnerable atheromatous plaques are at risk for rupture, thrombosis or embolization due to their composition (thin fibrous cap, large lipid core, dense inflammation).

Clinical complications of atherosclerosis are protean; these complications include ischemic heart disease (myocardial infarctions); cerebrovascular accidents (CVA); atheroemboli (transient ischemic attacks [TIAs] and renal infarcts); aneurysm formation; peripheral vascular disease; and mesenteric artery occlusion.

HYPERTENSION (HTN)

Hypertension is an elevated blood pressure leading to end-organ damage, or a sustained diastolic pressure >90 mm Hg and/or systolic pressure >140 mm Hg.

Hypertension is very common, affecting 25% of the U.S. population. African Americans tend to be more seriously affected than Caucasians, and the risk increases with age. Approximately 95% of cases of hypertension are idiopathic (essential); the remainder are due to secondary hypertension related to renal disease, pheochromocytoma, or other disease processes.

Mild to moderate elevations in blood pressure cause end-organ damage by damaging arterioles with hyaline arteriolosclerosis. Late manifestations of hypertension include concentric left ventricular hypertrophy; congestive heart failure; accelerated atherosclerosis; myocardial infarction; aneurysm formation, rupture, and dissection; intracerebral hemorrhage; and chronic renal failure.

Malignant (accelerated) hypertension accounts for 5% of the cases and is characterized by markedly elevated pressures (e.g., systolic pressure >180 mm Hg and/or diastolic >120 mm Hg), which can rapidly cause end-organ damage. Funduscopic examination may demonstrate retinal hemorrhages, exudates, and papilledema. See chapter 15 for a discussion of renal pathology. Malignant hypertension is a medical emergency; if untreated, most patients will die within 2 years from renal failure, intracerebral hemorrhage, or chronic heart failure.

ANEURYSMS AND ARTERIOVENOUS FISTULAS

Aneurysms are congenital or acquired weakness of the vessel wall media, resulting in a localized dilatation or outpouching. Complications include thrombus formation, thromboembolism, and compression of nearby structures. Rupture or dissection may cause sudden death.

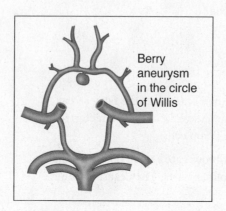

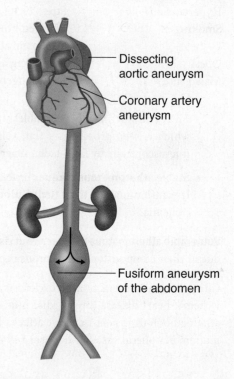

Figure 12-1. Location of Aneurysms

Atherosclerotic aneurysms are due to weakening of the media secondary to atheroma formation, and typically occur in the abdominal aorta below the renal arteries. They are associated with hypertension. Half of aortic aneurysms >6 cm in diameter will rupture within 10 years. Those >5 cm are treated surgically.

Syphilitic aneurysms involve the ascending aorta in tertiary syphilis (late stage). Syphilitic (luetic) aortitis causes an obliterative endarteritis of the vasa vasorum, leading to ischemia and smooth-muscle atrophy of the aortic media. Syphilitic aneurysms may dilate the aortic valve ring, causing aortic insufficiency.

Aortic dissecting aneurysm occurs when blood from the vessel lumen enters an intimal tear and dissects through the layers of the media. The etiology usually involves degeneration (cystic medial degeneration) of the tunica media. Aortic dissecting aneurysm presents with severe tearing pain. The dissecting aneurysm may compress and obstruct the aortic branches (e.g., renal or coronary arteries). Hypertension and Marfan syndrome are predisposing factors.

Berry aneurysm is a congenital aneurysm of the circle of Willis.

Microaneurysms are small aneurysms commonly seen in hypertension and diabetes.

Mycotic aneurysms are aneurysms usually due to bacterial or fungal infections.

Arteriovenous (AV) fistulas are a direct communication between a vein and an artery without an intervening capillary bed. They may be congenital or acquired (e.g., trauma). Potential complications include shunting of blood which may lead to high-output heart failure and risk of rupture and hemorrhage.

VENOUS DISEASE

Deep vein thrombosis (DVT) usually affects deep leg veins (90%), with iliac, femoral, and popliteal veins being particularly commonly affected. It is often asymptomatic and is consequently a commonly missed diagnosis. When symptomatic, it can produce unilateral leg swelling with warmth, erythema, and positive Homan sign (increased resistance to passive dorsiflexion of the ankle by the examiner). The diagnosis can be established with doppler "duplex" ultrasound. The major complication is pulmonary embolus.

Varicose veins are dilated, tortuous veins caused by increased intraluminal pressure. A variety of veins can be affected.

- **Superficial veins of the lower extremities** are particularly vulnerable due to a lack of structural support from superficial fat and/or incompetent valve(s). Varicosities of these superficial veins are very common (15% of the U.S. population); occur more frequently in females than males; and are common in pregnancy.

- **Esophageal varices** are due to portal hypertension (usually caused by cirrhosis) and may be a source of life-threatening hemorrhage.

- Varices of the anal region are commonly called **hemorrhoids**; are associated with constipation and pregnancy; and may be complicated by either bleeding (streaks of red blood on hard stools) or thrombosis (painful).

Venous insufficiency is more common in women than men, and the incidence increases with age. Lower extremities demonstrate edema, hyperpigmentation and ulceration due to venous hypertension and incompetent valves.

Vascular ectasias:

- **Nevus flammeus nuchae** is a neck "birthmark" or "stork bite" that regresses.

- **Port wine stain** is a vascular birthmark that does not regress.

- **Spider telangiectasias** occur on the face, blanch with pressure, and are associated with pregnancy.

VASCULAR NEOPLASMS

Hemangiomas are extremely common, benign vascular tumors. They are the most common tumor in infants appearing on the skin, mucous membranes, or internal organs. The major types are capillary and cavernous hemangiomas. Hemangiomas may spontaneously regress.

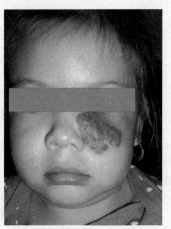

© Richard P. Usatine, M.D.
Used with permission.

Figure 12-2. Hemangioma

Hemangioblastomas are associated with von Hippel-Lindau disease, which may cause multiple hemangioblastomas involving the cerebellum, brain stem, spinal cord, and retina, as well as renal cell carcinoma.

Glomus tumors (glomangioma) are benign, small, painful tumors of the glomus body that usually occur under fingernails.

Kaposi sarcoma is a malignant tumor of endothelial cells associated with Kaposi-sarcoma–associated virus (HHV8). The condition causes multiple red-purple patches, plaques, or nodules that may remain confined to the skin or may disseminate. Microscopically, there is a proliferation of spindle-shaped endothelial cells with slit-like vascular spaces and extravasated erythrocytes.

- The **classic European form** occurs in older men of Eastern European or Mediterranean origin, who develop red-purple skin plaques on the lower extremities.

- The **transplant-associated form** occurs in patients on immunosuppression for organ transplants; involves skin and viscera; may regress with reduction of immunosuppression.

- The **African form** occurs in African children and young men in whom generalized lymphatic spread is common.

- The **AIDS-associated form** is most common in homosexual male AIDS patients; it is an aggressive form with frequent widespread visceral dissemination. Common sites of involvement include skin, GI tract, lymph nodes, and lungs. This form of Kaposi sarcoma is responsive to chemotherapy and interferon-alpha, and only rarely causes death.

Angiosarcoma (hemangiosarcoma) is a malignant vascular tumor with a high mortality that most commonly occurs in skin, breast, liver, and soft tissues. Liver angiosarcomas are associated with vinyl chloride, arsenic, and thorotrast.

Chapter Summary

- Polyarteritis nodosa is a segmental necrotizing vasculitis. The symptoms vary with the organ involved.

- Eosinophilic granulomatosis with polyangiitis is a medium-vessel vasculitis with bronchial asthma, granuloma formation, and eosinophilia.

- Granulomatosis with polyangiitis is a necrotizing vasculitis with granulomas that classically involves the nose, sinuses, lungs, and kidneys.

- Giant cell arteritis is a segmental granulomatous vasculitis with a predilection for involving cranial arteries. Headache, facial pain, and visual disturbances occur. Untreated temporal arteritis may cause blindness.

- Takayasu arteritis is a granulomatous vasculitis with massive intimal fibrosis that tends to involve the aortic arch and its major branches. It may produce blindness or loss of pulse in the upper extremities.

- Thromboangiitis obliterans tends to involve the extremities of young men who smoke heavily.

- Kawasaki disease is a febrile lymphadenopathy with rash with an associated segmental necrotizing vasculitis with a predilection for the coronary arteries.

- Raynaud disease is an idiopathic small artery vasospasm that causes blanching and cyanosis of the fingers and toes; the term *secondary Raynaud phenomenon* is used when similar changes are observed secondary to a systemic disease such as scleroderma or systemic lupus erythematosus.

- Arteriolosclerosis refers to small artery and arteriolar changes leading to luminal narrowing, most often seen in patients with diabetes, hypertension, and aging.

- Atherosclerosis is lipid deposition and intimal thickening of large and medium-sized arteries, resulting in fatty streaks and atheromatous plaques. Clinical complications of atherosclerosis include ischemic heart disease, cerebrovascular accidents, atheroemboli, aneurysm formation, peripheral vascular disease, and mesenteric artery occlusion.

- Hypertension is defined as elevated BP leading to end-organ damage or sustained diastolic pressure >90 mm Hg and/or systolic pressure >140 mm Hg. Hypertension is a common, initially silent disease that may eventually produce cardiac disease, accelerated atherosclerosis, aneurysm formation, and renal and CNS damage. Malignant hypertension is defined as markedly elevated pressures (e.g., systolic pressure >180 mm Hg or diastolic >120 mm Hg) causing rapid end-organ damage. Untreated patients often die within 2 years from renal failure, intracerebral hemorrhage, or chronic heart failure.

- An aneurysm is a congenital or acquired weakness of the vessel wall media, resulting in a localized dilation or outpouching. Complications include thrombus formation, compression of adjacent structures, and rupture with risk of sudden death.

- Atherosclerotic aneurysms are associated with hypertension and tend to involve the abdominal aorta.

- Syphilitic aneurysms tend to involve the ascending aorta and develop secondary to an obliterative endarteritis of the vasa vasorum, which is the blood supply of the aortic media.

(continued)

Chapter Summary *(cont'd)*

- Aortic dissecting aneurysms occur when blood from the vessel lumen enters an intimal tear and dissects through the layers of the media, which have often previously been damaged by cystic medial degeneration.

- Berry aneurysms are congenital aneurysms of the vessels near the circle of Willis.

- Deep vein thrombosis usually involves the deep leg veins and may be asymptomatic. The major complication is pulmonary embolus.

- Varicose veins are dilated, tortuous veins caused by increased intraluminal pressure. Common sites include the superficial veins of the lower extremities, esophageal varices, and hemorrhoids.

- Hemangiomas are extremely common, benign vascular tumors that may involve the skin, mucous membranes, or internal organs.

- Hemangioblastomas are vascular tumors associated with von Hippel-Lindau disease that tend to involve the central nervous system and retina.

- Glomus tumors are small, painful vascular tumors most often found under the fingernails.

- Kaposi sarcoma is a low-grade malignant tumor of endothelial cells that appears to have a viral etiology (HHV8) and in the United States is found most often in AIDS patients.

- Angiosarcoma is a malignant vascular tumor with a high mortality that occurs most commonly in skin, breast, liver, and soft tissues.

Cardiac Pathology 13

Learning Objectives

❏ Demonstrate understanding of the vasculitides

❏ Differentiate Raynaud disease from phenomenon

❏ Answer questions about arteriosclerosis, hypertension, aneurysms, and arteriovenous fistulas

❏ Explain information related to venous disease

❏ Demonstrate understanding of vascular neoplasms

ISCHEMIC HEART DISEASE

Cardiac ischemia is usually secondary to coronary artery disease (CAD); it is the most common cause of death in the United States. It is most often seen in middle-age men and postmenopausal women.

Angina pectoris is due to transient cardiac ischemia without cell death resulting in substernal chest pain.

- **Stable angina** (most common type) is caused by coronary artery atherosclerosis with luminal narrowing >75%. Chest pain is brought on by increased cardiac demand (exertional or emotional), and is relieved by rest or nitroglycerin (vasodilation). Electrocardiogram shows ST segment depression (subendocardial ischemia).

- **Prinzmetal variant angina** is caused by coronary artery vasospasm and produces episodic chest pain often at rest; it is relieved by nitroglycerin (vasodilatation). Electrocardiogram shows transient ST segment elevation (transmural ischemia).

- **Unstable or crescendo angina** is caused by formation of a nonocclusive thrombus in an area of coronary atherosclerosis, and is characterized by increasing frequency, intensity, and duration of episodes; episodes typically occur at rest. This form of angina has a high risk for myocardial infarction.

Myocardial infarction (MI) occurs when a localized area of cardiac muscle undergoes coagulative necrosis due to ischemia. It is the most common cause of death in the United States. The mechanism leading to infarction is coronary artery atherosclerosis (90% of cases). Other causes include decreased circulatory volume, decreased oxygenation, decreased oxygen-carrying capacity, or increased cardiac workload, due to systemic hypertension, for instance.

- **Distribution of coronary artery thrombosis.** The left anterior descending artery (LAD) is involved in 45% of cases; the right coronary artery (RCA) is involved in 35% of cases; and the left circumflex coronary artery (LCA) is involved in 15% of cases.

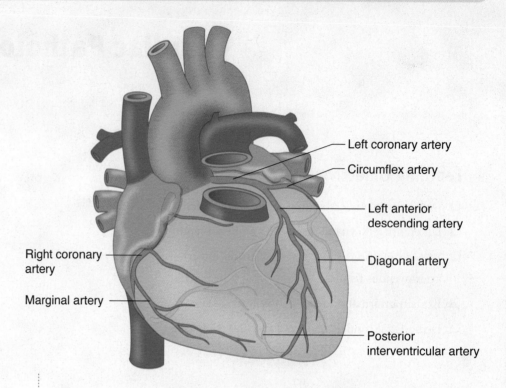

Figure 13-1. Arterial Supply to the Heart

Infarctions are classified as transmural, subendocardial, or microscopic.

- **Transmural** infarction (most common type) is considered to have occurred when ischemic necrosis involves >50% of myocardial wall. It is associated with regional vascular occlusion by thrombus. It causes ST elevated MIs (STEMIs) due to atherosclerosis and acute thromobosis.

- **Subendocardial** infarction is considered to have occurred when ischemic necrosis involves <50% of myocardial wall. It is associated with hypoperfusion due to shock. ECG changes are not noted. This type of infarction occurs in a setting of coronary artery disease with a decrease in oxygen delivery or an increase in demand.

- **Microscopic** infarction is caused by small vessel occlusion due to vasculitis, emboli, or spasm. ECG changes are not noted.

Clinical Correlate

Atypical presentation of MI with little or no chest pain is seen most frequently in elderly patients, diabetics, women, and postsurgical patients.

The clinical presentation of MI is classically a sudden onset of severe "crushing" substernal chest pain that radiates to the left arm, jaw, and neck. The pain may be accompanied by chest heaviness, tightness, and shortness of breath; diaphoresis, nausea, and vomiting; jugular venous distension (JVD); anxiety and often "feeling of impending doom." Electrocardiogram initially shows ST segment elevation. Q waves representing myocardial coagulative necrosis develop in 24–48 hours.

Table 13-1. Serum Markers Used to Diagnose Myocardial Infarctions

	Elevated by	Peak	Returns to Normal by
CK-MB	4–8 h	18 h	2–3 days
Cardiac-specific troponin I & T	3–6 h	16 h	7–10 days
LDH	24 h	3–6 days	8–14 days

- **Gross and microscopic sequence of changes.** The microscopic and gross changes represent a spectrum that is preceded by biochemical changes going from aerobic metabolism to anaerobic metabolism within minutes. The time intervals are variable and depend on the size of the infarct, as well as other factors.

Table 13-2. Gross Sequence of Changes

Time Post-Infarction	Gross Appearance
0–12 h	No visible gross change
12–24 h	Vague pallor and softening
1–7 days	Yellow pallor
7–10 days	Central pallor with a red border
6–8 wks	White, firm scar

Table 13-3. Microscopic Sequence of Changes

Time Post-Infarction	Microscopic Appearance
1–4 h	None or wavy myocyte fibers at border or contraction band necrosis
4 h–3 days	Coagulative necrosis
1–3 days	Neutrophilic infiltrate
3–7 days	Macrophages
7–10 days	Granulation tissue
3–8 wks	Remodeled type III collagen becoming dense, collagenous scar

Complications of MI include cardiac arrhythmias that may lead to sudden cardiac death; congestive heart failure; cardiogenic shock (>40–50% myocardium is necrotic); mural thrombus and thromboembolism; fibrinous pericarditis; ventricular aneurysm; and cardiac rupture. Cardiac rupture most commonly occurs 3–7 days after MI, and has effects that vary with the site of rupture: ventricular free wall rupture causes cardiac tamponade; interventricular septum rupture causes left to right shunt; and papillary muscle rupture causes mitral insufficiency.

Clinical Correlate

Auscultation of a friction rub is characteristic of pericarditis. Pericarditis is most common 2–3 days after infarction but may also occur several weeks later (Dressler syndrome—a rare autoimmune reaction (type II) where the necrotic heart muscle induces the immune system to generate autoantibodies to cardiac self-antigens).

Clinical Correlate

Clinically, the degree of orthopnea is often quantified in terms of the number of pillows the patient needs in order to sleep comfortably (e.g., "three-pillow orthopnea").

Note

Cor pulmonale = right-sided heart failure caused by pulmonary hypertension from intrinsic lung disease:

- Lung disease → pulmonary HTN →↑ right ventricular pressure → right ventricular hypertrophy → right-sided heart failure.

Sudden cardiac death is defined to be death within 1 hour of the onset of symptoms. The mechanism is typically a fatal cardiac arrhythmia (usually ventricular fibrillation).

Coronary artery disease is the most common underlying cause (80%); other causes include hypertrophic cardiomyopathy, mitral valve prolapse, aortic valve stenosis, congenital heart abnormalities, and myocarditis.

Chronic ischemic heart disease is the insidious onset of progressive congestive heart failure. It is characterized by left ventricular dilation due to accumulated ischemic myocardial damage (replacement fibrosis) and functional loss of hypertrophied non-infarcted cardiac myocytes.

CONGESTIVE HEART FAILURE

Congestive heart failure (CHF) refers to the presence of insufficient cardiac output to meet the metabolic demand of the body's tissues and organs. It is the final common pathway for many cardiac diseases and has an increasing incidence in the United States. Complications include both **forward failure** (decreased organ perfusion) and **backward failure** (passive congestion of organs). Right- and left-sided heart failure often occur together.

- **Left heart failure** can be caused by ischemic heart disease, systemic hypertension, myocardial diseases, and aortic or mitral valve disease. The heart has increased heart weight and shows left ventricular hypertrophy and dilatation. The lungs are heavy and edematous. Left heart failure presents with dyspnea, orthopnea, paroxysmal nocturnal dyspnea, rales, and S3 gallop.

  Microscopically, the heart shows cardiac myocyte hypertrophy with "enlarged pleiotropic nuclei," while the lung shows pulmonary capillary congestion and alveolar edema with intra-alveolar hemosiderin-laden macrophages ("heart failure cells"). Complications include passive pulmonary congestion and edema, activation of the renin-angiotensin-aldosterone system leading to secondary hyperaldosteronism, and cardiogenic shock.

- **Right heart failure** is most commonly caused by left-sided heart failure, with other causes including pulmonary or tricuspid valve disease and *cor pulmonale*. Right heart failure presents with JVD, hepatosplenomegaly, dependent edema, ascites, weight gain, and pleural and pericardial effusions. Grossly, right ventricular hypertrophy and dilatation develop. Chronic passive congestion of the liver may develop and may progress to cardiac sclerosis/cirrhosis (only with long-standing congestion).

VALVULAR HEART DISEASE

Degenerative calcific aortic valve stenosis is a common valvular abnormality characterized by age-related dystrophic calcification, degeneration, and stenosis of the aortic valve. It is common in congenital bicuspid aortic valves. It can lead to concentric left ventricular hypertrophy (LVH) and congestive heart failure with increased risk of sudden death. The calcifications are on the outflow side of the cusps. Treatment is aortic valve replacement.

Mitral valve prolapse has enlarged, floppy mitral valve leaflets that prolapse into the left atrium and microscopically show myxomatous degeneration. The condition affects individuals with Marfan syndrome. Patients are asymptomatic and a mid-systolic click can be heard on auscultation. Complications include infectious endocarditis and septic emboli, rupture of chordae tendineae with resulting mitral insufficiency, and rarely sudden death.

Rheumatic valvular heart disease/acute rheumatic fever

Rheumatic fever is a systemic recurrent inflammatory disease, triggered by a pharyngeal infection with Group A β-*hemolytic streptococci*. In genetically susceptible individuals, the infection results in production of antibodies that cross-react with cardiac antigens (type II hypersensitivity reaction). Rheumatic fever affects children (ages 5–15 years), and there is a decreasing incidence in the United States. Symptoms occur 2–3 weeks after a pharyngeal infection; laboratory studies show elevated anti-streptolysin O (ASO) titers. The Jones criteria are illustrated below.

Diagnosis of rheumatic fever requires **2 major** OR **1 major and 2 minor criteria**, plus a preceding group A strep infection.

Table 13-4. WHO Criteria for Rheumatic Fever Based on Revised Jones Criteria

Major Criteria	Minor Criteria
Carditis	Fever
Polyarthritis	Polyarthralgia
Chorea	Labs: elevated ESR or leukocyte count
Erythema marginatum	ECG: prolonged P-R interval
Subcutaneous nodules	

- **Acute rheumatic heart disease** affects myocardium, endocardium, and pericardium. The myocardium can develop myocarditis, whose most distinctive feature is the Aschoff body, in which fibrinoid necrosis is surrounded by macrophages (Anitschkow cells), lymphocytes, and plasma cells. Fibrinous pericarditis may be present. Endocarditis may be a prominent feature that typically involves mitral and aortic valves (forming fibrin vegetations along the lines of closure) and may also cause left atrial endocardial thickening (MacCallum plaques).

- **Chronic rheumatic heart disease** is characterized by mitral and aortic valvular fibrosis, characterized by valve thickening and calcification; fusion of the valve commissures; and damaged chordae tendineae (short, thickened, and fused). Complications can include mitral stenosis and/or regurgitation, aortic stenosis and/or regurgitation, congestive heart failure, and infective endocarditis.

Clinical Correlate

Endocarditis involving the tricuspid valve is highly suggestive of IV drug use or central line bacteremia.

Infectious bacterial endocarditis refers to bacterial infection of the cardiac valves, characterized by vegetations on the valve leaflets. Risk factors include rheumatic heart disease, mitral valve prolapse, bicuspid aortic valve, degenerative calcific aortic stenosis, congenital heart disease, artificial valves, indwelling catheters, dental procedures, immunosuppression, and intravenous drug use.

- **Acute endocarditis** is typically due to a *high virulence organism* that can colonize a normal valve, such as *Staphylococcus aureus*. Acute endocarditis produces large destructive vegetations (fibrin, platelets, bacteria, and neutrophils). The prognosis is poor, with mortality of 10–40%.

- **Subacute endocarditis** is typically due to a low virulence organism, such as *Streptococcus group viridians*, which usually colonizes a previously damaged valve. The disease course is typically indolent with <10% mortality.

Clinically, endocarditis presents with fever, chills, weight loss, and cardiac murmur. Embolic phenomena may occur, and may affect systemic organs; retina (Roth spots); and distal extremities (Osler nodes [painful, red subcutaneous nodules on the fingers and toes], Janeway lesions [painless, red lesions on the palms and soles], and splinter fingernail hemorrhages). Diagnosis is by serial blood cultures. Complications include septic emboli, valve damage resulting in insufficiency and congestive heart failure, myocardial abscess, and dehiscence of an artificial heart valve.

Marantic endocarditis (nonbacterial thrombotic endocarditis [NBTE]) is characterized by small, sterile vegetations along the valve leaflet line of closure in patients with a debilitating disease. The major complications are embolism and secondary infection of the vegetations.

MYOCARDITIS

Myocarditis is caused by infectious (coxsackie A and B viruses, Chagas disease) and immune causes. Clinically, the patient may be asymptomatic or may suffer from acute heart failure or even dilated cardiomyopathy.

CONGENITAL HEART DISEASE

Congenital heart disease is the most common cause of childhood heart disease in the United States; 90% of cases are idiopathic and 5% are associated with genetic disease (trisomies, cri du chat, Turner syndrome, etc.), viral infection (especially congenital rubella), or drugs and alcohol.

Coarctation of the aorta is a segmental narrowing of the aorta.

- **Preductal coarctation** (infantile-type) is associated with Turner syndrome and causes severe narrowing of aorta proximal to the ductus arteriosus. It is usually associated with a patent ductus arteriosus (PDA), which supplies blood to aorta distal to the narrowing, and right ventricular hypertrophy (secondary to the need for the right ventricle to supply the aorta through the patent ductus arteriosus). It presents in infancy with congestive heart failure that is accompanied by weak pulses and cyanosis in the lower extremities; the prognosis is poor without surgical correction.

Bridge to Microbiology

Viridans streptococci

- Alpha-hemolytic
- Bile-resistant
- Optochin-resistant

Clinical Correlate

S. bovis endocarditis or septicemia is associated with a higher incidence of occult colorectal tumors.

Colonoscopy should be performed in all patients with *S. bovis* bacteremia or endocarditis.

- **Postductal coarctation** (adult-type) causes stricture or narrowing of the aorta distal to the ductus arteriosus. It can present in a child or an adult with hypertension in the upper extremities, and hypotension and weak pulses in the lower extremities. Some collateral circulation may be supplied via the internal mammary and intercostal arteries; the effects of this collateral circulation may be visible on chest x-ray with notching of the ribs due to bone remodeling as a consequence of increased blood flow through the intercostal arteries.

Complications can include congestive heart failure (the heart is trying too hard), intracerebral hemorrhage (the blood pressure in the carotid arteries is too high), and dissecting aortic aneurysm (the blood pressure in the aortic route is too high).

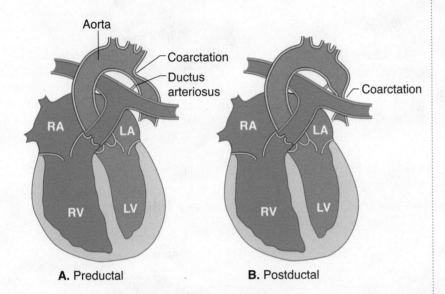

Figure 13-2. Coarctation of the Aorta

Table 13-5. Left Versus Right Shunt Congenital Disease

Right ⟶ Left Shunt	Left ⟶ Right Shunt
Early cyanosis (blue babies)	Late cyanosis (blue kids)
Blood shunted past the lungs	Secondary pulmonary HTN → reversal of shunt (Eisenmenger syndrome)
• Tetralogy of Fallot • Transposition of the great vessels • Truncus arteriosus • Tricuspid atresia	• Ventricular septal defect • Atrial septal defect • Patent ductus arteriosus

Note

"Overriding aorta" refers to the location of the aorta relative to the VSD.

Tetralogy of Fallot is the most common cause of congenital cyanotic heart disease. The classic tetrad includes **right ventricular outflow obstruction/stenosis; right ventricular hypertrophy; ventricular septal defect;** and **overriding aorta**. Clinical findings include cyanosis, shortness of breath, digital clubbing, and polycythemia. Progressive pulmonary outflow stenosis and cyanosis develop over time; treatment is surgical correction.

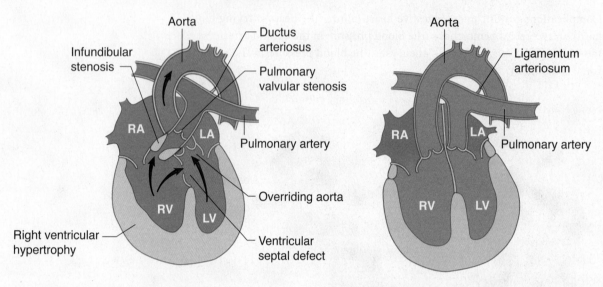

A. Tetralogy of Fallot

B. Transposition of the Great Vessels

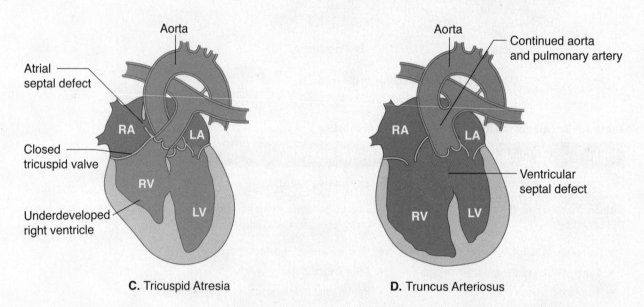

C. Tricuspid Atresia

D. Truncus Arteriosus

Figure 13-3. Common Forms of Cyanotic Congenital Heart Disease

Transposition of the great vessels is an abnormal development of the truncoconal septum whereby the aorta arises from the right ventricle, and the pulmonary artery arises from the left ventricle. The risk is increased in infants of diabetic mothers. Affected babies develop early cyanosis and right ventricular hypertrophy. To survive, infants must have mixing of blood by a VSD, ASD, or PDA. The prognosis is poor without surgery.

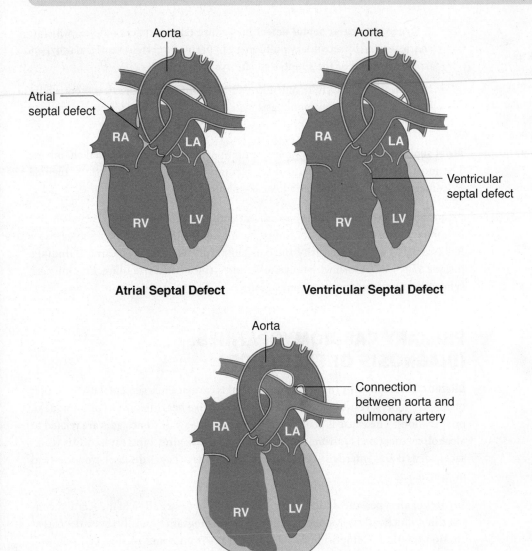

Atrial Septal Defect

Ventricular Septal Defect

Patent Ductus Arteriosus

Figure 13-4. Common Forms of Acyanotic Congenital Heart Disease

Truncus arteriosus is a failure to develop a dividing septum between the aorta and pulmonary artery, resulting in a common trunk. Blood flows from the pulmonary trunk to the aorta. Truncus arteriosus causes early cyanosis and congestive heart failure, with a poor prognosis without surgery.

Tricuspid atresia refers to the absence of a communication between the right atrium and ventricle due to developmental failure to form the tricuspid valve. Associated defects include right ventricular hypoplasia and an ASD. The prognosis is poor without surgery.

Ventricular septal defect (VSD), which consists of a direct communication between the ventricular chambers, is the second most common congenital heart defect (the most common is a bicuspid aortic valve).

- A **small ventricular septal defect** may be asymptomatic and close spontaneously, or it may produce a jet stream that damages the endocardium and increases the risk of infective endocarditis.

Bridge to Pharmacology

To keep PDA open: prostaglandin E2

To close PDA: indomethacin

Bridge to Embryology

In utero the ductus arteriosus is kept open by low arterial oxygen saturation and elevated prostaglandin E2 (PGE2) levels. Functional closure occurs in the first 2 days of life due to increased oxygen saturation and decreased PGE2. The ductus arteriosus becomes the ligamentum arteriosum.

- A **large ventricular septal defect** may cause Eisenmenger complex, which is characterized by secondary pulmonary hypertension, right ventricular hypertrophy, reversal of the shunt, and late cyanosis.

- In **both types**, a systolic murmur can be heard on auscultation. Ventricular septal defects are commonly associated with other heart defects. Large ventricular septal defects can be surgically corrected.

Atrial septal defect (ASD) is a direct communication between the atrial chambers. The most common type is an ostium secundum defect. Complications include Eisenmenger syndrome and paradoxical emboli.

Patent ductus arteriosus (PDA) is a direct communication between the aorta and pulmonary artery due to the continued patency of the ductus arteriosus after birth. It is associated with prematurity and congenital rubella infections. Clinical findings include machinery murmur, late cyanosis, and congestive heart failure. Eisenmenger syndrome may develop as a complication.

PRIMARY CARDIOMYOPATHIES (DIAGNOSIS OF EXCLUSION)

Dilated cardiomyopathy (most common form) is cardiac enlargement with dilatation of all 4 chambers, resulting in progressive congestive heart failure (typical mode of presentation). The cause is genetic in 20–50% of cases, but some cases are related to alcohol, medications (Adriamycin [doxorubicin]), cocaine, viral myocarditis (Coxsackievirus B and enteroviruses), parasitic infections (Chagas disease), iron overload or pregnancy.

In cases of all types, the underlying etiology leads to destruction of myocardial contractility, which affects systolic function. Echocardiogram typically shows decreased ejection fraction. Complications include mural thrombi and cardiac arrhythmias; prognosis is poor with 5-year survival of 25%. Treatment is heart transplantation. There is myocyte hypertrophy with interstitial fibrosis on microscopy, and eccentric hypertrophy seen on gross examination.

Hypertrophic cardiomyopathy (also called asymmetrical septal hypertrophy, and idiopathic hypertrophic subaortic stenosis [IHSS]) is a common cause of sudden cardiac death in young athletes. The condition is an asymmetrical hypertrophy of cardiac muscle that causes decreased compliance affecting diastolic function. Hypertrophic cardiomyopathy can be an autosomal dominant disorder (>50% of cases) or idiopathic. The muscle hypertrophy is due to the increased synthesis of actin and myosin, and on microscopic examination, the cardiac muscle fibers are hypertrophied and in disarray. Hypertrophic cardiomyopathy is most prominent in the ventricular septum, where it can obstruct the ventricular outflow tract. This can potentially lead to death during severe exercise when the cardiac outflow tract collapses, preventing blood from exiting the heart.

Restrictive cardiomyopathy (uncommon form) is caused by diseases which produce restriction of cardiac filling during diastole; etiologies include amyloidosis, sarcoidosis, endomyocardial fibroelastosis, and Loeffler endomyocarditis. In all of these diseases, increased deposition of material leads to decreased compliance, affecting diastolic function. On gross examination, the ventricles are not enlarged and the cavities are not dilated. Microscopy will reflect the underlying cause.

Arrhythmogenic right ventricular cardiomyopathy causes thinning of the right ventricle due to autosomal dominant mutations that encode desmosomal junctional proteins. On microscopy, there is fatty infiltration of the myocardium.

CARCINOID HEART DISEASE

Carcinoid heart disease is right-sided endocardial and valvular fibrosis secondary to serotonin exposure in patients with carcinoid tumors that have metastasized to the liver. It is a plaque-like thickening (endocardial fibrosis) of the endocardium and valves of the right side of the heart. Many patients experience carcinoid syndrome (also related to secretion of serotonin and other metabolically active products of the tumors), characterized by skin flushing, diarrhea, cramping, bronchospasm, wheezing, and telangiectasias. The diagnosis can be established by demonstrating elevated urinary 5-hydroxyindoleacetic acid (5-HIAA), a metabolite of the breakdown of serotonin via monoamine oxidase.

CARDIAC TUMORS

Primary cardiac tumors are rare. The majority are benign; the malignant tumors are sarcomas. Treatment is excision.

- **Cardiac myxoma** is a benign tumor usually arising within the left atrium near the fossa ovalis in decades 3-6 of life; it can present like mitral valve disease. In 10% of cases there is an autosomal dominant condition known as Carney complex (myxomas with endocrine abnormalities and lentigines or pigmented nevi). Cardiac myxoma is characterized microscopically by stellate-shaped cells within a myxoid background. Complications include tumor emboli and "ball-valve" obstruction of the valves.

- **Cardiac rhabdomyoma** is a benign tumor usually arising within the myocardium that is associated with tuberous sclerosis.

In a Nutshell

Tuberous Sclerosis Complex

- Autosomal dominant
- Mutation in genes *TSC1* and *TSC2*, which encode tumor suppressor proteins hamartin and tuberin, respectively
- Multiple hamartomas
- Cortical tubers
- Renal angiomyolipomas
- Cardiac rhabdomyomas
- Pulmonary hamartomas

PERICARDIAL DISEASE

Pericarditis. There are 2 kinds of pericarditis, acute and chronic.

- **Acute pericarditis** is characterized by a fibrinous exudate (viral infection or uremia) or by a fibrinopurulent exudate (bacterial infection).

- **Chronic pericarditis** can occur when acute pericarditis does not resolve and adhesions form.

Pericardial effusion may be serous (secondary to heart failure or hypoalbuminemia), serosanguineous (due to trauma, malignancy, or rupture of the heart or aorta) or chylous (due to thoracic duct obstruction or injury).

Tumors of the lung and breast may spread by **direct extension** to the pericardia.

Chapter Summary

- Ischemic heart disease, the most common cause of death in the United States, is usually secondary to coronary artery disease.

- Angina pectoris refers to transient cardiac ischemia (without cell death) resulting in substernal pain. Variants of angina include stable angina, Prinzmetal variant angina, and unstable angina.

- Myocardial infarction is a localized area of cardiac muscle coagulative necrosis due to ischemia. It often presents with sudden onset of severe "crushing" substernal chest pain that may radiate to the left arm, jaw, and neck. EKG changes and elevation of cardiac-specific troponin I and T in the serum to confirm the diagnosis.

- Congestive heart failure is insufficient cardiac output to meet the metabolic demands of the body's tissues and organs. Left heart failure can complicate ischemic heart disease, hypertension, myocardial diseases, and aortic or mitral valve disease. It is associated with left ventricular hypertrophy and dilatation, passive pulmonary congestion and edema, activation of the renin-angiotensin-aldosterone system leading to hyperaldosteronism, and cardiogenic shock. Right heart failure can complicate left heart failure, pulmonary or tricuspid valvular disease, and cor pulmonale. It causes jugular venous distension, hepatosplenomegaly, dependent edema, and ascites.

- Degenerative calcific aortic valve stenosis, the most common valvular abnormality, is an age-related dystrophic calcification, degeneration, and stenosis of the aortic valve that can cause concentric left ventricular hypertrophy, congestive heart failure, and an increased risk of sudden death.

- Mitral valve prolapse is a myxomatous degeneration of the mitral valve that causes the valve leaflets to become enlarged and floppy.

- Rheumatic fever is a systemic inflammatory disease, triggered by a pharyngeal infection with Group A beta-hemolytic streptococci, that in genetically susceptible individuals results in the production of antibodies that cross-react with cardiac antigens. Acute rheumatic heart disease can produce myocarditis, pericarditis, and endocarditis. Chronic rheumatic heart disease can damage the mitral and aortic valves, secondarily predisposing for mitral stenosis, congestive heart disease, and infective endocarditis.

- Infective bacterial endocarditis is a bacterial infection of the cardiac valves, characterized by vegetations on the valve leaflets. Acute endocarditis is caused by high-virulence organisms, notably *Staphylococcus aureus*, and produces large destructive lesions with a high mortality rate. Subacute endocarditis is caused by low-virulence organisms, notably *Viridans streptococci*, and usually involves previously damaged valves.

- Marantic endocarditis refers to the formation of small, sterile fibrin vegetations along the valve leaflet line of closure in patients with debilitating diseases.

- Congenital heart disease is the most common cause of childhood heart disease in the United States and may be idiopathic or associated with genetic disease, infection, or drug and alcohol use.

(continued)

Chapter Summary *(cont'd)*

- Coarctation of the aorta is a segmental narrowing of the aorta that is subclassified, depending upon the level at which the narrowing occurs, into preductal coarctation (poorer prognosis, association with Turner syndrome) and postductal coarctation (late onset).

- Tetralogy of Fallot is the most common cause of congenital cyanotic heart disease and is characterized by a classic tetrad of right ventricular outflow obstruction/stenosis, right ventricular hypertrophy, ventricular septal defect, and overriding aorta.

- Transposition of the great arteries is an abnormal development of the truncoconal septum that results in inversion of the aorta and pulmonary arteries with respect to the ventricles. Transposition of the great arteries has a poor prognosis without surgery.

- Truncus arteriosus is a failure to develop a dividing septum between the aorta and the pulmonary artery, resulting in a common trunk. Truncus arteriosus has a poor prognosis without surgery.

- Tricuspid atresia is the absence of a communication between the right atrium and ventricle due to developmental failure to form the tricuspid valve. Tricuspid atresia has a poor prognosis without surgery.

- Ventricular septal defect is the second most common congenital heart defect and consists of a direct communication between the ventricular chambers. The prognosis varies with the size of the defect.

- Atrial septal defect is a direct communication between the atrial chambers whose most common type involves the ostium secundum.

- Patent ductus arteriosus is a direct communication between the aorta and pulmonary artery due to the continued patency of the ductus arteriosus after birth.

- Dilated cardiomyopathy is the most common form of primary cardiomyopathy and consists of cardiac enlargement with dilatation of all 4 chambers due to diminished contractility.

- Hypertrophic cardiomyopathy is an asymmetric cardiac hypertrophy that is most prominent in the ventricular septum, where it may obstruct the ventricular outflow tract, with resulting increased risk of sudden cardiac death, particularly in young athletes.

- Restrictive cardiomyopathy is an uncommon form of cardiomyopathy caused by diseases such as amyloidosis and sarcoidosis that produce restriction of cardiac filling during diastole.

- Carcinoid heart disease is a right-sided endocardial and valvular fibrosis secondary to exposure to serotonin in patients with carcinoid tumors that have metastasized to the liver.

- Cardiac myxoma is a benign tumor, usually arising within the left atrium near the fossa ovalis.

- Cardiac rhabdomyoma is a benign tumor, usually arising within the myocardium. It is associated with tuberous sclerosis.

Learning Objectives

❑ Explain information related to congenital cystic lung lesions

❑ Demonstrate understanding of atelectasis

❑ Solve problems concerning pulmonary infections

❑ Demonstrate understanding of sarcoidosis

❑ Answer questions about obstructive versus restrictive lung disease

❑ Answer questions about vascular disorders of the lungs

❑ Demonstrate understanding of pulmonary and laryngeal neoplasias

❑ Explain information related to diseases of the pleural cavity

CONGENITAL CYSTIC LUNG LESIONS

The 2 most common malformations of the lung are **congenital cystic adenomatoid malformation** (CCAM) and **bronchopulmonary sequestration** (BPS). CCAM is a hamartomatous lesion, and BPS is a nonfunctioning bronchopulmonary segment separate from the tracheobronchial tree.

These conditions are followed by serial ultrasonography. Some resolve spontaneously, though minimally invasive surgery may be required.

ATELECTASIS

Atelectasis refers to an area of collapsed or nonexpanded lung. It is reversible, but areas of atelectasis predispose for infection due to decreased mucociliary clearance.

The major types are as follows:

- **Obstruction/resorption atelectasis** is collapse of lung due to resorption of air distal to an obstruction; examples include aspiration of a foreign body, chronic obstructive pulmonary disease (COPD), and postoperative atelectasis.

- **Compression atelectasis** is atelectasis due to fluid, air, blood, or tumor in the pleural space.

- **Contraction (scar) atelectasis** is due to fibrosis and scarring of the lung.

- **Patchy atelectasis** is due to a lack of surfactant, as occurs in hyaline membrane disease of newborn or acute (adult) respiratory distress syndrome (ARDS).

Bridge to Anatomy

Pores of Kohn are collateral connections between alveoli through which infections and neoplastic cells can spread.

PULMONARY INFECTIONS

In **bacterial pneumonia,** acute inflammation and consolidation (solidification) of the lung are due to a bacterial agent. Clinical signs and symptoms include fever and chills; productive cough with yellow-green (pus) or rusty (bloody) sputum; tachypnea; pleuritic chest pain; and decreased breath sounds, rales, and dullness to percussion.

Studies typically show elevated white blood cell count with a left shift (an increase in immature leukocytes). Chest x-ray for lobar pneumonia typically shows lobar or segmental consolidation (opacification), and for bronchopneumonia typically shows patchy opacification. Pleural effusion may also be picked up on chest x-ray.

In general, the keys to effective therapy are identification of the organism and early treatment with antibiotics.

Lobar pneumonia is characterized by consolidation of an entire lobe. The infecting organism is typically *Streptococcus pneumoniae* (95%) or *Klebsiella*. The lancet-shaped diplococcus *Streptococcus pneumoniae* is alpha-hemolytic, bile soluble, and optochin sensitive.

The **4 classic phases** of lobar pneumonia are **congestion** (active hyperemia and edema); **red hepatization** (neutrophils and hemorrhage); **grey hepatization** (degradation of red blood cells); and **resolution** (healing). In today's antibiotic era, these changes are not generally observed in practice.

Bronchopneumonia is characterized by scattered patchy consolidation centered on bronchioles; the inflammation tends to be bilateral, multilobar, and basilar, and particularly susceptible populations include the young, old, and terminally ill. Infecting organisms exhibit more variation than in lobar pneumonia, and include *Staphylococci, Streptococci, Haemophilus influenzae, Pseudomonas aeruginosa,* etc. Microscopic examination of tissue shows acute inflammation of bronchioles and surrounding alveoli. The diagnosis can often be established with sputum gram stain and sputum culture, but will sometimes require blood cultures.

Complications of pneumonia include fibrous scarring and pleural adhesions, lung abscess, empyema (pus in a body cavity), and sepsis.

Treatment of pneumonia is generally initial empiric antibiotic treatment, modified by the results of cultures and organism sensitivities.

Lung abscess is a localized collection of neutrophils (pus) and necrotic pulmonary parenchyma. The etiology varies with the clinical setting. **Aspiration** is the most common cause. It tends to involve right lower lobe and typically has mixed oral flora (often both anaerobic and aerobic) for infecting organisms.

Lung abscess may also occur following a pneumonia, especially one due to *S. aureus* or *Klebsiella*. Lung abscesses may also occur following airway obstruction (postobstructive) or deposition of septic emboli in the lung.

Complications of lung abscess include empyema, pulmonary hemorrhage, and secondary amyloidosis.

Atypical pneumonia is the term used for interstitial pneumonitis without consolidation. It is more common in children and young adults.

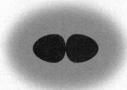

Streptococcus pneumoniae

Infecting organisms that can cause atypical pneumonia include *Mycoplasma pneumoniae, influenza virus, parainfluenza virus, respiratory syncytial virus* (RSV) (which is especially important in young children), *adenovirus, cytomegalovirus* (CMV) (which is especially important in the immunocompromised), *varicella virus,* and many others.

Diagnosis. Chest x-ray typically shows diffuse interstitial infiltrates. An elevated cold agglutinin titer specifically suggests *Mycoplasma* as a cause, which is important to identify since antibiotic therapy for *Mycoplasma* exists. Lung biopsy, if performed, typically shows lymphoplasmacytic inflammation within the alveolar septa.

Complications include superimposed bacterial infections and Reye syndrome (potentially triggered by viral illness [influenza/varicella] treated with aspirin).

Tuberculosis (TB). The number of cases of TB is declining in the United States, but the proportion of cases in people born outside the country is rising. In this clinical setting, a positive PPD skin test may demonstrate that the person has been exposed to the mycobacterial antigens. Individuals who have received the BCG vaccine in some foreign countries may have a positive PPD test without being infected. In such cases chest x-ray and sputum smears and cultures are done.

Infection is usually acquired by inhalation of aerosolized bacilli.

The **clinical presentation** of *Mycobacterium tuberculosis* includes fevers and night sweats, weight loss, cough, and hemoptysis.

Primary pulmonary TB develops on initial exposure to the disease. The Ghon focus of primary TB is characterized by subpleural caseous granuloma formation, either above or below the interlobar fissure. The term *Ghon complex* refers to the combination of the Ghon focus and secondarily-involved hilar lymph nodes with granulomas. Most primary pulmonary tuberculosis lesions (95%) will undergo fibrosis and calcification.

Progressive pulmonary TB can take several forms, including cavitary tuberculosis, miliary pulmonary tuberculosis, and tuberculous bronchopneumonia.

Secondary pulmonary TB (also known as postprimary or reactivation TB) occurs either with reactivation of an old, previously quiescent infection or with reinfection secondary to a second exposure to the mycobacteria. In secondary pulmonary TB, the infection often produces a friable nodule at the lung apex (Simon focus) secondary to the high oxygen concentration present at that site, since the upper parts of the lung typically ventilate more efficiently than the lower parts. Biopsy of affected tissues will typically show AFB-positive caseating granulomas.

Additionally, **dissemination to other organ systems** can occur in advanced TB via a hematogenous route that often results in a miliary pattern within each affected organ. Sites that may become involved include meninges; cervical lymph nodes (scrofula) and larynx; liver/spleen, kidneys, adrenals, and ileum; lumbar vertebrae bone marrow (Pott disease); and fallopian tubes and epididymis.

Nontuberculous mycobacteria. ***M. avium* complex (MAC)** typically occurs in AIDS patients with CD4 counts <50 cells/mm^3 and presents as disseminated disease.

The diagnosis of TB requires identification of the bacilli. Positive sputum smear necessitates culture for species identification. Adequate treatment requires drug susceptibility testing.

Note

BCG (Bacillus Calmette-Guérin) is a tuberculosis vaccine prepared from a strain of attenuated live bovine tuberculosis bacillus, *Mycobacterium bovis.*

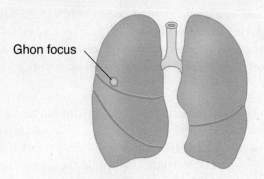

Figure 14-1. Primary Tuberculosis

SARCOIDOSIS

Sarcoidosis is a systemic granulomatous disease of uncertain etiology. The disease affects females more than males, with typical age 20–60. It is most common in African American women. Clinical presentation varies. It may be asymptomatic, or presenting symptoms may include cough and shortness of breath; fatigue and malaise; skin lesions; eye irritation or pain; and fever or night sweats. Most often, the disease is first detected on chest x-ray as bilateral hilar lymphadenopathy or parenchymal infiltrates.

The noncaseating granulomas that are characteristic of sarcoidosis may occur in **any organ of the body**. In the lung, they typically form diffuse scattered granulomas; lymph node involvement may cause hilar and mediastinal adenopathy. Skin, liver and/or spleen, heart, central nervous system, bone marrow, and gastrointestinal tract are also frequent targets of the disease. Eye involvement can be seen in Mikulicz syndrome (involvement of the uvea and parotid).

The diagnosis of sarcoidosis can be suggested by clinical studies. In the laboratory, serum angiotensin converting enzyme (ACE), which is synthesized by endothelial cells and macrophages, may be elevated. X-ray studies frequently show bilateral hilar lymphadenopathy.

Sarcoidosis is considered to be a **diagnosis of exclusion**. In practice, this means that the diagnosis is considered when a biopsy shows features characteristic of sarcoidosis (such as noncaseating granulomas, Schaumann bodies [laminated dystrophic calcification], and asteroid bodies [stellate giant cell cytoplasmic inclusions]). There are no pathognomonic microscopic features though, and the diagnosis requires clinicopathologic correlation.

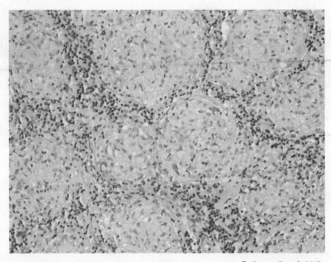

© Gregg Barré, M.D.
Used with permission.

Figure 14-2. Noncaseating Sarcoid Granulomas

The prognosis is favorable with a variable clinical course. Most patients completely recover but some succumb to respiratory compromise.

OBSTRUCTIVE VERSUS RESTRICTIVE LUNG DISEASE

Table 14-1. Obstructive Versus Restrictive Lung Disease

Obstructive Airway Disease	Restrictive Lung Disease
Definition: Increased resistance to airflow secondary to obstruction of airways	Decreased lung volume and capacity
Pulmonary function tests (spirometry) FEV_1/FVC ratio is decreased	Decreased TLC and VC
Examples: Chronic obstructive airway disease • Asthma • Chronic bronchitis • Emphysema • Bronchiectasis	Chest wall disorders • Obesity, kyphoscoliosis, polio, etc. Interstitial/infiltrative diseases • ARDS, pneumoconiosis • Pulmonary fibrosis

Table 14-2. Summary of Obstructive Versus Restrictive Pattern

Variable	Obstructive Pattern, e.g., Emphysema	Restrictive Pattern, e.g., Fibrosis
Total lung capacity	increased	decreased
FEV_1	decreased	decreased
Forced vital capacity	normal or slightly decreased	decreased
FEV_1/FVC	decreased	increased or normal
Peak flow	decreased	decreased
Functional residual capacity	increased	decreased
Residual volume	increased	decreased

OBSTRUCTIVE PULMONARY DISEASE

Chronic obstructive pulmonary disease (COPD) is a general term used to indicate chronic decreased respiratory function due to chronic bronchitis or emphysema. Both diseases are associated with smoking.

Chronic bronchitis is a clinical diagnosis made when a patient has a persistent cough and copious sputum production for at least 3 months in 2 consecutive years. It is highly associated with smoking (90%). Clinical findings include cough, sputum production, dyspnea, frequent infections, hypoxia, cyanosis, and weight gain.

Microscopic examination demonstrates hypertrophy and hyperplasia of bronchial mucous glands (Reid index equals the submucosal gland thickness divided by the bronchial wall thickness between the pseudostratified columnar epithelium and the perichondrium; normal ratio is ≤0.4).

Complications include increased risk for recurrent infections; secondary pulmonary hypertension leading to right heart failure (cor pulmonale) and lung cancer.

Emphysema is the term used when destruction of alveolar septa results in enlarged air spaces and a loss of elastic recoil. The 4 types of emphysema are named for the anatomical distribution of the septal damage.

- In **centrilobular emphysema**, the damage is in the proximal portion of the acinus and the cause is cigarette smoking.

- In **panacinar emphysema**, the damage affects the entire acinus and the common cause is alpha-1 antitrypsin deficiency.

- In **distal acinar emphysema** (unknown cause), extension to the pleura causes pneumothorax.

- In **irregular emphysema**, post-inflammatory scarring involves the acinus in an irregular distribution.

The etiology of emphysema involves a **protease/antiprotease imbalance**. On gross examination, the lungs are overinflated and enlarged, and have enlarged, grossly visible air spaces. Clinical findings include progressive dyspnea, pursing of lips and use of accessory respiratory muscles to breathe, barrel chest (increased anterior-posterior diameter), and weight loss.

Table 14-3. Manifestations Related to Area of Involvement

Centriacinar (Centrilobular)	Panacinar (Panlobular)
Proximal respiratory bronchioles involved, distal alveoli spared	Entire acinus involved
Most common type (95%)	
Associated with smoking, air pollution	α-1-antitrypsin deficiency
Distribution: worse in apical segments of upper lobes	Distribution: entire lung; worse in bases of lower lobes

Asthma is due to hyperreactive airways, which undergo episodic bronchospasm when triggered by certain stimuli.

- **Atopic (type I IgE-mediated hypersensitivity reaction) asthma** (most common form) usually affects children and young adults. There is often a positive family history.

- **Nonatopic asthma** is triggered by processes including respiratory infections (usually viral), stress, exercise, or cold temperatures.

- **Drug-induced asthma** affects about 10% of adults with a diagnosis of asthma. Aspirin is a key example of a precipitating drug.

- **Occupational asthma** is caused by workplace triggers including fumes and dusts.

An asthma attack is characterized by wheezing, severe dyspnea, and coughing. Problems with expiration cause lung overinflation. Status asthmaticus is a potentially fatal unrelenting attack of asthma.

Microscopic examination of sputum cytology may show Curschmann spirals (twisted mucus plugs admixed with sloughed epithelium), eosinophils, or Charcot-Leyden crystals (protein crystalloids from broken down eosinophils).

In patients dying from disease, autopsy findings include mucus plugs, increased mucous glands with goblet cell hyperplasia, inflammation (especially with eosinophils), edema; hypertrophy and hyperplasia of bronchial wall smooth muscle, and thickened basement membranes.

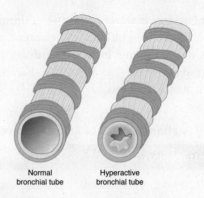

Normal
bronchial tube

Hyperactive
bronchial tube

Figure 14-3. Bronchial Changes in Asthma

Bronchiectasis is an abnormal permanent airway dilatation due to chronic necrotizing inflammation. Clinical findings include cough, fever, malodorous purulent sputum, and dyspnea. Causes are diverse, and include bronchial obstruction by foreign body, mucus, or tumor, necrotizing pneumonias, cystic fibrosis, and Kartagener syndrome.

- **Kartagener syndrome** is an autosomal recessive condition caused by immotile cilia due to a defect of dynein arms (primary ciliary dyskinesia). It is characterized clinically by bronchiectasis, chronic sinusitis, and situs inversus (a congenital condition where the major visceral organs are anatomically reversed compared with their normal anatomical positions).

On gross examination, bronchiectasis shows dilated bronchi and bronchioles extending out to the pleura. These changes may also be appreciated on chest x-ray. Complications include abscess, septic emboli, cor pulmonale, and secondary amyloidosis.

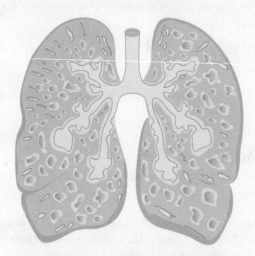

Figure 14-4. Cross-Section of Bronchiectasis

INFILTRATIVE RESTRICTIVE LUNG DISEASES (DIFFUSE INTERSTITIAL DISEASES)

Acute respiratory distress syndrome (ARDS) refers to diffuse damage of alveolar epithelium and capillaries, resulting in progressive respiratory failure that is unresponsive to oxygen treatment. Clinicians use the term *ARDS*, while pathologists use the term *diffuse alveolar damage (DAD)* to describe the pathologic changes.

ARDS may be caused by shock, sepsis, trauma, gastric aspiration, radiation, oxygen toxicity, drugs, or pulmonary infection. Activated neutrophils mediate cell damage. Clinically, patients show dyspnea, tachypnea, hypoxemia, cyanosis, and use of accessory respiratory muscles. X-rays show bilateral lung opacity ("white out").

On gross pathologic examination affected lungs are heavy, stiff, and noncompliant. Microscopically, there is intra-alveolar edema, and hyaline membranes line the alveolar spaces. In resolving cases there is proliferation of type II pneumocytes and interstitial inflammation and fibrosis.

Treatment is based on treating the underlying cause and on supporting respiration with mechanical ventilation. The prognosis is problematic even with good care, with overall mortality 40%.

Respiratory distress syndrome of the newborn (hyaline membrane disease of newborns) is caused by a deficiency of surfactant. It is associated with prematurity (gestational age of <28 weeks has a 60% incidence), maternal diabetes, multiple births, male gender, and cesarean section delivery. Clinically, infants are normal at birth but within a few hours develop increasing respiratory effort, tachypnea, nasal flaring, use of accessory muscles of respiration, an expiratory grunt, and cyanosis. Chest radiograph may demonstrate bilateral "ground-glass" reticulogranular densities. Autopsy findings include atelectasis and hyaline membranes.

Treatment is surfactant replacement, mechanical ventilation, and continuous positive airway pressure (CPAP). Respiratory distress syndrome of the newborn can sometimes be prevented if labor can be delayed and if corticosteroids are used to mature the lung. With improved therapies, now >90% of babies survive.

Chronic interstitial lung disease is a term describing heterogeneous lung disorders which share similar symptomology but vary in prognosis. Patients present with dyspnea and cough. Lung biopsy findings can be paired with clinical information to aid in therapeutic management/palliative care.

- **Idiopathic pulmonary fibrosis (IPF)** is a fatal disease. It shows patchy interstitial fibrosis and inflammation. "Honeycomb fibrosis" refers to dilated cystic spaces lined with type II pneumocytes; this histology is consistent with end-stage lung. Pathologists use the term *usual interstitial pneumonia* for IPF.

- **Nonspecific interstitial pneumonia** has a better prognosis than IPF. There is a cellular pattern and a fibrosing pattern.

- **Cryptogenic organizing pneumonia** responds to steroids. Histologically, there are plugs of connective tissue inside the alveolar spaces.

- **Collagen vascular disease pneumonitis** has varied patterns of parenchymal and pleural involvement. The prognosis is poor.

Bridge to Anatomy

Type II pneumocytes repopulate the alveolar epithelium in response to injury.

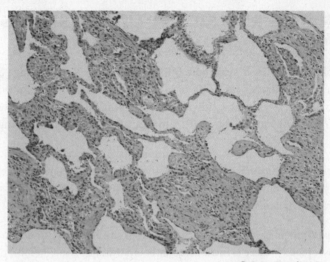

© Gregg Barré, M.D.
Used with permission.

Figure 14-5. Honeycomb Lung (Idiopathic Pulmonary Fibrosis)

- **Smoking-related pneumonitis.** Several entities have been identified.

  ○ Desquamative interstitial pneumonia features alveolar macrophages.

  ○ Respiratory bronchiolitis features bronchiolocentric macrophages.

  ○ Smoking-related interstitial fibrosis shows septal collagen deposition without significant associated inflammation.

- **Hypersensitivity pneumonitis.** After exposure to a sensitizing agent such as moldy hay, patients present with a febrile acute reaction or a chronic disease with weight loss. Biopsy shows peribronchiolar acute and chronic interstitial inflammation +/- noncaseating granulomas. The disease is immunologically mediated.

- **Eosinophilic pneumonia** describes a group of diseases with varying clinical features but a common histologic finding of a mixed septal inflammatory infiltrate and eosinophils within alveolar spaces. **Loeffler's syndrome** is a self-limiting type of eosinophilic pneumonia with peripheral blood eosinophilia.

Occupation-associated pneumoconiosis is a common cause of chronic interstitial lung disease. It is considered separately here to show the full spectrum of disease since neoplasia may occur during its course.

- **Pneumoconioses** are fibrosing pulmonary diseases caused by inhalation of an aerosol (mineral dusts, particles, vapors, or fumes). Key factors affecting their development include the type of aerosol and its ability to stimulate fibrosis; the dose and duration of exposure; and the size of the particle, with only particles <10 microns entering the alveolar sac.

  ○ **Coal worker's pneumoconiosis** is an important pneumoconiosis that is due to anthracosis, in which carbon pigment (anthracotic pigment) from coal mining accumulates in macrophages along the pleural lymphatics and interstitium. Clinically, the disease may progress through several stages. The earliest stage is asymptomatic.

  ○ **Simple coal worker's pneumoconiosis** (black lung disease) is characterized by coal-dust macules and nodules in the upper lobes that produce little pulmonary dysfunction.

- **Complicated coal worker's pneumoconiosis** is characterized by progressive massive fibrosis that is accompanied by increasing respiratory distress, secondary pulmonary hypertension, and cor pulmonale.

- **Caplan syndrome** is the term when pneumoconiosis (of any type) accompanies rheumatoid arthritis.

- **Asbestosis** is caused by members of a family of crystalline silicates. Occupations in which asbestos exposure may occur include shipyard work, insulation and construction industries, brake-lining manufacture.

  - **Serpentine asbestos** is composed of curved, flexible fibers, with the most common type of serpentine asbestos being chrysotile.

  - **Amphibole asbestos** is composed of straight, brittle fibers. Important types include crocidolite, tremolite, and amosite. Amphibole asbestos is more pathogenic than serpentine asbestos, and is highly associated with mesotheliomas.

  - **The pulmonary pathology of asbestosis** is a diffuse interstitial fibrosis that begins in the lower lobes; it causes slowly progressive dyspnea which may eventually be complicated by secondary pulmonary hypertension and cor pulmonale. Pulmonary biopsy may demonstrate asbestos bodies that have become coated with iron (ferruginous bodies). Otherwise, the findings are the same as usual interstitial pneumonia.

  - **Pleural involvement** may take the form of parietal pleural plaques (acellular type I collagen deposition) in a symmetrical distribution involving the domes of the diaphragm and posterolateral chest walls on chest x-ray. The apices and costophrenic angles are spared. Plaques on the anterior chest wall may be seen on CT. Fibrous pleural adhesions may occur on the visceral pleura.

  - **Lung cancer** is the most common tumor in asbestos-exposed individuals; there is a strong synergistic effect between smoking and asbestos exposure.

  - **Malignant mesothelioma** is a rare, highly malignant neoplasm associated with occupational exposure to asbestos in 90% of cases. It presents with recurrent pleural effusions, dyspnea, and chest pain. The tumor grossly encases and compresses the lung; microscopic exam exhibits carcinomatous and sarcomatous elements (biphasic pattern), while electron microscopy shows long, thin microvilli on some tumor cells. The prognosis of mesothelioma is poor. Other problems include increased risk of laryngeal, stomach, and colon cancers. Family members also have increased risk of cancer due to the worker bringing home clothing covered with asbestos fibers.

- **Silicosis** is due to exposure to silicon dioxide (silica). It is seen most frequently with occupational exposure (sandblasters, metal grinders, miners). The **pulmonary pathology** shows dense nodular fibrosis of the upper lobes which may progress to massive fibrosis; birefringent silica particles can be seen with polarized light.

  Patients present with insidious onset of dyspnea that is slowly progressive despite cessation of exposure. X-ray shows fibrotic nodules in the upper zones of the lungs. There is an increased risk of TB.

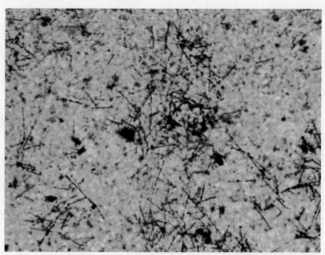

© Colin M. Bloor, M.D.
Used with permission.

Figure 14-6. Asbestos Fibers in Lung Tissue

- **Berylliosis** is an allergic granulomatous reaction due to workplace exposure to beryllium in the nuclear, electronics, and aerospace industries. Genetic susceptibility appears to play a role, as does a type IV hypersensitivity reaction, resulting in granuloma formation. Clinically, acute exposure causes acute pneumonitis, while chronic exposure causes pulmonary noncaseating granulomas and fibrosis, hilar lymph node granulomas, and systemic granulomas

VASCULAR DISORDERS

Pulmonary edema is fluid accumulation within the lungs, usually due to imbalance of Starling forces or endothelial injury.

- Pulmonary edema due to **increased hydrostatic pressure** can be seen in left-sided heart failure, mitral valve stenosis, high altitude pulmonary edema, and fluid overload.

- Pulmonary edema due to **decreased oncotic pressure** can be seen in nephrotic syndrome and liver disease.

- Pulmonary edema due to **increased capillary permeability** can be due to infections, drugs (bleomycin, heroin), shock, and radiation.

The pathology grossly shows wet, heavy lungs (usually worse in lower lobes), while microscopic examination shows intra-alveolar fluid, engorged capillaries, and hemosiderin-laden macrophages (heart-failure cells).

Pulmonary emboli (PE) and pulmonary infarction (*See* Circulatory Pathology, chapter 5.)

Pulmonary hypertension is increased pulmonary artery pressure, usually due to increased vascular resistance or blood flow.

The etiology varies and can include chronic obstructive pulmonary disease and interstitial disease (hypoxic vasoconstriction); multiple ongoing pulmonary emboli; mitral stenosis and left heart failure; congenital heart disease with left to right shunts (atrial septal defect, ventricular septal defect, patent ductus arteriosus); and primary (idiopathic) pulmonary hypertension, typically in young women.

Note

High altitude pulmonary edema is a hydrostatic-type pulmonary edema. Symptoms (i.e., cough and shortness of breath) resolve with descent and administration of oxygen.

Clinical Correlate

Dietary drugs fenfluramine and phentermine have been associated with primary pulmonary hypertension.

The pathology includes pulmonary artery atherosclerosis, small artery medial hypertrophy and intimal fibrosis, and plexogenic pulmonary arteriopathy. Pulmonary hypertension may also damage the heart, leading to right ventricular hypertrophy and then failure (cor pulmonale).

PULMONARY NEOPLASIA

Lung cancer is the leading cause of cancer death among both men and women; it has been increasing in women (increased smoking) in the past few decades. It occurs most commonly age 50–80. Major risk factors include cigarette smoking, occupational exposure (asbestosis, uranium mining, radiation, etc.), passive smoking, and air pollution. Clinical features include cough, sputum production, weight loss, anorexia, fatigue, dyspnea, hemoptysis, and chest pain. Obstruction may produce focal emphysema, atelectasis, bronchiectasis, or pneumonia.

Common genetic mutations in lung cancer involve the oncogenes *MYCL* (small cell carcinomas) and *KRAS* (adenocarcinomas); tumor suppressor genes: *TP53* and *RB1*.

Adenocarcinoma is more commonly seen in women and nonsmokers. Grossly, it causes a peripheral gray-white mass, and the tumor may develop in areas of parenchymal scarring (scar carcinoma). Microscopically, common patterns include acinar, papillary, mucinous, and solid. The precursor lesion—atypical adenomatous hyperplasia—progresses to adenocarcinoma in situ (noninvasive well-differentiated tumor <3 cm) and to minimally invasive tumor (invasion no more than 5 mm) before progressing to invasive adenocarcinoma.

Squamous cell carcinoma (SCC) is strongly related to smoking and affects males more than females. Squamous cell carcinoma arises from bronchial epithelium after a progression:

metaplasia → dysplasia → carcinoma *in situ* → invasive carcinoma

Pathologically, the tumor grossly causes a gray-white bronchial mass, usually centrally located. Microscopically, well-differentiated tumors show invasive nests of squamous cells with intercellular bridges (desmosomes) and keratin production ("squamous pearls").

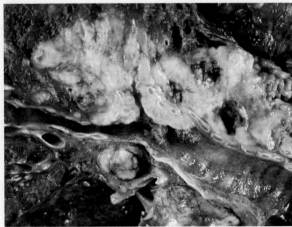

© Katsumi M. Miyai, M.D., Ph.D.; Regents of the University of California.
Used with permission.

Figure 14-7. Squamous Cell Carcinoma of the Lung

Small cell carcinoma has a strong association with smoking, and affects males more than females. This neuroendocrine tumor is very aggressive, with rapid growth and early dissemination. Small cell carcinoma is commonly associated with paraneoplastic syndromes.

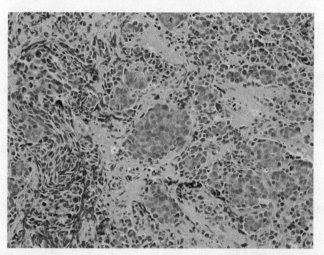

© Gregg Barré, M.D.
Used with permission.

Figure 14-8. Small Cell Carcinoma with Crush Artifact in the Lower Left Field

Pathologically, gross examination demonstrates central, gray-white masses. Microscopic examination shows small round or polygonal cells in clusters, and electron microscopy shows cytoplasmic dense-core neurosecretory granules.

Large cell carcinoma has large anaplastic cells without evidence of differentiation.

Intrathoracic spread of lung cancer is to lymph nodes, particularly hilar, bronchial, **tracheal, and mediastinal; pleura (adenocarcinoma);** and lung apex causing **Horner syndrome (Pancoast tumor).**

- Obstruction of the superior vena cava by tumor causes **superior vena cava syndrome,** characterized by distended head and neck veins, plethora, and facial and upper arm edema.

- **Esophageal obstruction** can cause dysphagia.

- Recurrent laryngeal **nerve involvement** causes hoarseness, while phrenic nerve damage causes diaphragmatic paralysis.

Extrathoracic sites of metastasis include adrenal (>50%), liver, brain, and bone.

Note

Horner Syndrome causes ipsilateral:

- Ptosis
- Miosis
- Anhidrosis
- Enophthalmos

Paraneoplastic syndromes

- Endocrine/metabolic syndromes include Cushing syndrome secondary to ACTH production, SIADH secondary to ADH production, and hypercalcemia secondary to PTH production (squamous cell carcinoma).

- Eaton-Lambert syndrome (*See* Skeletal Muscle and Peripheral Nerve Pathology chapter.)

- Acanthosis nigricans (*See* Skin Pathology chapter.)

- Hypertrophic pulmonary osteoarthropathy is characterized by periosteal new bone formation with clubbing and arthritis.

Treatment of non–small cell lung cancer is with surgery, and treatment of small cell lung cancer is with chemotherapy and radiation. Despite treatment, the prognosis is poor, with overall 5-year survival 16%.

Bronchial carcinoids occur in a younger age group (mean age 40 years) and typically produce a polypoid intrabronchial mass or plaque; it is characterized on light microscopy by small, round, uniform cells growing in nests (organoid pattern), and on electron microscopy by cytoplasmic dense-core neurosecretory granules. Atypical carcinoid is more aggressive than typical carcinoid.

Metastatic carcinoma is the most common malignant neoplasm in the lung. It typically causes multiple, bilateral, scattered nodules; common primary sites include breast, stomach, pancreas, and colon.

Hamartomas are benign tumors; they occur more commonly in middle-aged adults but also occur in children. They can appear as coin lesions on chest x-ray. Microscopically, they are comprised of nonencapsulated fibromyxoid tissue. Carney triad is the finding of a hamartoma with a predominantly cartilaginous component (pulmonary chondroma), an extra-adrenal paraganglioma and a gastric gastrointestinal stromal tumor.

LARYNGEAL CANCER

Laryngeal squamous cell carcinoma causes hoarseness, difficulty swallowing, pain, hemoptysis, and eventual respiratory compromise. Risk factors include smoking, alcohol, and frequent cord irritation (professional singing or lecturing). Complications include direct extension, metastases, and infection.

Bridge to Pharmacology

Erlotinib (Tarceva®) is used to treat non–small cell lung cancer, pancreatic cancer, and other types of cancers that have failed a prior trial of chemotherapy. It is a tyrosine-kinase inhibitor which inhibits the epidermal growth factor receptor (EGFR). The drug targets EGFR tyrosine kinase which is highly expressed and sometimes mutated in various forms of cancer.

DISEASES OF THE PLEURAL CAVITY

Pleural effusion is the accumulation of fluid in the pleural cavity.

- *Empyema* refers to pus in pleural space.

- *Chylothorax* refers to chylous fluid in the pleural space secondary to obstruction of the thoracic duct, usually by tumor.

Pneumothorax is the term used for air in the pleural cavity. It can be due to traumatic penetrating chest wall injuries or spontaneous rupture of apical blebs in typically tall young adults (spontaneous pneumothorax). The term **tension pneumothorax** is used if a life-threatening shift of thoracic organs across midline occurs.

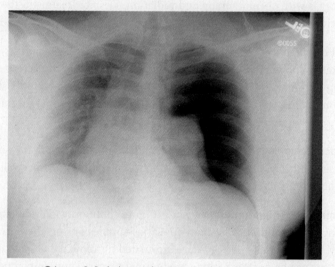

© James G. Smirniotopoulos, M.D.; Uniformed Services University.
Used with permission.

Figure 14-9. Densely Black Appearance on Chest X-Ray of a Pneumothorax

Hemothorax is the presence of blood in the pleural cavity. Trauma is a common cause. There may be hypotension and shift of the trachea to the unaffected side.

Chylothorax is lymphatic fluid in the pleural cavity. Malignancy is a common cause.

Mesothelioma (*See* section on asbestosis earlier in this chapter.)

Chapter Summary

- The 2 most common lung malformations are congenital cystic adenomatoid malformation and bronchopulmonary sequestration.

- Atelectasis is an area of collapsed or unexpanded lung and can occur secondary to obstruction, compression, contraction, or lack of surfactant.

- Bacterial pneumonia is an acute inflammation and consolidation (solidification) of the lung due to a bacterial agent. Lobar pneumonia causes consolidation of an entire lobe and is most commonly caused by infection with *Streptococcus pneumoniae*. Bronchopneumonia causes scattered patchy consolidation centered around bronchioles and can be due to a wide variety of bacterial agents.

- Lung abscess is a localized collection of neutrophils (pus) and necrotic pulmonary parenchyma and may occur following aspiration, pneumonia, obstruction, or septic emboli.

- Atypical pneumonia causes interstitial pneumonitis without consolidation and can be due to viral agents and *Mycoplasma pneumoniae*.

- TB causes caseating granulomas containing acid-fast mycobacteria. Primary TB can produce a Ghon complex, characterized by a subpleural caseous granuloma above or below the lobar fissure accompanied by hilar lymph node granulomatous inflammation. Secondary TB tends to involve the lung apex. Progressive pulmonary TB can take the forms of cavitary TB, miliary pulmonary TB, and TB bronchopneumonia. Miliary TB can also spread to involve other body sites.

- Sarcoidosis is a granulomatous disease of unknown etiology that produces clinical disease somewhat resembling TB.

- Obstructive airway disease is characterized by increased resistance to airflow secondary to obstruction of airways, whereas restrictive lung disease is characterized by decreased lung volume and capacity.

- COPD includes chronic bronchitis, emphysema, asthma, and bronchiectasis.

- Chronic bronchitis is a clinical diagnosis made when persistent cough and copious sputum production have been present for at least 3 months in 2 consecutive years.

- Emphysema is associated with destruction of respiratory bronchioles or alveolar septa, resulting in enlarged air spaces and a loss of elastic recoil, and producing overinflated, enlarged lungs.

- Asthma is due to hyperreactive airways, resulting in episodic bronchospasm when triggered by stimuli that may include allergens, respiratory infections, stress, exercise, cold temperatures, and drugs.

- Bronchiectasis is an abnormal permanent airway dilatation due to chronic necrotizing infection; most patients have underlying lung disease such as bronchial obstruction, necrotizing pneumonias, cystic fibrosis, or Kartagener syndrome.

- Acute respiratory distress syndrome is due to diffuse damage to the alveolar epithelium and capillaries, resulting in progressive respiratory failure that is unresponsive to oxygen treatment. Causes include shock, sepsis, trauma, gastric aspiration, radiation, oxygen toxicity, drugs, pulmonary infections, and many others.

(continued)

Chapter Summary *(cont'd)*

- Respiratory distress syndrome of the newborn causes respiratory distress within hours of birth and is seen in infants with deficiency of surfactant secondary to prematurity, maternal diabetes, multiple births, or C-section delivery.

- Pulmonary edema is fluid accumulation within the lungs that can be due to many causes, including left-sided heart failure, mitral valve stenosis, fluid overload, nephrotic syndrome, liver disease, infections, drugs, shock, and radiation. Most pulmonary emboli arise from deep vein thrombosis in the leg and may be asymptomatic, cause pulmonary infarction, or cause sudden death.

- Pulmonary hypertension is increased pulmonary artery pressure, usually due to increased vascular resistance or blood flow. Pulmonary hypertension can be primary (idiopathic) or related to underlying COPD, interstitial disease, pulmonary emboli, mitral stenosis, left heart failure, and congenital heart disease with left to right shunt.

- Lung cancer is the leading cause of cancer deaths among both men and women. Major risk factors are cigarette smoking, occupational exposures, air pollution, and "scarring." Histologic types include adenocarcinoma, squamous cell carcinoma, small cell carcinoma, and large cell carcinoma.

- Pleural effusion is the accumulation of fluid in the pleural cavity. Pneumothorax is air in the pleural cavity.

- Mesotheliomas are rare, highly malignant neoplasms that can involve the pleura and are closely related to prior asbestos exposure.

- Pneumoconiosis is a fibrosing pulmonary disease caused by inhalation of an aerosol, such as mineral dust, particles, vapors, or fumes.

- Coal worker's pneumoconiosis (black lung disease) can range in severity from slight pulmonary dysfunction to progressive massive fibrosis leading to increasing respiratory distress and cor pulmonale. Caplan syndrome is the term used for the combination of pneumoconiosis (due to many different agents) and rheumatoid arthritis.

- Asbestosis can cause pulmonary fibrosis, bronchogenic carcinoma, and malignant mesotheliomas. Silicosis can cause pulmonary fibrosis and an increased risk of TB. Berylliosis can cause an acute pneumonitis or granulomatous disease with fibrosis of the lungs.

Learning Objectives

- ❏ Demonstrate understanding of congenital anomalies of the kidney
- ❏ Use knowledge of cystic disease to solve problems
- ❏ Answer questions about nephritic/nephrotic syndrome, secondary/chronic glomerulonephritis, tubulointerstitial nephritis, and acute tubular injury
- ❏ Describe epidemiology and course of urolithiasis
- ❏ Solve problems concerning chronic renal failure
- ❏ Solve problems concerning tumors of the kidney
- ❏ Explain information related to ureteral disorders
- ❏ Explain information related to urinary bladder pathology

CONGENITAL ANOMALIES OF THE KIDNEY

Renal agenesis

- **Bilateral agenesis** is incompatible with life. Ultrasound shows oligohydramnios.
- Affected fetuses typically also have Potter facies (flattened nose, posteriorly rotated ears, and recessed chin); talipes equinovarus (talus [ankle]+ pes [foot] and equino [heel] + varus [turned upward] = clubfoot); and pulmonary hypoplasia.
- In **unilateral agenesis**, the remaining kidney undergoes compensatory hypertrophy. Patients often have adequate renal function and are asymptomatic.

Hypoplasia is failure of a kidney (usually unilateral) to develop to normal weight; the hypoplastic kidney has a decreased number of calyces and lobes.

Horseshoe kidney is a common congenital anomaly that is found in 1 in 600 abdominal x-rays. The kidneys show fusion, usually at the lower pole; affected individuals have normal renal function but may be predisposed to renal calculi.

Abnormal locations. The most common abnormal location is a pelvic kidney. The ectopic kidney usually has normal function. Tortuosity of ureters may predispose to pyelonephritis.

In a Nutshell
Oligohydramnios (Potter) Sequence
Renal agenesis
↓
Oligohydramnios
↓
Fetal compression
↓
Flattened facies and positional abnormalities of hands and feet

CYSTIC DISEASE

Autosomal recessive polycystic kidney disease (also called infantile polycystic kidney disease or renal dysgenesis Potter type I) is a rare autosomal recessive disease that presents in infancy with progressive and often fatal renal failure. A mutation in the *PKHD1* gene is implicated.

The kidneys are bilaterally enlarged and have a spongelike cut surface. The liver may have multiple hepatic cysts and cirrhosis may develop in childhood. Pulmonary hypoplasia is present to varying degrees.

Autosomal dominant polycystic kidney disease (also called adult polycystic kidney disease or renal dysgenesis Potter type III) is an autosomal dominant disease that affects 1 in 1,000. There is most frequently a mutation of the *PKD1* gene on chromosome 16 which produces a transmembrane protein called polycystin 1. Other mutations involve *PKD2* and polycystin 2.

Clinically, patients are asymptomatic with normal renal function until middle age, and then present with renal insufficiency, renal stones, hematuria, and hypertension or with abdominal masses and flank pain. Diagnosis is established with U/S and CT scan. Most patients develop end-stage renal failure by decade 7.

On gross pathologic examination, the kidneys have massive bilateral enlargement with large bulging cysts filled with serous, turbid, or hemorrhagic fluid. Microscopic examination shows functioning nephrons present between the cysts; the cysts arise from the tubular epithelial cells of the kidney.

Extrarenal manifestations include cysts of the liver, pancreas, and lungs; berry aneurysms of the circle of Willis; mitral valve prolapse; and colonic diverticula.

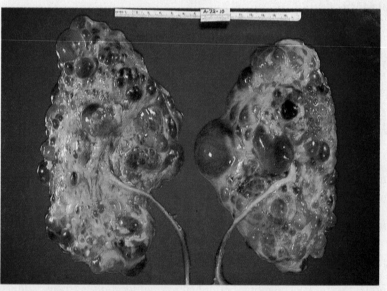

© cdc.gov.

Figure 15-1. Gross Pathology of Polycystic Kidneys

Renal dysplasia is the most common renal cystic disease in children, in whom it causes an enlarged renal mass with cartilage and immature collecting ducts. It may progress clinically to renal failure.

Acquired polycystic disease is seen in renal dialysis patients and is associated with a small risk of developing renal adenomas and renal cell carcinoma.

Simple retention cysts of the kidney are common in adults and occasionally cause hematuria.

Medullary diseases with cysts

- Medullary sponge kidney can cause nephrolithiasis but is otherwise innocuous.

- Nephronophthisis-medullary cystic disease complex presents as polyuria and polydipsia; it can progress to chronic renal failure in young adults. There are autosomal recessive forms. The cysts are in the cortex and the medulla.

GLOMERULAR DISEASES

Immune mechanisms play a role in the pathogenesis of most glomerular diseases, either via deposition of immune complexes or injury from antibodies. Glomerular diseases may be divided into those originating in the kidney and those caused by systemic disease (secondary).

Glomerular disease may present clinically as **nephrotic** or **nephritic syndrome**. Their clinical features are different.

Table 15-1. Clinical Syndromes in Glomerular Disease

Nephritic Syndrome	Nephrotic Syndrome
Hematuria (RBC casts)	Severe proteinuria (>3.5 g/day)
Hypertension	Hypoalbuminemia (<3 g/dL)
Azotemia	Generalized edema
Oliguria	Hyperlipidemia
Proteinuria (<3.5 g/day)	Lipiduria

Renal biopsy can yield a definitive diagnosis when light microscopy features are considered in concert with immunofluoresence (IF) and electron microscopy (EM).

Clinical Correlate

The cysts in autosomal dominant (adult) PKD involve <10% of nephrons, but they gradually expand and compress the rest of the kidney, interfering with its function. This is why kidney function can remain normal for many years.

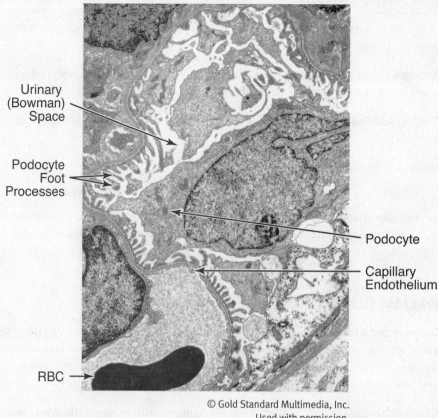

Urinary (Bowman) Space

Podocyte Foot Processes

Podocyte

Capillary Endothelium

RBC

© Gold Standard Multimedia, Inc.
Used with permission.

Figure 15-2. Transmission Electron Micrograph Demonstrating Podocytes

PRIMARY GLOMERULOPATHIES (NEPHRITIC SYNDROME)

Acute poststreptococcal glomerulonephritis (APSGN) (or acute proliferative glomerulonephritis or postinfectious glomerulonephritis) is an immune complex disease that typically occurs 2–4 weeks after a streptococcal infection of the throat or skin. There is a decreasing incidence in the United States; children are affected more often than adults.

The infecting organism is most commonly β-hemolytic group A *streptococci*, but APSGN can also be caused by other bacteria, viruses, parasites, and even systemic diseases (SLE and polyarteritis nodosa). Clinically, it presents with nephritic syndrome with elevated antistreptolysin O (ASO) titers (when related to streptococcal infection) and low C3.

Renal biopsy. Light microscopy shows an infiltrate of neutrophils in the glomeruli; the process is diffuse, that is, it involves all the glomeruli. Immunofluorescence shows granular deposits of IgG and C3 throughout the glomerulus within the capillary walls and some mesangial areas. Electron microscopy shows subepithelial immune complex deposits (humps).

Treatment is conservative fluid management. Most children (>95%) have a good prognosis, with complete recovery, but severe disease can also occur (RPGN 1% and chronic glomerulonephritis 2%). In adults, 15-50% develop end-stage disease.

Clinical Correlate

The classic presentation of APSGN is a young child with fever, malaise, periorbital edema, hypertension, smoky urine, and oliguria, beginning approximately 2 weeks after a streptococcal infection.

Note

The characteristic finding in RPGN is the formation of crescents within Bowman space. The crescents are composed of fibrin, parietal epithelial cells, monocytes, and macrophages.

Rapidly progressive glomerulonephritis (RPGN) (crescentic glomerulonephritis) is group of diseases characterized by glomerular crescents and a rapid deterioration of renal function.

- **Anti-glomerular basement membrane antibody-mediated crescentic glomerulonephritis** has a peak incidence at age 20-40, and males are affected more frequently than females.

Pulmonary involvement is called **Goodpasture syndrome**. These patients have pulmonary hemorrhage and hemoptysis.

Renal biopsy findings include hypercellularity, crescents, and fibrin deposition in glomeruli. Immunofluorescence shows a smooth and linear pattern of IgG and C3 in the glomerular basement membrane (GBM). By electron microscopy, there are no deposits, but there is glomerular basement membrane disruption.

Even with treatment (plasma exchange, steroids, and cytotoxic drugs), the prognosis is poor because of risks of severe and life-threatening pulmonary hemorrhage and renal failure. Early aggressive treatment may prevent end-stage renal failure.

Immune-complex mediated crescentic glomerulonephritis

- Any of the immune complex nephrites can cause crescent formation.
- IF shows a granular pattern and EM shows discrete deposits.

Pauci-immune crescentic glomerulonephritis

- Antineutrophilic cytoplasmic antibodies (ANCA) are present in serum.
- IF and EM are negative for immunoglobulins and complement components.

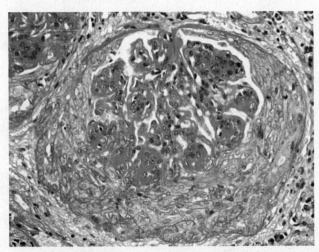

© Katsumi M. Miyai, M.D., Ph.D.; Regents of the University of California. Used with permission.

Figure 15-3. Crescent Formation in Rapidly Progressive Glomerulonephritis, as Seen with Trichrome Stain

IgA nephropathy (Berger disease) is the most common cause of glomerulonephritis in the world, being particularly common in France, Japan, Italy, and Austria. It affects children and young adults (mostly males).

IgA nephropathy is characterized by recurrent gross hematuria (a predominately nephritic presentation), whose onset may follow a respiratory infection. IgA nephropathy can be associated with celiac sprue and Henoch-Schönlein purpura or can be secondary to celiac sprue or liver disease.

The pathogenesis is unknown, but may be related to a possible entrapment of circulating immune complexes with activation of the alternate complement pathway; it may also be related to a genetic predisposition.

Renal biopsy. Light microscopy may show normal glomeruli or mesangial proliferation. Immunofluorescence shows mesangial deposits of IgA and C3. Electron microscopy shows mesangial immune complex deposits.

Many cases slowly progress to renal failure over 25 years.

Membranoproliferative glomerulonephritis (MPGN) is a form of glomerular disease that affects both the glomerular mesangium and the basement membranes; it occurs in 2 types, Type I and Type II (dense deposit disease).

The clinical presentation is variable, and may be nephritic, nephrotic, or mixed. MPGN may be secondary to many systemic disorders (systemic lupus erythematosus, endocarditis), chronic infections (HBV, HCV, HIV), and malignancies (chronic lymphocytic leukemia).

Laboratory studies show decreased serum C3 and the presence of C3 nephritic factor (MPGN type II).

Light microscopy demonstrates a lobulated appearance of the glomeruli due to mesangial and endothelial cell proliferation and/or deposition of subendothelial immune complex deposits. Splitting of the basement membrane ("tram-tracking") may be seen with a silver or periodic acid-Schiff (PAS) stain.

Immunofluorescence in type I MPGN shows a granular pattern of C3 often with IgG, C1q, and C4; in type II, immunofluorescence shows a granular and linear pattern of C3 deposition.

Electron microscopy in type I shows subendothelial and mesangial immune complex deposits, and in type II shows dense deposits within the glomerular basement membrane.

MPGN typically has a slowly progressive course, resulting in chronic renal failure over the course of 10 years. There is a high incidence of recurrence in transplants.

Alport syndrome is a rare X-linked disorder caused by a defect in type IV collagen. It is characterized by hereditary nephritis, hearing loss, and ocular abnormalities. The most common mutation causing Alport is in the *COL4A5* gene coding for the alpha-3, -4, and -5 chain of type IV collagen.

Gross or microscopic hematuria begins in childhood. Hearing loss (leading to sensorineural deafness) and various ocular abnormalities of the lens and cornea can occur. Alport is a progressive disease that ultimately results in renal failure.

Electron microscopy shows alternating thickening and thinning of basement membrane with splitting of the lamina densa, causing a "basketweave" appearance.

PRIMARY GLOMERULOPATHIES (NEPHROTIC)

Membranous glomerulonephritis is a common cause of nephrotic syndrome in adults that is mediated by immune complexes.

Most cases (85%) are idiopathic; in most of these cases, autoantibodies cross-react with podocyte antigens. Membranous glomerulonephritis may also be caused by drugs (penicillamine), infections (hepatitis virus B and C, syphilis, etc.), and systemic diseases (SLE, diabetes mellitus, etc.). It has also been associated with malignant carcinomas of the lung and colon, and there may be a genetic predisposition.

Renal biopsy shows diffuse thickening of the capillary walls. Basement membrane projections ("spikes") are seen on silver stains. Immunofluorescence shows a granular and linear pattern of IgG and C3. Electron microscopy shows subepithelial deposits along the basement membranes with effacement of podocyte foot processes.

The clinical course is variable and may lead to spontaneous remission, persistent proteinuria, or end-stage renal disease.

Minimal change disease (also called lipoid nephrosis and nil disease) is the most common cause of nephrotic syndrome in children. Peak incidence is age 2–6.

The diagnosis is one of exclusion. Light microscopy shows normal glomeruli with lipid accumulation in proximal tubule cells (lipoid nephrosis). Immunofluorescence is negative, with no immune deposits. Electron microscopy shows effacement of epithelial (podocyte) foot processes, microvillous transformation, and no immune complex deposits.

The prognosis is excellent because treatment with corticosteroids produces a dramatic response in children. The majority have a complete recovery.

Focal segmental glomerulosclerosis is a very common cause of nephrotic syndrome that occurs in all ages. African Americans are affected more frequently than Caucasians.

The condition may be idiopathic (primary), or it may be related to a wide variety of predisposing conditions including loss of renal tissue; preexisting glomerular diseases (such as IgA nephropathy); sickle cell anemia; heroin use; AIDS; or morbid obesity. Inherited and congenital forms occur.

Renal biopsy. Light microscopy shows focal segmental sclerosis and hyalinization of glomeruli; focal segmental glomerulosclerosis initially affects the glomeruli along the medullary border. Immunofluorescence shows IgM and C3 deposits in the sclerotic segments. Electron microscopy shows effacement of foot processes in nonsclerotic regions and increased mesangial matrix in sclerotic segments.

Clinical course. There is frequently a poor response to steroids, with the overall prognosis being poor (most progressing to chronic renal failure), though children do better than adults. There is a high rate of recurrence in renal transplants. A variant form, collapsing glomerulopathy, has a worse prognosis.

Note

Focal: only some of the glomeruli are affected

Segmental: only a portion of the glomerular tuft exhibits sclerosis

SECONDARY GLOMERULONEPHRITIS

Secondary glomerulonephritis is glomerular disease that is secondary to other disease processes.

Diabetes causes nodular glomerulosclerosis, hyaline arteriolosclerosis, and diabetic microangiopathy. Clinically, diabetic patients may develop microalbuminuria that can progress to nephrotic syndrome.

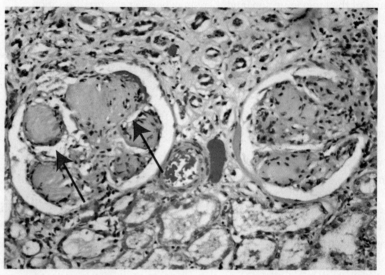

© cdc.gov.

Figure 15-4. Sclerotic Nodules (arrows) of Nodular Glomerulosclerosis (Kimmelstiel-Wilson Syndrome) Associated with Diabetes

Systemic lupus erythematosus can cause various patterns of damage to the kidney with clinical features that can include hematuria, nephritic syndrome, nephrotic syndrome, hypertension, and renal failure.

CHRONIC GLOMERULONEPHRITIS

End-stage renal disease is the final stage of many forms of glomerular disease. It is characterized by progressive renal failure, uremia, and ultimately death.

Clinical features include anemia, anorexia, malaise, proteinuria, hypertension, and azotemia. Urinalysis shows broad, waxy casts. On pathologic examination, the kidneys are grossly small and shrunken; microscopic exam shows hyalinization of glomeruli, interstitial fibrosis, atrophy of tubules, and a lymphocytic infiltrate.

Treatment is dialysis and renal transplantation.

TUBULOINTERSTITIAL NEPHRITIS

Tubulointerstitial nephritis is an acute or chronic inflammation of tubules and interstitium. It can be due to many causes, including medications, infections, acute pyelonephritis, systemic lupus erythematosus, lead poisoning, urate nephropathy, or multiple myeloma.

- **Acute pyelonephritis** refers to bacterial infections involving the renal pelvis, tubules, and interstitium. Pyelonephritis affects females much more than males, but the incidence increases in older males with prostatic hyperplasia.

  Ascending infection is the most common route of infection. Causative organisms include gram-negative enteric bacilli, *Escherichia coli*, *Proteus*, *Klebsiella*, and *Enterobacter*. Predisposing factors include urinary obstruction, vesicoureteral reflux, pregnancy, urethral instrumentation, diabetes mellitus, benign prostatic hyperplasia, and other renal pathology. Symptoms can include fever, chills, and malaise; dysuria, frequency, and urgency; and costovertebral angle tenderness. Urinalysis shows pyuria and white blood cell casts.

  The kidney may be enlarged, and the cortical surface may show abscesses. Microscopically there is a neutrophilic insterstitial infiltrate. **Parenchymal abscesses** may be present. The tubules contain neutrophil casts.

- **Chronic pyelonephritis** can occur from chronic obstruction or in the setting of vesicoureteral reflux. Scarring can be seen at the upper and lower poles of the kidney, with associated calyceal blunting. Microscopically there is interstitial fibrosis and inflammation with thyroidization of the tubule. Some patients develop glomerulosclerosis. Renal insufficiency develops gradually.

- **Drug-induced tubular interstitial nephritis** is commonly caused by penicillins, other antibiotics, diuretics, and NSAIDs. Interstitial inflammation is characteristic and granulomas may be seen. This hypersensitivity reaction presents a couple of weeks after drug exposure with fever, eosinophilia, rash, and hematuria. Minimal proteinuria may be present. Recovery is expected after withdrawal of the drug.

- **Urate nephropathy** is caused by a deposition of urate crystals (secondary to leukemia treatment, lead poisoning, and gout) in renal tubules and interstitium. It may produce acute renal failure.

ACUTE TUBULAR INJURY

Acute tubular injury (ATI) is acute renal failure associated with potentially reversible injury to the tubular epithelium. It is the most common cause of acute renal failure in the United States. It is characterized by oliguria with elevation of blood urea nitrogen (BUN) and creatinine; metabolic acidosis and hyperkalemia; and dirty brown granular casts and epithelial casts on urinalysis.

- **Ischemic acute tubular necrosis** is the most common cause of ATI. The condition is due to decreased blood flow caused by severe hemorrhage, severe renal vasoconstriction, hypotension, dehydration, or shock.

- **Nephrotoxic ATN** has a large number of causes, including drugs (e.g., polymyxin, methicillin, gentamicin, sulfonamides); radiographic contrast agents; heavy metals (e.g., mercury, lead, gold); organic solvents (e.g., carbon tetrachloride, chloroform, methyl alcohol); ethylene glycol (antifreeze); mushroom poisoning; phenol; pesticides; and myoglobin.

The **prognosis** is excellent if the patient survives the underlying disease, and if the patient had no preexisting kidney disease.

Clinical Correlate

It may be difficult to distinguish cystitis from pyelonephritis. The presence of fever, costovertebral angle tenderness, and WBC casts in the urine are helpful clues to the diagnosis of pyelonephritis.

UROLITHIASIS

Renal calculi occur in up to 6% of the population; men are affected more often than women.

- **Stone composition.** Most (75%) stones are calcium oxalate stones. Magnesium ammonium phosphate ("struvite") stones are associated with infection by urea-splitting bacteria (proteus), and these stones often form large staghorn calculi. Uric acid stones are seen in gout, leukemia, and in patients with acidic urine. Cystine stones are uncommon.

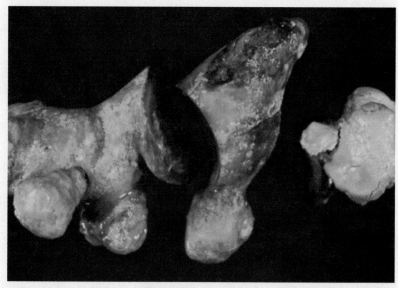

© Katsumi M. Miyai, M.D., Ph.D.; Regents of the University of California. Used with permission.

Figure 15-5. Struvite (Magnesium Ammonium Phosphate) Stone Forming Staghorn Calculi

- **Pathology.** Most stones are unilateral stones that are formed in the calyx, pelvis, and urinary bladder.

- **Clinical features.** Calcium stones are radiopaque and can be seen on x-ray. Renal colic may occur if small stones pass into the ureters. Stones may cause hematuria, urinary obstruction, and predispose to infection.

- **Treatment of stones** is with lithotripsy or endoscopic removal.

CHRONIC RENAL FAILURE

Chronic renal failure is the end stage of many different renal diseases. It is characterized pathologically by bilaterally shrunken kidneys. Clinically, it causes progressive irreversible azotemia, normocytic anemia, platelet dysfunction, renal osteodystrophy, and hypertension.

VASCULAR DISORDERS OF THE KIDNEY

Renal artery stenosis of any etiology causes decreased blood flow to the involved kidney, with resulting secondary hypertension that is often not responsive to antihypertensive medications. Treatment is usually surgical.

- Atheromatous plaque is the most common cause of renal artery stenosis.

- Dysplastic lesions ("fibromuscular dysplasia") are an important additional cause of renal artery stenosis.

  All 3 lesion types occur in middle-aged adults.

  - Medial fibroplasia with aneurysms (most common) causes alternating stenosis and aneurysms in "string of beads" pattern on arteriography

  - Perimedial fibroplasia involves the outer media

  - Medial hyperplasia

- Miscellaneous diseases that can affect the renal arteries (with or without stenosis) include congenital anomalies, Takayasu arteritis, and radiation injuries.

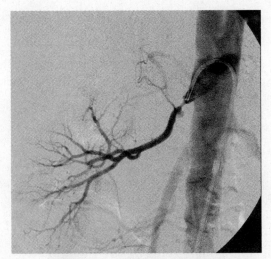

© Lily Chu, National Naval Medical Center Bethesda.
Used with permission.

Figure 15-6. Renal Artery Stenosis as Demonstrated by Angiogram

Benign nephrosclerosis is caused by hypertension. The kidneys have a finely granular external surface and on microscopy show hyaline arteriolosclerosis, tubular atrophy, interstitial fibrosis, and glomerulosclerosis. Lab findings include mild proteinuria, hematuria, and azotemia.

Malignant (accelerated) hypertension can damage the kidney, causing fibrinoid necrosis of arterioles, glomerulitis, and hyperplastic arteriolosclerosis. Clinically, it causes cerebral edema, papilledema, retinal hemorrhage, intracerebral hemorrhage, and oliguric acute renal failure. The cortical surface shows pinpoint petechial hemorrhages ("flea-bitten" look).

Renal infarction is due to thrombi from the left side of the heart, atheroembolic disease, and vasculitis. It presents with sudden onset of flank pain and hematuria. Small infarcts may be asymptomatic.

Sickle cell anemia can cause medullary infarctions due to blockage of blood flow in the medullary vessels, which can result in asymptomatic hematuria, loss of urine concentrating ability, renal papillary necrosis, and pyelonephritis.

Diffuse cortical necrosis can cause anuria; the condition can occur with obstetric emergencies and disseminated intravascular coagulation.

TUMORS OF THE KIDNEY

Benign tumors of the kidney are as follows:

- **Cortical adenomas** are small, encapsulated cortical nodules measuring <3 cm; they are a common finding at autopsy. They may be composed of tubular or papillary structures. The papillary adenomas share the same chromosomal gains as papillary renal cell carcinoma.

- **Angiomyolipomas** are hamartomas composed of fat, smooth muscle, and blood vessels, common in patients with tuberous sclerosis.

- **Oncocytomas** are large, benign tumors that are resected to rule out renal cell carcinoma when they are found incidentally on imaging studies. They are brown on cut surface and have abundant pink cytoplasm on microscopy.

Renal cell carcinoma (RCC) is most common age 50–70, with males affected more than females.

Risk factors include cigarette smoking, chronic analgesic use, asbestos exposure, chronic renal failure, acquired cystic disease, and von Hippel-Lindau disease (VHL tumor suppressor gene).

In 10% of cases, the "classic" triad occurs:

- Hematuria
- Palpable mass
- Flank pain

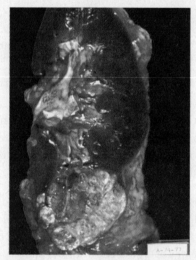

© Katsumi M. Miyai, M.D., Ph.D.; Regents of the University of California. Used with permission.

Figure 15-7. Renal Cell Carcinoma

A variety of paraneoplastic syndromes from ectopic hormone production can occur:

- Polycythemia (erythropoietin production)
- Hypertension (renin production)
- Cushing syndrome (corticosteroid synthesis)
- Hypercalcemia (PTH-like hormone)
- Feminization or masculinization (gonadotropin release)

Renal cell carcinoma may also cause secondary amyloidosis, a leukemoid reaction, or eosinophilia.

There is a high incidence of metastasis on initial presentation. The clinical course is unpredictable.

Gross examination typically demonstrates a large, solitary yellow mass found most commonly in the upper pole. Areas of necrosis and hemorrhage are commonly present. The tumor often invades the renal vein and may extend into the inferior vena cava and heart.

Histologic types of RCC are as follows:

- **Clear cell RCC (most common)**
  - Often invades renal venous system
  - May have loss of genetic material in 3p
  - A small percent occur in association with von Hippel-Lindau disease
  - Microscopically, there is an alveolar growth pattern with microcysts
  - Tumor is resistant to chemotherapy and radiotherapy

- **Papillary RCC**
  - Tends to be bilateral and multifocal
  - Cut surface is granular
  - Microscopically, the papillae have a single layer of cells
  - Gains of chromosome 7 and 17 are common
  - Duplications of chromosome 7 increase dosage of protooncogene *MET*

- **Chromophobe RCC (rare)**
  - Have cells that stain more darkly than clear cell RCC
  - Have loss of multiple chromosomes
  - Least aggressive of the RCCs

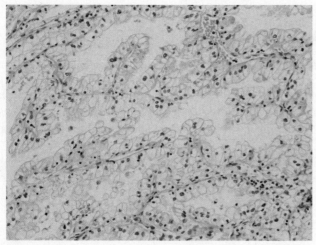

© Gregg Barré, M.D.
Used with permission.

Figure 15-8. Renal Cell Carcinoma

Wilms tumor (nephroblastoma) typically presents age 2-5 as a large abdominal mass. Patients with WAGR, DDS, or BWS syndrome are at increased risk of Wilms tumor.

- WAGR syndrome is the cluster of Wilms tumor, aniridia, genital anomalies, and mental retardation.
- Beckwith-Wiedemann syndrome (BWS) is an overgrowth disorder with characteristic features and an attendant increased risk of cancer.
- Denys-Drash syndrome (DDS) affects the genitalia and kidneys.

Both WAGR and DDS are associated with deletions and mutations, respectively, of the *WT1* gene. BWS arises through imprinting abnormalities at the *WT2* locus.

Pathologically, Wilms tumor causes a large, solitary tan mass. Microscopic examination reveals a tumor containing 3 elements: metanephric blastema, epithelial elements (immature glomeruli and tubules), and stroma.

Treatment is surgery, chemotherapy, and radiation, which as a combined therapy yields an excellent prognosis. Long-term survival rate is 90%.

Transitional cell carcinomas can involve the renal pelvis as well as the urinary bladder.

OBSTRUCTIVE DISORDERS OF THE URINARY SYSTEM

Hydronephrosis is a common complication of urinary tract obstruction. It is characterized by dilation of the ureter and renal pelvis. Specific causes include renal stones, retroperitoneal fibrosis, benign prostatic hyperplasia, and cervical cancer.

- In **unilateral hydronephrosis**, the kidney may enlarge to 20 cm. It may be found incidentally on physical exam. The parenchyma becomes compressed. If complete obstruction occurs suddenly, **necrosis of the renal papillae** may result.
- **Bilateral obstruction** that is complete presents as anuria; incomplete bilateral obstruction may present as polyuria.

URETERAL DISORDERS

Congenital anomalies include double ureters and congenital megaureter.

Ureteropelvic junction (UPJ) obstruction is the most common cause of hydronephrosis in infants and children. **Congenital UPJ obstruction** can also be identified in adults. It is often seen with other congenital anomalies. Treatment is surgical.

Ureteritis cystica describes chronic inflammation which causes formation of small mucosal cysts in the ureter. This condition can predispose for adenocarcinoma of the ureter.

Renal stones commonly lodge in the ureters.

Retroperitoneal fibrosis is usually an idiopathic condition causing severe fibrosis of the retroperitoneal area, which can entrap the ureters. Some cases show sclerosing conditions in other body sites and are associated with elevated serum IgG4.

Transitional cell carcinoma is the most common ureteral carcinoma.

URINARY BLADDER PATHOLOGY

Congenital anomalies of the bladder. Exstrophy of the bladder is a developmental failure of the formation of the abdominal wall and bladder which leaves the bladder open at the body surface. Urachal cyst remnants may permit drainage of urine from a newborn's umbilicus, and may also be a cause of bladder adenocarcinoma.

Cystitis. The etiology of cystitis varies, with important causes including organisms, notably from fecal flora (*Escherichia coli, Proteus, Klebsiella, Enterobacter*); radiation cystitis (may follow radiation therapy); and chemotherapy agents such as cyclophosphamide (hemorrhagic cystitis).

Clinically, it affects females far more than males. Symptoms include frequency, urgency, dysuria, and suprapubic pain; systemic signs such as fever and malaise are uncommon. Predisposing factors include benign prostatic hypertrophy, bladder calculi, and cystocele.

Malakoplakia is a bladder inflammatory pattern associated with a defect in macrophage function. The cause is unknown. Macrophages contain **Michaelis-Gutmann bodies**, laminated basophilic structures.

Urinary bladder tumors are most commonly due to transitional cell carcinoma. There is an increasing incidence of urinary bladder tumors; males are affected more than females, and peak incidence is age 40-60. Risk factors include:

- Cigarette smoking and occupational exposure to azo dye production (transitional cell carcinoma) (both due to 2-naphthylamine)

- Chronic bladder infection with *Schistosoma haemotobium* (squamous cell carcinoma) (Africa including Egypt and the Middle East)

Bladder cancer usually presents with painless hematuria, but it may also cause dysuria, urgency, frequency, hydronephrosis, and pyelonephritis.

Prognosis of bladder cancer depends on the tumor grade and stage. There is a high incidence of recurrence.

Precursors of invasive transitional cell carcinoma can arise from a flat or papillary lesion.

- **Carcinoma in situ (CIS)** is a high-grade lesion with cytologic atypia in the full thickness of the epithelium. It is frequently multifocal. In 50-75% of untreated cases, it progresses to invasive cancer.

- Papillary precursors to invasive carcinoma include **papilloma ⇒ papillary urothelial neoplasia of low malignant potential ⇒ low-grade urothelial carcinoma ⇒ high-grade urothelial carcinoma.**

Other bladder tumors include papillomas, adenocarcinoma, and embryonal rhabdomyosarcoma.

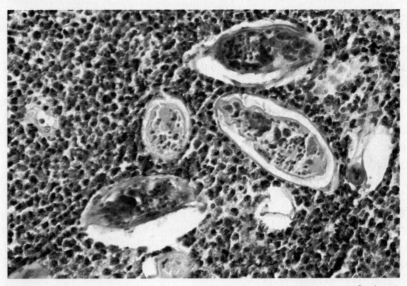

© cdc.gov.

Figure 15-9. Migratory Eggs of *Schistosoma haemotobium* Surrounded by Dense Inflammation in the Bladder Wall

Miscellaneous bladder conditions

- **Acquired diverticuli** can complicate urinary tract outlet obstruction due to benign prostatic hyperplasia or other causes.

- **Cystocele** is the term used for prolapse of the bladder into the vagina. It is common in middle-aged to elderly women.

- **Cystitis cystica et glandularis** causes formation of small cysts and glands in the bladder mucosa related to chronic inflammation. It is associated with an increased risk of adenocarcinoma.

Chapter Summary

- Renal agenesis is the failure of one or both kidneys to develop. Bilateral renal agenesis is incompatible with life, but persons with unilateral agenesis may have adequate renal function. Other congenital anomalies of the kidney include hypoplasia, horseshoe kidney, and abnormal locations.

- Autosomal recessive polycystic kidney disease presents in infancy with progressive renal failure. Autosomal dominant polycystic kidney disease presents in adulthood with renal insufficiency, hematuria, and hypertension. The kidneys may be massively enlarged by the time of diagnosis. Renal dysplasia is the most common renal cystic disease in children and may cause a renal mass and renal failure. Nephronophthisis-medullary cystic disease complex may progress to renal failure, but medullary sponge kidney is generally innocuous. Acquired polycystic disease is seen in renal dialysis patients. Simple retention cysts are common in adult kidneys.

- Glomerular diseases can present with either nephritic syndrome or nephrotic syndrome. Nephritic syndrome is characterized by hematuria, hypertension, azotemia, oliguria, and proteinuria <3.5 g/day. Nephrotic syndrome is characterized by severe proteinuria >3.5 g/day, hypoalbuminemia, generalized edema, hyperlipidemia, and lipiduria.

- Acute post-streptococcal glomerulonephritis is associated with subepithelial immune complex deposits (subepithelial humps) by electron microscopy, occurs 2–4 weeks after a streptococcal infection of the throat or skin, and usually causes nephritic syndrome in children.

- Anti-glomerular basement membrane antibody-mediated crescentic glomerulo-nephritis is characterized by a smooth and linear pattern of IgG and C3 by immunofluorescence. It is the result of damage by autoantibodies to the basement membrane. Lung involvement is called Goodpasture syndrome.

- Rapidly progressive glomerulonephritis is characterized microscopically by hypercellular glomeruli with crescent formation in Bowman space. Clinically, it is not a specific entity.

- IgA nephropathy is characterized by mesangial deposits of IgA and C3, is the most common cause of glomerulonephritis worldwide, and tends to produce recurrent gross hematuria in children and young adults.

- Membranoproliferative glomerulonephritis is characterized microscopically by mesangial proliferation and basement membrane splitting and clinically may produce a nephritic pattern, a nephrotic pattern, or a mixed pattern.

- Membranous glomerulonephritis is characterized by diffuse thickening of capillary walls and basement membrane projections (spikes) visible with silver stains and is a common cause of nephrotic syndrome in adults.

- Minimal change disease is characterized by effacement of epithelial (podocyte) foot processes visible with electron microscopy and is the most common cause of nephrotic syndrome in children.

- Focal segmental glomerulosclerosis is characterized by focal segmental sclerosis and hyalinization of glomeruli and is a cause of nephrotic syndrome that can occur idiopathically or secondary to other glomerular diseases, sickle cell anemia, heroin use, AIDS, and morbid obesity.

(continued)

Chapter Summary (cont'd)

- Secondary glomerulonephritis can be caused by DM and systemic lupus erythematosus.

- Chronic glomerulonephritis with small, shrunken kidneys is the final stage of many forms of glomerular diseases and is characterized by progressive renal failure, uremia, and ultimately death.

- Acute tubular injury is acute renal failure associated with reversible injury to the tubular epithelium and can be due to ischemia or nephrotoxins.

- Acute pyelonephritis is a bacterial infection involving the renal pelvis, tubules, and interstitium and is most commonly due to *E. coli*, *Proteus*, *Klebsiella*, or *Enterobacter*.

- Renal calculi are common and may be composed of calcium oxalate, struvite, uric acid, or cystine. Clinically, stones may cause renal colic, hematuria, urinary obstruction, and a predisposition for infection.

- Benign tumors of the kidney include cortical adenomas and angiomyolipomas. Renal cell carcinoma tends to produce a large solitary renal mass in middle-aged to older adults and may cause hematuria, palpable mass, flank pain, and paraneoplastic syndromes.

- Wilms tumor is a childhood malignancy that presents with a large abdominal mass. It now has an excellent long-term prognosis.

- Vascular diseases of the kidney include renal artery stenosis, benign nephrosclerosis, hyperplastic arteriolosclerosis, renal infarction, and diffuse cortical necrosis.

- Ureteral disorders include congenital anomalies, ureteritis cystica, stones lodged in a ureter, retroperitoneal fibrosis, and transitional cell carcinoma.

- Cystitis, or urinary bladder inflammation, can be due to bacterial infection, radiation, or chemotherapy.

- Transitional cell carcinoma is the most common type of bladder tumor and usually presents with painless hematuria. Other bladder tumors include papillomas, adenocarcinoma, and embryonal rhabdomyosarcoma.

- Congenital anomalies of the bladder include exstrophy and urachal cyst remnants.

- Other bladder conditions include acquired diverticuli, cystocele, and cystitis cystica et glandularis.

Gastrointestinal Tract Pathology 16

Learning Objectives

❑ Answer questions about esophagus, stomach, small and large intestines

❑ Solve problems concerning gastric lymphoma

ESOPHAGUS

Congenital and Mechanical Disorders

Tracheoesophageal fistula may arise as a congenital connection between the esophagus and trachea that is often associated with esophageal atresia. It is often discovered soon after birth because of aspiration. In adults the condition can occur secondary to malignancy, trauma, or iatrogenic causes.

Esophageal webs are web-like protrusions of the esophageal mucosa into the lumen which typically present with dysphagia. Plummer-Vinson syndrome is a disease of middle-aged women characterized by esophageal webs, iron deficiency anemia, and increased risk of carcinoma. Schatzki rings are web-like narrowings at the gastroesophageal junction.

Achalasia is a failure of the lower esophageal sphincter (LES) to relax with swallowing. The etiology is unknown in most cases; in South America, achalasia may be caused by Chagas disease. Presentation is with progressive dysphagia. The esophagus is characteristically dilated proximal to the lower esophageal sphincter; barium swallow shows a "bird-beak" sign. Microscopically, there is a loss of ganglion cells in the myenteric plexus. Treatment is LES balloon dilation or myotomy. Achalasia carries an increased risk for esophageal carcinoma.

Hematemesis and Esophageal Bleeding

Mallory-Weiss syndrome is esophageal bleeding due to linear lacerations at the gastroesophageal junction from severe prolonged vomiting; the most common cause is acute alcohol ingestion and/or chronic alcoholism. Esophageal rupture (Boerhaave syndrome) may result.

Esophageal varices are dilated submucosal veins in the lower third of the esophagus, usually secondary to portal hypertension. The most common cause is cirrhosis. Clinically, the presentation is asymptomatic, though there is massive hematemesis when the varices are ruptured. Complications include potentially fatal hemorrhage. Treatment is generally band ligation, sclerotherapy, or balloon tamponade.

Clinical Correlate

The most common type of tracheoesophageal fistula:

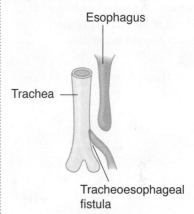

Clinical Correlate

Chagas disease, a tropical parasitic disease common in South America, is caused by *Trypanosoma cruzi*. It is transmitted by reduviid or "kissing" bugs. Chagas disease can cause:

- Romaña's sign (unilateral swelling of the eyelid)
- Cardiomyopathy
- Megaesophagus and megacolon

Esophagitis

Gastroesophageal reflux disease (reflux esophagitis) (GERD) is esophageal irritation and inflammation due to reflux of gastric secretions into the esophagus. Reflux typically presents with heartburn and regurgitation. Complications include bleeding, stricture, bronchospasm and asthma, and Barrett esophagus.

Barrett esophagus is a metaplasia of the squamous esophageal mucosa to a more protective columnar type (intestinal metaplasia). It occurs because of chronic exposure to gastric secretions, usually in the setting of GERD. The endoscopic appearance is of an irregular gastroesophageal junction with tongues of red granular mucosa extending up into the esophagus. Barrett has an increased risk for dysplasia and esophageal adenocarcinoma. The incidence of Barrett esophagus is increasing in the United States.

Esophageal Carcinoma

Squamous cell carcinoma (SCC) of the esophagus is the most common type of esophageal cancer in the world. It affects males more than females, and African Americans more than Caucasians; typical age is usually age >50. Risk factors include:

- Heavy smoking and alcohol use
- Achalasia
- Plummer-Vinson syndrome
- Tylosis
- Lye ingestion

The presentation of squamous cell carcinoma of the esophagus varies; it is often asymptomatic until late in the course. When symptoms do develop they may include progressive dysphagia, weight loss and anorexia, bleeding, hoarseness, and cough. Diagnosis is by endoscopy with biopsy. Treatment is surgery though the prognosis is poor.

Adenocarcinoma of the esophagus affects Caucasians more than African Americans. It arises in the distal esophagus. The progression from Barrett metaplasia to dysplasia and eventually to invasive carcinoma occurs due to the stepwise accumulation of genetic and epigenetic changes. The prognosis is poor.

In the United States, adenocarcinoma and squamous cell carcinoma of the esophagus occur with equal frequency.

STOMACH

Congenital Disorders

Pyloric stenosis is a congenital stenosis of the pylorus due to marked muscular hypertrophy of the pyloric sphincter, resulting in gastric outlet obstruction. It affects male infants more than females. It is associated with Turner and Edwards syndromes. Presentation is the onset of regurgitation and vomiting in week 2 of life; waves of peristalsis are visible on the abdomen and there is a palpable oval abdominal mass. Treatment is surgical.

Congenital diaphragmatic hernia occurs when a congenital defect is present in the diaphragm, resulting in herniation of the abdominal organs into the thoracic cavity. The stomach is the most commonly herniated organ due to left-sided congenital diaphragmatic hernia. Congenital diaphragmatic hernia is often associated with intestinal malrotation. It may be complicated by significant lung hypoplasia.

Hypertrophic Gastropathy

Ménétrier disease is a rare disease of middle-aged men. It is caused by profound hyperplasia of surface mucous cells, accompanied by glandular atrophy. It is characterized by enlarged rugal folds in the body and fundus; clinically, patients experience decreased acid production, protein-losing enteropathy, and increased risk of gastric cancer.

Zollinger-Ellison syndrome. See discussion of gastrinoma in the Pancreas chapter.

Acute Inflammation and Stress Ulcers

Acute hemorrhagic gastritis causes acute inflammation, erosion, and hemorrhage of the gastric mucosa, secondary to a breakdown of the mucosal barrier and acid-induced injury. The etiology is diverse, with initiating agents including chronic aspirin or NSAID use, alcohol use, smoking, recent surgery, burns, ischemia, stress, uremia, and chemotherapy. Patients present with epigastric abdominal pain, or with gastric hemorrhage, hematemesis, and melena.

Gastric stress ulcers are multiple, small, round, superficial ulcers of the stomach and duodenum. Predisposing factors include:

- NSAID use
- Severe stress
- Sepsis
- Shock
- Severe burn or trauma
- Elevated intracranial pressure (Cushing ulcers)

ICU patients have a high incidence of gastric stress ulcer. These ulcers may be complicated by bleeding.

Chronic Gastritis

Chronic gastritis is chronic inflammation of the gastric mucosa, eventually leading to atrophy (chronic atrophic gastritis).

Fundic type chronic gastritis is an autoimmune atrophic gastritis that involves the body and the fundus. It is caused by autoantibodies directed against parietal cells and/or intrinsic factor. The result is loss of parietal cells, decreased acid secretion, increased serum gastrin (G-cell hyperplasia), and pernicious anemia (megaloblastic anemia due to lack of intrinsic factor and B12 malabsorption). Women are affected more than men.

Grossly, one sees a loss of rugal folds in the body and fundus. Microscopically, mucosal atrophy is seen with loss of glands and parietal cells, chronic lymphoplasmacytic inflammation, and intestinal metaplasia. Patients are at increased risk for gastric carcinoma.

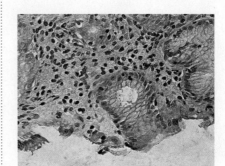

Helicobacter pylori, Warthin-Starry stain.
Bradley Gibson, M.D.
Used with permission.

Antral type chronic gastritis (also called *Helicobacter pylori* gastritis) is the most common form of chronic gastritis in the United States. The *H. pylori* organisms are curved, gram-negative rods which produce urease. The risk of infection increases with age. Infection is also associated with duodenal/gastric peptic ulcer, and gastric carcinoma with intestinal type histology.

Microscopically, *H. pylori* organisms are visible in the mucous layer of the surface epithelium. Other microscopic features include foci of acute inflammation, chronic inflammation with lymphoid follicles, and intestinal metaplasia.

Chronic Peptic Ulcer (Benign Ulcer)

Peptic ulcers are ulcers of the distal stomach and proximal duodenum caused by gastric secretions (hydrochloric acid and pepsin) and impaired mucosal defenses. Predisposing factors include the following:

- Chronic NSAID and aspirin use
- Steroid use
- Smoking
- *H. pylori* infection

Patients present with burning epigastric pain. Diagnosis is by endoscopy with or without biopsy. Treatment is acid suppression (H2 blocker, proton pump inhibitor, etc.) and eradication of *H. pylori*.

Complications of peptic ulcer include hemorrhage, iron deficiency anemia, penetration into adjacent organs, perforation (x-ray shows free air under the diaphragm), and pyloric obstruction.

Duodenal peptic ulcers are more common than gastric peptic ulcers. Associations include the following:

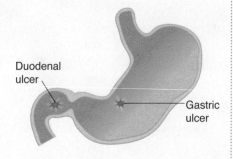

Duodenal ulcer

Gastric ulcer

- *H. pylori* (~100%)
- Increased gastric acid secretion
- Increased rate of gastric emptying
- Blood group O
- Multiple endocrine neoplasia (MEN) type I
- Zollinger-Ellison syndrome
- Cirrhosis
- Chronic obstructive pulmonary disease

Most duodenal peptic ulcers are located in the anterior wall of the proximal duodenum.

Gastric peptic ulcers are associated with *H. pylori* (75%). Most are located in the lesser curvature of the antrum. Grossly, they are small (<3 cm), sharply demarcated ('punched out'), solitary with round/oval shape, smooth borders, and radiating mucosal folds.

Gastric Carcinoma (Malignant Ulcer)

Gastric carcinoma is more common in Japan than in the United States, and has a decreasing incidence in the United States. Dietary factors can be risk factors:

- Smoked fish and meats
- Pickled vegetables

- Nitrosamines
- Benzpyrene
- Reduced intake of fruits and vegetables

Other risk factors include *H. pylori* infection, chronic atrophic gastritis, smoking, blood type A, bacterial overgrowth in the stomach, prior subtotal gastrectomy, and Ménétrier disease.

Gastric carcinoma is often (90%) asymptomatic until late in the course, when it can produce weight loss and anorexia. It can also present with epigastric abdominal pain mimicking a peptic ulcer, early satiety, and occult bleeding with iron deficiency anemia.

Most gastric carcinomas are located in the lesser curvature of the antrum. They are large (>3 cm) ulcers with heaped-up margins and a necrotic ulcer base. They may also occur as a flat or polypoid mass. Several histological types occur.

- The **intestinal type** shows gland-forming adenocarcinoma microscopically.
- The **diffuse type** shows diffuse infiltration of stomach by poorly differentiated tumor cells, numerous signet-ring cells (whose nuclei are displaced to the periphery by intracellular mucin), and *linitis plastica* (thickened "leather bottle"–like stomach) gross appearance.

Gastric carcinoma may specifically metastasize to the left supraclavicular lymph node (Virchow sentinel node) and to the ovary (Krukenberg tumor).

Diagnosis is by endoscopy with biopsy; treatment is gastrectomy. The prognosis is poor, with overall 5-year survival ~30%.

GASTRIC LYMPHOMA

Marginal zone B-cell lymphoma and diffuse large B-cell lymphoma occur in the stomach.

SMALL AND LARGE INTESTINES

Mechanical Obstruction

Volvulus is a twisting of a segment of bowel on its vascular mesentery, causing intestinal obstruction and infarction. It is often associated with congenital abnormalities such as intestinal malrotation. Common locations include the sigmoid colon and small bowel; complications include infarction and peritonitis.

Intussusception is the telescoping of a proximal segment of the bowel into the distal segment. It is most common in infants and children. Children present with vomiting, abdominal pain, passage of blood per rectum, and lethargy; a sausage-shaped mass is often palpable in the right hypochondrium.

In adults, intussusception may be caused by a mass or tumor. The intussuscepted segment can become infarcted.

Incarcerated hernia is a segment of bowel that is imprisoned within a hernia; the condition can become complicated by intestinal obstruction and infarction.

Note

Acquired megacolon may be caused by Chagas disease or ulcerative colitis (toxic megacolon).

Hirschsprung disease (or congenital aganglionic megacolon) is caused by congenital absence of ganglion cells in the rectum and sigmoid colon, resulting in intestinal obstruction. The condition affects males more than females, and can be associated with Down syndrome. Hirschsprung may present with delayed passage of meconium, or with constipation, abdominal distention, and vomiting.

Grossly, the affected segment is narrowed, and there is dilation proximal to the narrow segment (megacolon). Microscopically, there is an absence of ganglion cells in Auerbach and Meissner plexuses, and the diagnosis is established when rectal biopsy demonstrates the absence of ganglion cells. Treatment is resection of the affected segment.

Malabsorption Syndromes

Celiac sprue (or gluten-sensitive enteropathy and nontropical sprue) is caused by hypersensitivity to gluten (and gliadin), resulting in loss of small bowel villi and malabsorption. HLA-DQ2 and/or -DQ8 are carried by most patients. Microscopic exam demonstrates a loss of villi, with increased intraepithelial lymphocytes and increased plasma cells in the lamina propria.

Clinically, it often presents in childhood with malabsorption. Symptoms include abdominal distention, bloating, and flatulence, along with diarrhea, steatorrhea, and weight loss. Dermatitis herpetiformis may occur age >20. In adults, celiac presents between decades 4-7. Treatment is dietary restriction of gluten. There is an increased risk of gastrointestinal cancer.

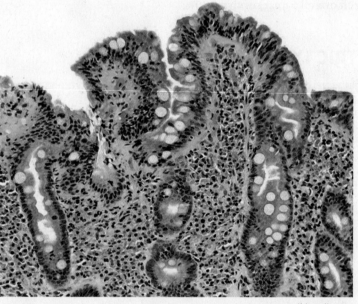

wikimedia.org.

Figure 16-1. Celiac Disease

Environmental enteropathy (previously known as **tropical sprue**) is a maladaptive disease of unknown etiology (infection and/or nutritional deficiency). If affects residents of low-income countries. Biopsy shows blunting of villi and a lymphocytic infiltrate.

Whipple disease is a rare infectious disease involving many organs, including small intestines, joints, lung, heart, liver, spleen, and central nervous system. It typically affects Caucasian males age 30-50.

The infecting organism is *Tropheryma whipplei*. Microscopically, the small bowel lamina propria is filled with macrophages stuffed with the PAS-positive, gram-positive, rod-shaped bacilli. Patients present with malabsorption, weight loss, and diarrhea. Treatment is antibiotics.

Inflammatory bowel disease (IBD). There are 2 categories of IBD:

- **Crohn's disease (CD)** (or regional enteritis)
- **Ulcerative colitis (UC)**

Colitis of indeterminate type describes cases that cannot be clearly classified.

Caucasians develop IBD more frequently than non-Caucasians. The incidence of IBD is increasing.

Age distribution varies with the disease:

- CD has a bimodal distribution with peaks at age 10–30 and 50–70
- UC peaks at age 20–30

IBD can present with episodes of bloody diarrhea or stools with mucus, crampy lower abdominal pain, or fever. CD may present with malabsorption or extraintestinal manifestations. It may mimic appendicitis. CD may cause perianal fistulas.

Diagnosis of IBD requires endoscopic biopsy and clinicopathologic correlation.

New studies indicate that risk of colorectal carcinoma (CRC) in CD and UC are equivalent for similar extent and duration of disease; the risk of CRC is not as high as previous studies suggested.

Note

Damage to the ileal mucosa can cause deficiencies of vitamin B12 and folate.

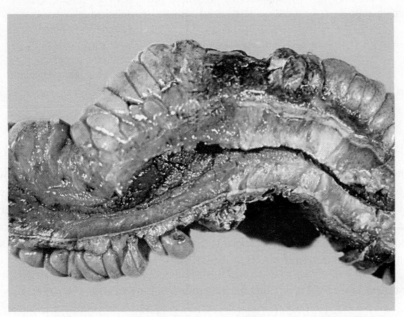

© Katsumi M. Miyai, M.D., Ph.D.; Regents of the University of California.
Used with permission.

Figure 16-2. Narrowed Colon Segment in Crohn's Disease

Table 16-1. Crohn's Disease Versus Ulcerative Colitis

	Crohn's Disease	Ulcerative Colitis
Most common site	Terminal ileum	Rectum
Distribution	Mouth to anus	Rectum → colon "back-wash" ileitis
Spread	Discontinuous/"skip"	Continuous
Gross features	• Focal aphthous ulcers with intervening normal mucosa • Linear fissures • Cobblestone appearance • Thickened bowel wall • "Creeping fat"	Extensive ulceration Pseudopolyps
Micro	Noncaseating granulomas	Crypt abscesses
Inflammation	Transmural	Limited to mucosa and submucosa
Complications	• Strictures • "String sign" on barium studies • Obstruction • Abscesses • Fistulas • Sinus tracts	Toxic megacolon
Genetic association		HLA-B27
Extraintestinal manifestations	Common (e.g., migratory polyarthritis, ankylosing spondylitis, primary sclerosing cholangitis, erythema nodosum, pyoderma gangrenosum, uveitis)	Common (e.g., migratory arthritis, ankylosing spondylitis, primary sclerosing cholangitis, erythema nodosum, pyoderma gangrenosum, uveitis)

Miscellaneous Conditions

Ischemic bowel disease is caused by decreased blood flow and ischemia of the bowel, secondary to atherosclerosis with thrombosis, thromboembolism, or reduced cardiac output from shock. It is most common in older individuals. Typical presentation is with abdominal pain and bloody diarrhea. The disease distribution tends to involve watershed areas (e.g., splenic flexure), and affected areas typically show hemorrhagic infarction.

Treatment is surgical resection, but the prognosis is poor, with >50% mortality.

Hemorrhoids are tortuous, dilated anal submucosal veins caused by increased venous pressure. Risk factors include constipation and prolonged straining during bowel

Bridge to Anatomy

The splenic flexure of the colon receives blood from both the superior and inferior mesenteric arteries.

movements, pregnancy, and cirrhosis. Complications include painful thrombosis and streaks of bright red blood on hard stool.

Angiodysplasia is arteriovenous malformations of the intestines. It occurs in the cecum and right colon. Individuals age >55 are most commonly affected, presenting with multiple episodes of rectal bleeding. It is associated with Osler-Weber-Rendu and CREST syndromes. Treatment is surgical resection.

Melanosis coli is common with laxative abuse; it causes black pigmentation of the colon due to the ingestion of the laxative pigment by macrophages in the mucosal and submucosa. It can mimic colitis or malignancy.

Pseudomembranous colitis (antibiotic-associated colitis) is an acute colitis characterized by the formation of inflammatory pseudomembranes in the intestines. It is usually caused by *Clostridium difficile* infection (often brought on by a course of broad-spectrum antibiotics, especially clindamycin and ampicillin), but it can be caused by ischemic bowel disease.

Gross examination shows yellow-tan mucosal membranes. Microscopic exam shows the pseudomembranes are composed of an adherent layer of acute inflammatory cells, mucus and necrotic debris overlying sites of colonic mucosal injury. Presentation is with diarrhea, fever, and abdominal cramps. Diagnosis is established with detection of *C. difficile* toxin in the stool. Treatment of clostrial pseudomembranous colitis is vancomycin or metronidazole.

Appendicitis is most commonly caused by obstruction of the appendix by a fecalith. It often starts with periumbilical pain that subsequently localizes to the right lower quadrant. Nausea, vomiting, and fever may also be present. Lab studies show an elevated white blood cell count. A complication is appendiceal rupture leading to peritonitis. Grossly, a fibrinopurulent exudate may be seen on the appendiceal serosa; microscopically, neutrophils are present within the mucosa and muscular wall (muscularis propria) of the appendix.

Diverticula

Meckel diverticulum is a congenital small bowel diverticulum caused by persistance of a remnant of the vitelline (omphalomesenteric) duct (*see* Anatomy Lecture Notes). With Meckel, the "rule of 2s" applies:

- 2% of the normal population
- 2 feet from the ileocecal valve
- Length 2 cm
- Age ≤2 years at time of diagnosis

Most Meckel diverticula are asymptomatic but they may contain rests of ectopic gastric mucosa and present with intestinal bleeding.

Colonic diverticulosis is an acquired outpouching of the bowel wall, characterized by herniation of the mucosa and submucosa through the muscularis propria (pseudodiverticulum). It is extremely common in the United States.

- Incidence increases with age
- Major risk factor is a low-fiber diet, which leads to increased intraluminal pressure
- Most common location is sigmoid colon

In a Nutshell

Osler-Weber-Rendu Syndrome

- a.k.a. Hereditary hemorrhagic telangiectasia
- Autosomal dominant
- Telangiectasias of skin and mucous membranes
- Common on lips, tongue, and fingertips
- May develop iron deficiency anemia

Note

Given that only 2 layers of the bowel wall are involved, these acquired outpouchings are technically pseudodiverticula.

Many cases are asymptomatic and picked up on screening colonoscopy. When symptomatic, it can cause constipation alternating with diarrhea, left lower quadrant abdominal cramping and discomfort, occult bleeding and an iron deficiency anemia, or lower gastrointestinal tract hemorrhage. Complications include diverticulitis, fistulas, and perforation with accompanying peritonitis.

Polyps

Hamartomatous polyps include nonfamilial juvenile polyps and polyps associated with a familial (Peutz-Jeghers) syndrome. Nonsyndromic polyps do not have malignant potential.

Hyperplastic polyps are the most common histologic type; they occur most often in the left colon and are usually <5 mm. Although previously considered not to have malignant potential, newer studies suggest they are part of a group of polyps with serrated histology and risk of progression to cancer. **Serrated polyps** occur more often in the right colon.

Tubular and villous adenomas have long been known to have malignant potential. Microscopically, they show cellular dysplasia and either pure tubular, pure villous or tubulovillous histology.

Familial Syndromes

Familial adenomatous polyposis (FAP), also called adenomatous polyposis coli (APC), is due to an autosomal dominant mutation of the *APC* gene on chromosome 5q21.

Affected individuals may develop **thousands of colonic adenomatous polyps**; the diagnosis is made with discovery of >100 adenomatous polyps on endoscopy. **Complications:** by age 40, virtually 100% will develop an invasive adenocarcinoma and increased risks for developing duodenal adenocarcinoma and adenocarcinoma of the papilla of Vater.

Gardner syndrome is an autosomal dominant variant of familial adenomatous polyposis characterized by numerous colonic adenomatous polyps, multiple osteomas, fibromatosis, and epidermal inclusion cysts.

Turcot syndrome is a rare variant of familial adenomatous polyposis characterized by numerous colonic adenomatous polyps and central nervous system tumors (gliomas).

Hereditary nonpolyposis colorectal cancer (HNPCC), or Lynch syndrome, is due to an autosomal dominant mutation of a DNA nucleotide mismatch repair gene that predisposes for colon cancer. It is associated with an increased risk of cancer at other sites, including the endometrium and the ovary.

Peutz-Jeghers syndrome is an autosomal dominant condition characterized by multiple hamartomatous polyps (primarily in the small intestine); melanin pigmentation of the oral mucosa; and increased risk of cancer at numerous sites including the lung, pancreas, breast, and uterus.

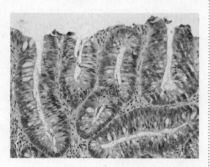

Tubular Adenoma
© Gregg Barré, M.D.
Used with permission.

Neoplasia

Colonic adenocarcinoma is the third most common tumor in the United States, in terms of incidence and mortality. Risk factors include:

- Dietary factors (low fiber, low fruits/vegetables and high in red meat and animal fat)
- Colon polyps (isolated adenomatous polyps, hereditary polyposis syndromes)
- Other colon disease (Lynch syndrome, ulcerative colitis)

Diagnosis is established via endoscopy with biopsy.

Cancer genetics: Mutations of the *APC* gene cause activation of the Wnt pathway, leading β-catenin to translocate to the nucleus where it causes the overexpression of growth-promoting genes. DNA mismatch repair causes microsatellite instability, which is another genetic carcinogenesis pathway.

The pattern of spread in colonic adenocarcinoma includes lymphatic spread to mesenteric lymph nodes, with distant spread to liver, lungs, and bone. Staging is with the TNM system. Treatment can include surgical resection and chemotherapy (for metastatic disease); CEA levels can be used to monitor for disease recurrence.

Screening is recommended for the general population beginning age 50. Current guidelines suggest:

- Colonoscopy every 10 years or annual fecal occult blood test (FOBT), or
- Combination of FOBT (every 3 years) and sigmoidoscopy (every 5 years)

Table 16-2. Right-Sided Cancer Versus Left-Sided Cancer

	Right-Sided Cancer	Left-Sided Cancer
Gross	Polypoid mass	Circumferential growth producing a "napkin-ring" configuration
Barium studies	Polypoid mass	"Apple-core" lesion
Presentation	Bleeding • Occult blood in stool • Iron deficiency anemia	Change in bowel habits • Constipation or diarrhea • Reduced caliber stools • Obstruction

Carcinoid tumors are neuroendocrine tumors that often produce serotonin. Locations include the appendix (most common) and the terminal ileum. Metastasis to the liver may result in carcinoid heart disease.

Carcinoid syndrome is characterized by diarrhea, cutaneous flushing, bronchospasm and wheezing, and fibrosis. The diagnosis is substantiated by demonstrating elevated urinary 5-HIAA (5-hydroxyindoleacetic acid).

Gastrointestinal stromal tumor (GIST) is the most common sarcoma of the GI tract. Most cases have a *KIT* mutation. The peak incidence is in decade 7. Treatment is resection and a tyrosine-kinase inhibitor.

In a Nutshell

TNM Staging of Colorectal Cancer

Stage I (T1-2N0M0): tumors that do not penetrate through mucosa (T1) or muscularis (T2)

Stage II (T3N0M0): tumors that have penetrated through the muscularis but have not spread to the lymph nodes

Stage III (TXN1M0): regional lymph node involvement

Stage IV (TXNXM1): metastasis to distant sites

Note

Histologically, carcinoid tumors appear similar to other neuroendocrine tumors, with nests of small uniform cells.

Bridge to Biochemistry

Serotonin is converted to 5-HIAA by monoamine oxidase.

Chapter Summary

- Congenital and mechanical disorders of the esophagus include tracheoesophageal fistula, esophageal webs, and achalasia. Achalasia is due to failure of the lower esophageal sphincter to relax with swallowing.

- Esophageal bleeding can be due to laceration at the gastroesophageal junction produced by severe vomiting (Mallory-Weiss syndrome), or esophageal varices that develop secondary to portal hypertension.

- GERD is esophageal irritation and inflammation due to reflux of gastric secretions into the esophagus. Barrett esophagus is metaplasia of the squamous esophageal mucosa to a more protective columnar type because of chronic exposure to gastric secretions.

- Esophageal carcinoma may be squamous cell carcinoma or adenocarcinoma. Squamous cell carcinoma is the most common form in the world and is associated with heavy smoking, heavy alcohol use, achalasia, and Plummer-Vinson syndrome. Adenocarcinoma involves the distal esophagus and usually arises in areas of Barrett esophagus.

- Pyloric stenosis is a congenital stenosis of the pylorus due to marked muscular hypertrophy of the pyloric sphincter, resulting in gastric outlet obstruction. Congenital diaphragmatic hernia is a congenital defect in the diaphragm, resulting in herniation of the abdominal organs into the thoracic cavity.

- Ménétrier disease is a form of hypertrophic gastropathy with enlarged rugal folds that can produce decreased acid production, a protein-losing enteropathy, and increased risk of cancer. Zollinger-Ellison syndrome is a form of hypertrophic gastropathy with enlarged rugal folds that occurs secondary to gastrin stimulation by a pancreatic gastrinoma.

- Acute hemorrhagic gastritis is acute inflammation, erosion, and hemorrhage of the gastric mucosa due to a breakdown of the mucosal barrier and acid-induced injury. Gastric stress ulcers are multiple, small, round, superficial ulcers of the stomach and duodenum.

- Chronic gastritis is a chronic inflammation of the gastric mucosa resulting in eventual atrophy. Chronic gastritis is subdivided into a fundic type, which is related to autoantibodies to parietal cells and/or intrinsic factor, and an antral type, which is related to *H. pylori* gastritis.

- Peptic ulcers are ulcers of the distal stomach and proximal duodenum caused by gastric secretions (hydrochloric acid and pepsin) and impaired mucosal defenses. Duodenal peptic ulcers are more common than gastric ulcers.

- Gastric carcinomas tend to be asymptomatic until late in their course and may show a variety of histologic patterns.

- Volvulus is twisting of a segment of bowel on its vascular mesentery, resulting in intestinal obstruction and infarction.

- Intussusception is telescoping of a proximal segment of bowel into the distal segment.

- Incarcerated hernia is a segment of bowel that becomes imprisoned within a hernia.

- Hirschsprung disease is a congenital absence of ganglion cells in the rectum and sigmoid colon resulting in intestinal obstruction.

(continued)

Chapter Summary *(cont'd)*

- Celiac sprue is a hypersensitivity to gluten, resulting in loss of small bowel villi and malabsorption.

- Environmental enteropathy is a malabsorptive disease of unknown etiology affecting travelers to tropical regions, such as the Caribbean and South America.

- Whipple disease is a rare infectious disease involving many organs, including small intestines, joints, lung, heart, liver, spleen, and CNS.

- IBD includes Crohn's disease, ulcerative colitis, and colitis of indeterminate type. Crohn's disease has "skip" lesions, has transmural involvement with formation of granulomas, and tends to form fistulas, abscesses, and sinuses. Ulcerative colitis is confined to the rectum and colon, has inflammation limited to the mucosa and submucosa with crypt abscesses, and can cause toxic megacolon.

- Ischemic bowel disease is the result of decreased blood flow and ischemia of the bowel secondary to atherosclerosis with thrombosis, thromboembolism, or reduced cardiac output from shock.

- Hemorrhoids are tortuous dilated submucosal veins caused by increased venous pressure.

- Angiodysplasia is arteriovenous malformation of the intestines.

- Melanosis coli is a black pigmentation of the colon that is common with laxative abuse.

- Pseudomembranous colitis is characterized by formation of inflammatory pseudomembranes in the intestine following infection by *Clostridium difficile*, and/ or ischemic bowel disease.

- Meckel diverticulum is a congenital small bowel diverticulum that is a remnant of the vitelline duct.

- Colonic diverticulosis is common in the elderly and features acquired outpouchings of the bowel wall, characterized by herniation of the mucosa and submucosa through the muscularis propria.

- Hyperplastic colon polyps are the most common benign colon polyps. They typically arise in the left colon.

- Adenomatous colonic polyps are benign neoplasms of the colonic mucosa that have the potential to progress to colonic adenocarcinoma. Familial adenomatous polyposis is a genetic condition in which patients develop thousands of colonic adenomatous polyps and have a virtually 100% chance of developing colon cancer by age 40 unless the affected colon is resected. **Gardner syndrome** is a variant of familial adenomatous polyposis with associated osteomas, fibromatosis, and epidermal inclusion cysts. **Turcot syndrome** is a rare variant of familial adenomatous polyposis associated with CNS gliomas. **Hereditary nonpolyposis colorectal cancer** has increased risks of colon, endometrial, and ovarian cancers, but it is not associated with multiple adenomatous polyps. **Peutz-Jeghers** syndrome has multiple hamartomatous polyps with increased risk of cancers of the lung, pancreas, breast, and uterus, but not colon.

- Colonic adenocarcinoma is the third most common cancer and a leading cause of cancer mortality in the United States. It tends to produce a polypoid mass when it involves the right side of the colon and a napkin ring lesion when it involves the left side. The TNM system is used for staging colon cancer.

- Carcinoid tumors are neuroendocrine tumors that can involve the appendix and terminal ileum and may produce carcinoid syndrome with diarrhea, flushing, bronchospasms, fibrosis, and sometimes carcinoid heart disease.

Pancreatic Pathology 17

Learning Objectives

❏ Demonstrate understanding of congenital anomalies of the pancreas

❏ Use knowledge of inflammation of the pancreas or tumors of the pancreas to solve problems

CONGENITAL ANOMALIES OF THE PANCREAS

- **Pancreatic agenesis** is incompatible with life.

- **Pancreatic divisum** is a variant of pancreatic duct anatomy.

- **Annular pancreas** encircles the duodenum and presents as obstruction.

- **Ectopic pancreatic tissue** can hemorrhage, become inflamed, or give rise to a neuroendocrine tumor. These rests most often arise in the stomach, duodenum, or jejunum.

INFLAMMATION OF THE PANCREAS

Acute pancreatitis is acute inflammation caused by injury to the exocrine portion of the pancreas. The etiology is diverse:

- Gallstones
- Alcohol
- Hypercalcemia
- Drugs
- Shock
- Infections
- Trauma
- Scorpion stings

Pancreatic acinar cell injury results in activation of pancreatic enzymes and enzymatic destruction of the pancreatic parenchyma.

Symptoms include stabbing epigastric abdominal pain radiating to the back. Severe acute pancreatitis can also cause shock. Lab studies show elevated serum amylase and lipase. Complications include acute respiratory distress syndrome (ARDS), disseminated intravascular coagulation (DIC), pancreatic pseudocyst; pancreatic calcifications, and hypocalcemia. Severe cases have a 30% mortality rate.

In a Nutshell

Pancreatic pseudocyst is a fluid-filled sac adjacent to the pancreas. The wall of granulation tissue lacks an epithelial lining.

- Gross pathologic examination shows focal hemorrhage and liquefication in the pancreas, accompanied by chalky, white-yellow fat necrosis of adjacent adipose tissue.

- Microscopically there is liquefactive necrosis of the pancreatic parenchyma with acute inflammation and enzymatic fat necrosis.

- Necrosis of blood vessels causes hemorrhage.

Chronic pancreatitis refers to irreversible changes in pancreatic function with accompanying chronic inflammation, atrophy, and fibrosis of the pancreas secondary to repeated bouts of pancreatitis. Manifestations include abdominal pain, pancreatic insufficiency and malabsorption, pancreatic calcifications, pseudocyst, and secondary diabetes mellitus (late complication).

It is common in middle-aged male alcoholics. Pathology shows grossly firm, white, and fibrotic pancreas. Microscopically there is extensive fibrosis with parenchymal atrophy and chronic inflammation.

Autoimmune pancreatitis can occur in association with IgG4-associated fibrosing disorders; this variant responds to steroid therapy.

PANCREATIC TUMORS

Pancreatic neuroendocrine tumors (islet cell tumors) are less common than exocrine tumors. Most are considered low grade malignancies. Some patients lack laboratory evidence of hormone overproduction. These tumors are not distinguishable from each other on the basis of gross appearance or histology.

- **Insulinoma (β-cell tumor)** (most common type of islet cell tumor)
    - Produces insulin
    - Can cause hypoglycemia, sweating, hunger, confusion, and insulin coma
    - Surgical excision is curative

- **Gastrinoma (G-cell tumor)**
    - Produces gastrin
    - Excess gastrin manifests as Zollinger-Ellison syndrome, which is characterized by thick gastric folds, elevated serum gastrin, gastric hyperacidity, and intractable peptic ulcers
    - Gastrinomas may arise outside the pancreas
    - May be associated with MEN I

- **Glucagonoma (α-cell tumor)**
    - Produces glucagon
    - Excess glucagon causes hyperglycemia (diabetes), anemia, and skin rash

- **Somatostatinoma** (δ-cell tumor)
    - Produces somatostatin
    - Excess somatostatin inhibits insulin secretion, leading to diabetes
    - Can also inhibit gastrin secretion (leading to hypochlorhydria) and cholecystokinin secretion (leading to gallstones and steatorrhea)
    - Prognosis is poor

- **VIPoma**
  ○ Produces vasoactive intestinal peptide (VIP)
  ○ Excess VIP causes WDHA syndrome: watery diarrhea, hypokalemia, and achlorhydria

Pancreatic carcinoma is the fifth most common cause of cancer death in the United States, and the incidence is rising.

- Most common ages 60-80
- Smoking is a risk factor
- Presents with only vague signs and symptoms until late in course
- When more definitive signs and symptoms develop, they can include abdominal pain, migratory thrombophlebitis, and obstructive jaundice

The tumor may occur in the head (60%), body (15%), and tail (5%). Microscopically, the adenocarcinoma arises from the duct epithelium. Tumor desmoplasia and perineural invasion are common. Tumor markers for pancreatic carcinoma include CEA and CA19-9, but they are not useful screening assays.

Treatment is surgical excision (Whipple procedure). The prognosis is very poor, with 5-year survival only ~5%.

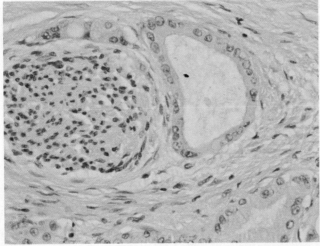

© Gregg Barré, M.D.
Used with permission.

Figure 17-1. Pancreatic Adenocarcinoma with Perineural Invasion

Pancreatic cystic neoplasms: Serous neoplasms account for 25% of pancreatic cystic neoplasms; most are benign (cystadenomas) and the tumors carry a mutation of *VHL*.

Mucinous neoplasms: Mucinous cystic neoplasms are common in women and can harbor dysplasia or carcinoma; distal pancreatectomy is curative in most cases. **Intraductal papillary mucinous neoplasms** are common in men and tend to arise in the head of the pancreas; *GNAS* mutations are common and carcinoma may arise in the neoplasm.

Chapter Summary

- In acute pancreatitis, pancreatic acinar cell injury results in activation of pancreatic enzymes and enzymatic destruction of the pancreatic parenchyma. Acute pancreatitis can be seen in a variety of clinical settings, notably associated with gallstones or alcohol use. Pancreatic pseudocysts may arise as a complication. Chronic pancreatitis reflects permanent damage to the organ; fibrosis is a histologic hallmark.

- Pancreatic islet cell tumors may secrete insulin, gastrin, glucagon, somatostatin, or vasoactive intestinal peptide.

- Pancreatic cystic neoplasms may be serous (usually benign) or mucinous.

- Pancreatic carcinoma is the fifth most common cause of cancer death in the United States and has a very poor prognosis.

Learning Objectives

❏ Use knowledge of gallstones (cholelithiasis), inflammatory conditions of the gallbladder, and miscellaneous conditions to solve problems

❏ Explain information related to biliary tract cancer

GALLSTONES (CHOLELITHIASIS)

Gallstones are frequently asymptomatic but can cause biliary colic (right upper quadrant pain due to impacted stones). Diagnosis is by U/S; the majority of stones are not radiopaque. Complications include cholecystitis, choledocholithiasis (calculi within the biliary tract), biliary tract obstruction, pancreatitis, and cholangitis.

Cholesterol stones are composed mostly of cholesterol monohydrate. The incidence increases with age. Risk factors include female gender, obesity, pregnancy, oral contraceptives, and hormone replacement therapy. Native American Pima and Navajo Indians have an increased incidence of cholesterol gallstones.

Pigmented bilirubinate stones are composed of calcium salts and unconjugated bilirubin. Risk factors are chronic hemolytic anemias, cirrhosis, bacterial infection, and parasites (*Ascaris* or *Clonorchis* [*Opisthorchis*] *sinensis*).

INFLAMMATORY CONDITIONS

Acute cholecystitis is an acute inflammation of the gallbladder, usually caused by cystic duct obstruction by gallstones. It can present with biliary colic, right upper quadrant tenderness on palpation, nausea and vomiting, low-grade fever, and leukocytosis. Complications include gangrene of the gallbladder, perforation and peritonitis, fistula formation and gallstone ileus (small bowel obstruction by a large gallstone). Acute acalculous cholecystitis is associated with surgery, trauma, and sepsis.

Chronic cholecystitis is ongoing chronic inflammation of the gallbladder, usually caused by gallstones. Well-developed examples show stromal and mural lymphocytic and plasmacytic infiltrates. Macrophages and granulomas may also be present. The wall is thickened.

Note

Formation of cholesterol stones involves the precipitation of cholesterol from supersaturated bile.

Clinical Correlate

Murphy's sign is inspiratory arrest in response to palpation of the right subcostal area during deep inspiration. It is seen in patients with pain due to cholecystitis.

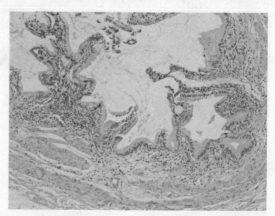

© Gregg Barré, M.D.
Used with permission.

Figure 18-1. Chronic Cholecystitis

Ascending cholangitis is a bacterial infection of the bile ducts ascending up to the liver, usually associated with obstruction of bile flow oftentimes from bile duct stones. It presents with biliary colic, jaundice, high fever, and chills. The infecting organisms are usually gram-negative enteric bacteria.

MISCELLANEOUS CONDITIONS

Cholesterolosis refers to an accumulation of cholesterol-laden macrophages within the mucosa of the gallbladder wall. Gross examination shows yellow speckling of the red-tan mucosa ("strawberry gallbladder"). Microscopic examination shows lipid-laden macrophages within the lamina propria.

Hydrops of the gallbladder (mucocele) occurs when chronic obstruction of the cystic duct leads to the resorption of the normal gallbladder contents and enlargement of the gallbladder by the production of large amounts of clear fluid (hydrops) or mucous secretions (mucocele).

BILIARY TRACT CANCER

Gallbladder cancer is frequently asymptomatic until late in the course. When the tumor does present, it may be with cholecystitis, enlarged palpable gallbladder, or biliary tract obstruction (uncommon). X-ray may show a calcified "porcelain gallbladder." Microscopically, the tissues show adenocarcinoma. The prognosis for gallbladder cancer is poor; 5-year survival rate is ~12%.

Bile duct cancer. Bile duct carcinoma is carcinoma of the **extrahepatic** bile ducts, while cholangiocarcinoma is carcinoma of the **intrahepatic** bile ducts. Klatskin tumor is a carcinoma of the bifurcation of the right and left hepatic bile ducts. Risk factors for bile duct cancer include *Clonorchis (Opisthorchis) sinensis* (liver fluke) in Asia and primary sclerosing cholangitis. Bile duct cancer typically presents with biliary tract obstruction. Microscopic examination shows adenocarcinoma arising from the bile duct epithelium. The prognosis is poor.

Adenocarcinoma of the ampulla of Vater may exhibit duodenal, biliary, or pancreatic epithelium. Patients present with painless jaundice. The 5-year survival rate is <50% in spite of resection.

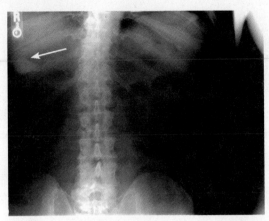

© Gloria Jicha: Tripler Army Medical Center.
Used with permission.

Figure 18-2. X-Ray Showing Calcified (Porcelain) Gallbladder

Chapter Summary

- Gallstones can take the form of cholesterol stones or pigmented bilirubinate stones. Cholesterol stones are composed of mostly cholesterol monohydrate. Pigmented bilirubinate stones are composed of calcium salts and unconjugated bilirubin.

- Gallstone disease is frequently asymptomatic, or may cause right upper quadrant pain due to impacted stones.

- Acute cholecystitis is an acute inflammation of the gallbladder usually caused by cystic duct obstruction with gallstones. Chronic cholecystitis is ongoing chronic inflammation of the gallbladder that is usually caused by gallstones.

- Ascending cholangitis is a bacterial infection of the bile ducts ascending up to the liver and is usually associated with obstruction of bile flow.

- Cholesterolosis is a clinically insignificant yellow-speckling of the gallbladder mucosa.

- Hydrops of the gallbladder occurs when chronic obstruction of the cystic duct leads to the resorption of the normal gallbladder contents and enlargement of the gallbladder, with production of large amounts of clear fluid (hydrops) or mucous secretions (mucocele).

- Gallbladder cancer has a very poor prognosis because it is frequently asymptomatic until late in the course. Bile duct cancer also has a poor prognosis.

Learning Objectives

❏ Solve problems concerning jaundice, cirrhosis, viral hepatitis, amebic liver abscess, and alcoholic liver disease

❏ Differentiate metabolic liver disease from hemodynamic liver disease

❏ Solve problems concerning liver tumors

LIVER DYSFUNCTION

Dysfunction of the liver may be divided into 4 categories that may coexist:

- **Hepatic failure** occurs in the setting of hepatic necrosis secondary to acute liver failure, chronic liver disease, and hepatocyte dysfunction.

- **Portal hypertension** occurs in the setting of cirrhosis or increased portal venous blood flow.

- **Cholestasis** occurs in the setting of impaired bile flow due to hepatocyte dysfunction or biliary obstruction.

- **Cirrhosis** occurs in the setting of hepatocyte injury and is usually an irreversible nodular regeneration that is end stage.

JAUNDICE

Clinical jaundice occurs with bilirubin levels >2–3 mg/dL. The classic presentation is yellow skin (jaundice) and sclera (icterus). Causes of jaundice include overproduction of bilirubin, defective hepatic bilirubin uptake, defective conjugation, and defective excretion.

Table 19-1. Unconjugated Versus Conjugated Bilirubinemia

Unconjugated (Indirect) Bilirubinemia	Conjugated (Direct) Bilirubinemia
Increased RBC turnover (hemolytic anemias)	Biliary tract obstruction
Physiologic (newborn babies)	Biliary tract disease (PSC and PBC)
Hereditary (Gilbert and Crigler-Najjar syndromes)	Hereditary (Dubin-Johnson and Rotor syndromes)
	Liver disease (cirrhosis and hepatitis)

Increased red blood cell (RBC) turnover. RBCs are the major source of bilirubin. Jaundice related to overproduction of bilirubin can be seen in hemolytic anemia and ineffective erythropoiesis (thalassemia, megaloblastic anemia, etc.). Laboratory studies show increased unconjugated bilirubin. Chronic hemolytic anemia patients often develop pigmented bilirubinate gallstones. The most common cause of marked jaundice in the newborn is blood group incompatibility (most commonly ABO) between mother and child, causing **hemolytic disease of the newborn**.

Physiologic jaundice of the newborn is a transient unconjugated hyperbilirubinemia due to the immaturity of the liver. Risk factors include prematurity and hemolytic disease of the newborn (erythroblastosis fetalis). Physiologic jaundice of the newborn can be complicated by kernicterus; treatment is phototherapy. Jaundice also occurs in newborns who have infections.

Hereditary hyperbilirubinemias

When hyperbilirubinemia is prolonged in the newborn, a mutation affecting bilirubin conjugation enters the differential diagnosis.

- **Gilbert syndrome** is a common benign inherited disorder that causes unconjugated hyperbilirubinemia due to bilirubin UDP-glucuronosyltransferase (UGT) deficiency. Kernicterus rarely occurs and the treatment is phenobarbital.

- **Crigler-Najjar syndrome** causes unconjugated hyperbilirubinemia due to bilirubin glucuronosyltransferase (UGT) absence or deficiency. Treatment for type 1 is gene replacement therapy and liver transplantation. For a milder type 2, phenobarbital is used.

- **Dubin-Johnson syndrome** is a benign autosomal recessive disorder characterized by decreased bilirubin excretion due to a defect in the canalicular cationic transport protein. It produces conjugated hyperbilirubinemia and a distinctive black pigmentation of the liver, but has no clinical consequences.

- **Rotor syndrome** is an autosomal recessive conjugated hyperbilirubinemia that is similar to Dubin-Johnson syndrome, but without liver pigmentation. There are no clinical consequences.

Biliary tract obstruction may have multiple etiologies, including gallstones; tumors (pancreatic, gallbladder, and bile duct); stricture; and parasites (liver flukes—*Clonorchis [Opisthorchis] sinensis*). The presentation can include jaundice and icterus; pruritus due to increased plasma levels of bile acids; abdominal pain, fever, and chills; dark urine (bilirubinuria); and pale clay-colored stools. Lab studies show elevated conjugated bilirubin, elevated alkaline phosphatase, and elevated 5′-nucleotidase.

Primary biliary cirrhosis (PBC) is a chronic liver disease that is characterized by inflammation and granulomatous destruction of intrahepatic bile ducts. Females have 10 times the incidence of primary biliary cirrhosis compared to males; the peak incidence is age 40–50.

Presentation includes obstructive jaundice and pruritus; xanthomas, xanthelasmas, and elevated serum cholesterol; fatigue; and cirrhosis (late complication). Most patients have another autoimmune disease (scleroderma, rheumatoid arthritis or systemic lupus erythematosis).

Laboratory studies show elevated conjugated bilirubin, elevated alkaline phosphatase, and elevated 5'-nucleotidase. Treatment with oral ursodeoxycholic acid slows disease progression. **Antimitochondrial autoantibodies** (AMA) are present in >90% of cases, which further supports an autoimmune basis. Microscopically, lymphocytic and granulomatous inflammation involves interlobular bile ducts.

Primary sclerosing cholangitis (PSC) is a chronic liver disease characterized by segmental inflammation and fibrosing destruction of intrahepatic and extrahepatic bile ducts. The exact etiologic mechanism is not known but growing evidence supports an immunologic basis.

The male to female ratio is 2:1; peak age 20–40. Most cases of PSC are associated with ulcerative colitis. The presentation is similar to PBC. Complications include biliary cirrhosis and cholangiocarcinoma.

Microscopically, there is periductal chronic inflammation with concentric fibrosis around bile ducts and segmental stenosis of bile ducts. Cholangiogram shows "beaded appearance" of bile ducts.

CIRRHOSIS

Cirrhosis is end-stage liver disease characterized by disruption of the liver architecture by bands of fibrosis which divide the liver into nodules of regenerating liver parenchyma.

Causes of cirrhosis include alcohol, viral hepatitis, biliary tract disease, hemochromatosis, cryptogenic/idiopathic, Wilson disease, and α-1-antitrypsin deficiency.

On gross Pathology, **micronodular** cirrhosis has nodules <3 mm, while **macronodular** cirrhosis has nodules >3 mm; mixed micronodular and macronodular cirrhosis can also occur. At the end stage, most diseases result in a mixed pattern, and the etiology may not be distinguished based on the appearance.

Cirrhosis has a multitude of **consequences**, including portal hypertension, ascites, splenomegaly/hypersplenism, esophageal varices, hemorrhoids, caput medusa, decreased detoxification, hepatic encephalopathy, spider angiomata, palmar erythema, gynecomastia, decreased synthesic function, hepatorenal syndrome and coagulopathy.

VIRAL HEPATITIS

Viral hepatitis can be asymptomatic or it can present with malaise and weakness, nausea and anorexia, jaundice, or dark urine. Lab studies show markedly elevated alanine aminotransferase (ALT) and aspartate aminotransferase (AST). Diagnosis is by serology.

Acute viral hepatitis is viral hepatitis with signs and symptoms for <6 months. It can be caused by any of the hepatitis viruses.

Microscopically, the liver shows lobular disarray, hepatocyte swelling (balloon cells), apoptotic hepatocytes (Councilman bodies), lymphocytes in portal tracts and in the lobule, hepatocyte regeneration, and cholestasis.

Clinical Correlate

Prothrombin time, not partial thromboplastin time, is used to assess the coagulopathy due to liver disease.

Clinical Correlate

Non-hepatitis viruses which may infect the liver include:

- *Epstein-Barr virus* (EBV)—infectious mononucleosis
- *Cytomegalovirus* (CMV)
- Herpes
- Yellow fever

Clinical Correlate

Hepatitis D requires hepatitis B to propagate.

Chronic viral hepatitis is viral hepatitis with signs and symptoms for >6 months. It can be caused by hepatitis viruses B, C, and D.

- Microscopically, **chronic persistent hepatitis** shows inflammation confined to portal tracts.

- **Chronic active hepatitis** shows inflammation spilling into the parenchyma, causing interface hepatitis (piecemeal necrosis of limiting plate).

Hepatitis B often has "ground glass" hepatocytes (due to cytoplasmic HBsAg).

Table 19-2. The Hepatitis Viruses

Common Virus Name	Hepatitis A (HAV)	Hepatitis B (HBV)	Hepatitis C (HCV)	Hepatitis D (HDV)	Hepatitis E (HEV)
Common disease name	"Infectious"	"Serum"	"Post-transfusion" or "non-A, non-B"	"Delta"	"Enteric"
Virus	*Hepatovirus* nonenveloped capsid RNA	*Hepadnavirus* enveloped DNA	*Flavivirus* enveloped RNA	Defective enveloped circular RNA	*Hepevirus* nonenveloped capsid RNA
Transmission	Fecal-oral	Parenteral, sexual, perinatal	Parenteral, sexual	Parenteral, sexual	Fecal-oral
Severity	Mild	Occasionally severe	Usually subclinical	Co-infection with HBV occasionally severe; super-infection with HBV often severe	Normal patients: mild; pregnant patients: severe
Chronicity or carrier state	No	Yes	Yes (high)	Yes	No
Clinical diseases	Acute hepatitis	• Acute hepatitis • Chronic hepatitis • Cirrhosis • Hepatocellular carcinoma (HCC)	• Chronic hepatitis • Cirrhosis • HCC	• Acute hepatitis • Chronic hepatitis • Cirrhosis • HCC	Acute hepatitis
Laboratory diagnosis	Symptoms and anti-HAV IgM	Symptoms and serum levels of HBsAg, HBeAg, and anti-HBc IgM	Symptoms and EIA for anti-HCV	Anti-HDV ELISA	Tests not routinely available
Prevention	Vaccine, hygiene	Vaccine			Hygiene
Treatment	Supportive	Antivirals, interferons, transplant	Antivirals, interferons, transplant	See hepatitis B	Supportive

Table 19-3. Hepatitis B Terminology and Markers

Abbreviation	Name and Description
HBV	Hepatitis B virus, a hepadnavirus (enveloped, partially double-stranded DNA virus); Dane particle = infectious HBV
HBsAg	Antigen found on surface of HBV; also found on spheres and filaments in patient's blood: positive during acute disease; continued presence indicates carrier state
HBsAb	Antibody to HBsAg; provides immunity to hepatitis B
HBcAg	Antigen associated with core of HBV
HBcAb	Antibody to HBcAg; positive during window phase; IgM HBcAb is an indicator of recent disease
HBeAg	A second, different antigenic determinant on the HBV core; important indicator of transmissibility
HBeAb	Antibody to e antigen; indicates low transmissibility
Delta agent	Small RNA virus with HBsAg envelope; defective virus that replicates only in HBV-infected cells

Table 19-4. Hepatitis A Serology

Acute or recent infection	anti-HAV IgM
Prior infection or immunization	anti-HAV IgG

Table 19-5. Hepatitis B Serology

	HBsAg HBeAg* HBV-DNA	HBcAb IgM	HBcAb IgG	HBsAb IgG
Acute infection	+	+	−	−
Window period	−	+	−	−
Prior infection	−	−	+	+
Immunization	−	−	−	+
Chronic infection	+	−	+	−

*HBeAg—correlates with viral proliferation and infectivity

AMEBIC LIVER ABSCESS

Amebic liver abscess is rare in the United States except in those who have traveled to/from tropical areas with poor sanitation. The causative organism is *Entamoeba histolytica*. The presentation, which may occur years after travel, includes RUQ pain, fever, and hepatic tenderness.

Detection of a space-occupying liver lesion with positive serology is diagnostic. Treatment is antibiotics. Drainage is rarely necessary.

ALCOHOLIC LIVER DISEASE

Fatty change (steatosis) is reversible with abstinence. The gross appearance is of an enlarged, yellow, greasy liver. Microscopically, the liver initially shows centrilobular macrovesicular steatosis (reversible) that can eventually progress to fibrosis around the central vein (irreversible).

Alcoholic hepatitis is an acute illness that usually follows a heavy drinking binge. Some patients have no symptoms and others develop RUQ pain, hepatomegaly, jaundice, malaise, anorexia, or even fulminant liver failure.

Microscopically, the liver shows hepatocyte swelling (ballooning) and necrosis, Mallory bodies (cytokeratin intermediate filaments), neutrophils, fatty change, and eventual fibrosis around the central vein. The prognosis can be poor, since each episode has a 20% risk of death, and repeated episodes increase the risk of developing cirrhosis.

Alcoholic cirrhosis develops in 15% of alcoholics, and is typically a micronodular or Laennec cirrhosis.

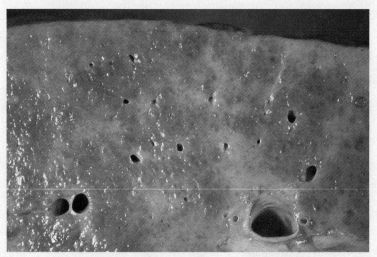

© cdc.gov.

Figure 19-1. Alcoholic Cirrhosis, Liver

METABOLIC LIVER DISEASE

Wilson disease (hepatolenticular degeneration) is a genetic disorder of copper metabolism resulting in the accumulation of toxic levels of copper in various organs. It affects the liver (fatty change, chronic hepatitis, and micronodular cirrhosis), cornea (Kayser-Fleischer rings [copper deposition in Descemet's membrane]), and brain (neurological and psychiatric manifestations, movement disorder).

Diagnosis is established by demonstrating decreased serum ceruloplasmin levels, increased tissue copper levels (liver biopsy), and increased urinary copper excretion. Treatment includes copper chelators (D-penicillamine); liver transplantation is curative.

The disease is autosomal recessive, and the WD gene (*ATP7B* on chromosome 13) codes for a hepatocyte canalicular copper-transporting ATPase. Damage to the gene leads to a decreased biliary excretion of copper. Wilson disease presents in children or adolescents with liver disease.

Hemochromatosis is a disease of increased levels of iron, leading to tissue injury. **Hereditary (primary) hemochromatosis** is a recessive disorder of the *HFE* gene on chromosome 6p. The most common mutation of the *HFE* gene is the C282Y mutation, which increases small intestine absorption of iron. **Secondary hemochromatosis** can follow transfusions for chronic anemias. Hemochromatosis affects 5 times as many males as females, and the disease is common in people of Northern European descent.

Hemochromatosis can cause micronodular cirrhosis and hepatocellular carcinoma (200 times the normal risk ratio); secondary diabetes mellitus; hyperpigmented skin ("bronzing"); congestive heart failure and cardiac arrhythmias; and hypogonadism. Diagnosis is established by demonstrating markedly elevated serum iron and ferritin or increased tissue iron levels (Prussian blue stain) on liver biopsy. Treatment is phlebotomy.

α-1-antitrypsin deficiency is an autosomal recessive disorder characterized by production of defective α-1-antitrypsin (α1-AT), which accumulates in hepatocytes and causes liver damage and low serum levels of α1-AT.

α1-AT is produced by the *SERPINA1* gene (chromosome 14); >75 gene variants are described. Normal individuals are homozygous *PiMM*. Heterozygotes have intermediate levels of the enzyme. Homozygous *PiZZ* have severe reductions (10% of normal) in enzyme levels.

α-1-antitrypsin deficiency affects the liver (micronodular cirrhosis and an increased risk of hepatocellular carcinoma) and lungs (panacinar emphysema). Microscopically, PAS positive, eosinophilic cytoplasmic globules are found in hepatocytes. Treatment includes smoking abstinence/cessation to prevent emphysema; liver transplantation is curative.

In a Nutshell

Protease-Antiprotease Imbalance

α-1-antitrypsin is an important protease inhibitor.

- Responsible for inhibiting neutrophil elastase
- Inhibits trypsin, chymotrypsin, and bacterial proteases

Reye syndrome is a rare, potentially fatal disease that occurs in young children with viral illness (varicella or influenza) treated with aspirin. The disease mechanism is unknown; mitochondrial injury and dysfunction play an important role. Reye causes hepatic fatty change (microvesicular steatosis) and cerebral edema/encephalopathy. There is complete recovery in 75% of patients, but those that do not recover may experience permanent neurologic deficits. Coma and death may result. Treatment is supportive.

Nonalcoholic fatty liver disease is a disease of lipids accumulating in hepatocytes that is not associated with heavy alcohol use. It occurs equally in men and women, and is strongly associated with obesity, hyperinsulinemia, insulin resistance, and type 2 diabetes mellitus.

The pathogenesis involves lipid accumulation in hepatocytes that can progress to steatohepatitis (NASH—nonalcoholic steatohepatitis) and finally cirrhosis. Nonalcoholic fatty liver disease is a diagnosis of exclusion.

HEMODYNAMIC LIVER DISEASES

Budd-Chiari syndrome (hepatic vein thrombosis) refers to occlusion of the hepatic vein by a thrombus, often resulting in death. While a few cases are idiopathic, more often there is an underlying process predisposing for the thrombosis e.g., polycythemia vera, pregnancy, oral contraceptives, paroxysmal nocturnal hemoglobinuria, or hepatocellular carcinoma. It presents with abdominal pain, hepatomegaly, ascites, jaundice, splenomegaly, and in some cases, death.

The initial diagnostic test is ultrasonography. Microscopically, the liver shows centrilobular congestion and necrosis. In the chronic form, fibrosis develops. Treatment includes supportive care and treatment of the underlying condition. Some patients require lifelong anticoagulation.

Chronic passive congestion of the liver refers to a "backup of blood" into the liver, usually due to right-sided heart failure. Grossly, the liver characteristically has a nutmeg pattern of alternating dark (congested central areas) and light (portal tract areas) liver parenchyma. Microscopically, the liver shows centrilobular congestion.

Complications include centrilobular necrosis, which is an ischemic necrosis of centrilobular hepatocytes. Long-standing congestion can lead to centrilobular fibrosis, which can eventually become cardiac cirrhosis (sclerosis).

LIVER TUMORS

Hemangioma is the most common primary tumor of the liver, mostly affecting women. It is a benign vascular tumor that typically forms a subcapsular, red, spongy mass. It is often asymptomatic and detected incidentally on CT or MRI. Resection is rarely indicated, and liver biopsy carries the risk of bleeding.

Hepatocellular adenoma (HCA) affects young women and is related to oral contraceptive use. Half of cases are asymptomatic. Symptoms include abdominal pain or spontaneous intraperitoneal hemorrhage (25% of cases). Due to the risk of transformation to HCC, resection is often recommended.

There are 3 subtypes of HCA:

- **H-HCA** is a solitary or multiple tan steatotic nodule with rare transformation into HCC
    - Mutation of hepatocyte nuclear factor 1
- **b-HCA** can resemble HCC histologically and transforms to HCC in some cases
    - Was named for the associated beta-catenin mutations
- **I-HCA** shows inflammatory infiltrates, sinusoidal dilatation, and thick-walled arteries
    - Acute inflammatory markers are elevated; malignant transformation occurs less frequently

Focal nodular hyperplasia is subcapsular lesion often discovered incidentally by the radiologist. Laboratory values are generally normal. It is a nodular proliferation in response to a vascular anomaly. There is a central, stellate scar. Excision is generally not required due to the characteristic appearance on imaging.

Hepatocellular carcinoma (HCC) is the most common primary malignant tumor of the liver in adults. The incidence is higher in Asia and Japan than in the United States. Risk factors include cirrhosis, hepatitis B and C viruses, alcohol, aflatoxin B1.

HCC has a tendency for hematogenous spread and invasion of portal and hepatic veins. The tumor marker is α-fetoprotein (AFP).

The fibrolamellar variant affects younger age, has fibrous bands, and has a better prognosis.

Angiosarcoma is a rare, fatal tumor associated with exposure to vinyl chloride.

Hepatoblastoma is the most common hepatic malignancy in infants and children. Lobectomy is the standard of care. Histology shows immature precursor cells.

Metastatic tumors are the most common tumors found within the liver. Common primary sites include the colon, breast, and lung. Metastatic tumors tend to occur as multiple well-circumscribed masses.

Chapter Summary

- Jaundice produces yellow skin and sclera and occurs with bilirubin levels
  >2–3 mg/dL.

- Increased red blood cell turnover, due to either hemolytic anemia or ineffective
  erythropoiesis, causes an unconjugated hyperbilirubinemia and may predispose
  for pigmented bilirubinate gallstones.

- Physiologic jaundice of the newborn is a transient unconjugated
  hyperbilirubinemia due to the immaturity of the liver.

- Gilbert syndrome and Crigler-Najjar syndrome are inherited causes of
  unconjugated hyperbilirubinemia due to bilirubin glucuronosyltransferase
  deficiency or absence. Gilbert disease is completely benign. Type I Crigler-Najjar
  syndrome is treated with liver transplant. The more mild type II Crigler-Najjar
  syndrome causes jaundice.

- Dubin-Johnson syndrome is a benign autosomal recessive disorder that causes
  conjugated hyperbilirubinemia secondary to decreased bilirubin excretion due
  to a defect in the canalicular transport protein. A distinctive feature of Dubin-
  Johnson syndrome is black pigmentation of the liver. Rotor syndrome is similar to
  Dubin-Johnson syndrome but does not have the liver pigmentation.

- Biliary tract obstruction can be due to gallstones, tumors, stricture, or parasite,
  and can present with jaundice, pruritus, abdominal pain, bilirubinuria, and
  pale stools.

- Primary biliary cirrhosis is a chronic liver disease of probable autoimmune
  etiology that is characterized by inflammation and granulomatous destruction of
  intrahepatic bile ducts.

- Primary sclerosing cholangitis is a chronic liver disease characterized by
  segmental inflammation and fibrosing destruction of intrahepatic bile ducts.

- Cirrhosis is an end-stage liver disease characterized by disruption of the liver
  architecture by bands of fibrosis that divide the liver into nodules of regenerating
  liver parenchyma.

- Acute viral hepatitis can be caused by any of the hepatitis viruses. Chronic viral
  hepatitis can be caused by hepatitis viruses B, C, and D.

- Hepatitis A virus is spread by the fecal-oral route and usually causes mild acute
  hepatitis.

- Hepatitis B virus is spread parenterally, sexually, and vertically (mother to child)
  and may cause acute hepatitis, chronic hepatitis, cirrhosis, and hepatocellular
  carcinoma.

- Hepatitis C is spread by the parenteral and sexual routes, and may cause acute
  hepatitis, chronic hepatitis, cirrhosis, and hepatocellular carcinoma.

- Hepatitis D is a defective virus that requires hepatitis B as a coinfection or
  superinfection to produce severe disease, which may take the form of acute
  hepatitis, chronic hepatitis, or cirrhosis.

- Hepatitis E virus is spread by the fecal-oral route and causes acute hepatitis that
  may be severe in infected pregnant women.

(continued)

Chapter Summary *(cont'd)*

- Amebic liver abscess is due to infection with *Entamoeba histolytica* and requires antibiotics for therapy.

- Alcoholic liver disease can produce steatosis, alcoholic hepatitis, or alcoholic cirrhosis.

- Wilson disease is a genetic disorder of copper metabolism resulting in accumulation of toxic levels of copper leading to liver disease, Kayser-Fleischer corneal rings, and neurologic and psychiatric manifestations.

- Hemochromatosis is characterized by increased levels of iron that can deposit into tissues, leading to cirrhosis, hepatocellular carcinoma, DM, bronze skin, congestive heart failure, cardiac arrhythmias, and hypogonadism.

- Alpha-1-antitrypsin deficiency is an autosomal recessive disorder characterized by production of defective alpha-1-antitrypsin, which accumulates in hepatocytes and causes liver damage and low serum levels of alpha-1-antitrypsin.

- Reye syndrome is a potentially fatal disease that occurs in young children with viral illnesses treated with aspirin. It can cause liver steatosis and cerebral edema.

- Nonalcoholic fatty liver disease is highly associated with obesity and type 2 DM leading to hepatic lipid accumulation, nonalcoholic steatohepatitis, and can progress to cirrhosis in 10–30% of patients.

- Budd-Chiari syndrome is occlusion of the hepatic vein by a thrombus, often resulting in death.

- Chronic passive congestion of the liver is a "backup of blood" into the liver, usually due to right-sided heart failure, and, in long-standing cases, may lead to cirrhosis (sclerosis).

- Benign tumors of the liver include hemangiomas and hepatic adenomas. Malignant tumors include hepatocellular carcinoma, cholangiocarcinoma, hepatoblastoma, angiosarcoma, and metastatic tumors.

- Metastatic tumors are more common than primary tumors.

Central Nervous System Pathology

20

Learning Objectives

❏ Solve problems concerning infections across the blood brain barrier

❏ Answer questions about cerebrovascular disease, CNS trauma, and brain herniation

❏ Use knowledge of developmental abnormalities and perinatal brain injury

❏ Explain information related to demyelinating disorders

❏ Solve problems concerning degenerative and dementing disorders

❏ Describe CNS tumors

INFECTIONS

Meningitis is inflammation of the 2 inner meningeal layers, the pia and the arachnoid.

Acute aseptic (viral) meningitis is caused by leptomeningeal inflammation due to viruses (enterovirus most frequent); the inflammation produces a lymphocytic infiltration of leptomeninges and superficial cortex. Patients present with fever, signs of meningeal irritation, and depressed consciousness. Mortality is low. Viral meningitis carries a better prognosis than bacterial meningitis.

Acute viral meningitis is the most common neurologic symptom associated with primary HIV infection; it presents around the time of seroconversion with an acute confusional state. Symptoms resolve after 1 month with supportive care.

Acute purulent (bacterial) meningitis is a purulent leptomeningeal inflammation.

- *Streptococcus pneumoniae* is the most common cause of meningitis in infants, young children, and adults.

- Neonates are infected most frequently with group B streptococci but *Eschericia coli* causes a greater number of fatalities.

- *Neisseria meningitidis* is seen in teens and young adults and is often associated with a maculopapular rash.

- The incidence of *Listeria monocytogenes* increases after age 50. This pathogen also tends to infect people with poor cell-mediated immunity.

The leptomeninges are opaque on gross examination. Microscopic examination shows neutrophilic infiltration of the leptomeninges, extending variably to cortex.

Diffuse cerebral edema carries a risk of fatal herniations. The classic triad of bacterial meningitis is fever, nuchal rigidity, and altered mental status.

Mycobacterial meningoencephalitis can be caused by *Mycobacterium tuberculosis* or atypical mycobacteria. It occurs in patients who have reactivation of latent infection and immunocompromised patients such as AIDS patients (*Mycobacterium avium-intracellulare*). Diagnosis requires microscopy/culture of large volumes of CSF. MRI is the imaging test of choice and shows basal meningeal enhancement and hydrocephalus. It usually involves the basal surface of the brain, and may cause characteristic tuberculomas within the brain and dura mater.

Table 20-1. CSF Parameters in Different Forms of Meningitis

Condition	Cells/µL	Glucose (µg/dL)	Proteins (mg/dL)	Pressure (mm H$_2$O)
Normal values	<5 lymphocytes	45–85 (50–70% glycemia)	15–45	70–180
Purulent (bacterial)	Up to 90,000 neutrophils	Decreased (<45)	Increased (>50)	Markedly elevated
Aseptic (viral)	100–1,000 most lymphocytes	Normal or decreased	Normal or slightly increased (>50)	Normal or slightly elevated
Granulomatous (mycobacterial/fungal)	100–1,000 most lymphocytes	Decreased (<45)	Increased (>50)	Moderately elevated

The **viral encephalitides** have common features of perivascular cuffs, microglial nodules, neuron loss, and neuronophagia. Clinical manifestations are variable, and can include mental status change, fever, and headache, often progressing to coma.

- Arthropod-borne forms can be due to St. Louis, Eastern and Western equine, and Venezuelan encephalitides.

- Herpes simplex type 1 produces a characteristic **hemorrhagic necrosis of temporal lobes**. Cowdry type A bodies are intranuclear inclusions seen in neurons and glial cells.

- **Rabies** has characteristic Negri bodies in the cytoplasm of hippocampal and Purkinje cells.

- **HIV encephalopathy** shows histopathology of microglial nodules and diagnostic multinucleated giant cells. Spinal involvement leads to vacuolar myelopathy, which is similar to vitamin B12 deficiency–associated subacute combined degeneration.

- **Progressive multifocal leukoencephalopathy (PML)** is caused by JC polyomavirus. It occurs in immunocompromised patients and patients taking immunomodulatory therapies. Neurologic symptoms are varied and include impairment of cognition and motor function. There is no specific antiviral drug and mortality is high. Tissue sections show areas of demyelination and enlarged oligodendrocytes.

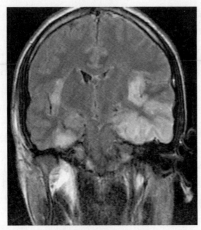

© Paul J. Shogan, National Capital Consortium.
Used with permission.

Figure 20-1. CT Scan Showing Edema of Bilateral Temporal Lobes, Related to Herpes Simplex Encephalitis

Fungal meningoencephalitides. *Candida, Aspergillus, Cryptococcus,* and *Mucor* species are the most frequent agents. *Aspergillus* and *Mucor* have a marked tropism for blood vessels, which leads to vasculitis, rupture of blood vessels, and hemorrhage. *Cryptococcus* causes diffuse meningoencephalitis, which leads to invasion of the brain through the Virchow-Robin space (a continuation of the subarachnoid space around blood vessels entering the neuropil) and soap bubble lesions.

Toxoplasmosis is caused by the protozoan parasite *Toxoplasma gondii.* It is common in AIDS patients, and the condition causes cerebral abscess with central necrosis and chronic inflammation. MRI/CT scan shows a characteristic ring-enhancing lesion.

Cerebral abscess can occur as a result of either hematogenous dissemination or direct spread from contiguous foci. **Systemic predisposing conditions** include acute bacterial endocarditis, cyanotic heart disease (right-to-left shunt), and chronic pulmonary abscesses. **Local predisposing conditions** include mastoiditis, paranasal sinusitis, acute otitis, open fracture, and previous neurosurgery. CT/MRI scan characteristically shows a ring-enhancing lesion. Clinical manifestations include signs of increased intracranial pressure (headache, vomiting, and papilledema). Focal neurological deficits vary depending on the site of lesion.

Subacute sclerosing panencephalitis is a rare complication of measles (rubeola) virus infection. Persistent immune-resistant measles virus infection causes slow-virus encephalitis. The typical scenario is a child who had measles age <2 and then 6–15 years later develops progressive mental deterioration with seizures. Subacute sclerosing panencephalitis may be fatal in 1–2 years once it develops.

Creutzfeldt-Jakob disease (CJD) is the most common human transmissible spongiform encephalopathy due to a prion (a protein with the capacity to be an infectious agent) that can change the conformation of normal prion protein(s). This can lead to rapidly progressive dementia, memory loss, personality changes, and hallucinations.

- The **prion protein** (PrP) is a 30-kD protein normally present in neurons. It is encoded by a single-exon gene on chromosome 20. Its normal conformation is an α-helix: PrP^c. In disease states, PrP^c changes to a β-pleated sheet conformation: PrP^{sc}. A low rate of spontaneous change results in sporadic cases of CJD. Mutations of PrP result in hereditary cases of CJD. PrP^{sc} facilitates conformational change of other PrP^c molecules into PrP^{sc}.

- PrP^{sc} is responsible for **cerebral pathologic changes**, characteristically resulting in spongiform change. This change is a fine vacuolization of the neuropil in the gray matter (especially cortex), which is due to large membrane-bound vacuoles within neuronal processes. There is an associated neuronal loss and astrogliosis. Kuru plaques are deposits of amyloid composed of altered PrP protein.

- About 85% of Creutzfeld-Jakob cases are sporadic, and 15% are familial. Affected patients are typically middle-aged to elderly patients who develop rapidly progressive dementia and memory loss with startle myoclonus or other involuntary movements. Typical EEG changes may be diagnostic. Death occurs within 6–12 months.

- Variant Creutzfeldt-Jacob disease occurs in younger patients and results from exposure to bovine spongiform encephalopathy.

Table 20-2. Prion Diseases

Disease	Infectious Agent	Host	Comments
Kuru	Prion	Human	Subacute spongiform encephalopathy (SSE); Fore Tribe in New Guinea; consuming infected brains
Creutzfeldt-Jakob	Prion	Human	SSE Genetic predisposition
Gerstmann-Straussler	Prion	Human	SSE
Fatal familial insomnia	Prion	Human	SSE
Scrapie	Prion	Sheep	SSE—scraping their wool off on fences

HIV-associated neurocognitive disorder (HAND) presents as cognitive decline with behavioral changes and motor symptoms. Diagnosis is based on clinical features and the exclusion of other etiologies.

CEREBROVASCULAR DISEASE

Cerebrovascular disease is the third most frequent cause of death in industrialized countries, and it is the leading cause of serious disability in the United States. Risk factors are similar to coronary artery disease.

- **Global cerebral ischemia** (diffuse ischemic encephalopathy) is caused by a fall in blood flow to the brain, due to processes such as shock, cardiac arrest, and hypotensive episodes. While the entire brain can be damaged, some regions have selective vulnerability, including Purkinje neurons, hippocampus, CA1 (Sommer sector), and pyramidal neurons of cortex. The pathology often includes infarcts in watershed areas, cortical laminar necrosis, and diffuse ischemic necrosis of neocortex. Global cerebral ischemia may lead to brain death.

Bridge to Anatomy

The brain is highly dependent on a constant supply of oxygen and glucose from the cerebral arteries, which have collateral blood flow at the circle of Willis.

- **Transient ischemic attack** (TIA) is due to small platelet thrombi or athero-emboli and is characteristically reversible, with symptoms lasting less than 24 hours.

- **Stroke** can be due to infarction (85% of all stroke cases) or hemorrhage (15% of all stroke cases).

- Infarction causes 85% of all stroke cases.

  ○ Can be due to **thrombotic occlusion** in the setting of atherosclerosis of the cerebral arteries; the thrombotic infarction is characteristically an anemic (white) infarct.

  ○ Can be due to **embolic occlusion**, most often due to thromboemboli from cardiac chambers and less frequently due to atheroemboli. Embolic infarction produces a hemorrhagic infarct. Small-vessel disease is a cause of small, lacunar infarcts or lacunae, and it is related to hypertension, resulting in hyaline arteriolosclerosis.

  ○ Atherosclerotic aneuryms are fusiform, involve the basilar artery, and present with infarction.

  ○ The pathology (i.e., morphological features of brain infarcts) of infarction is illustrated in Table 20-3. Clinical manifestations depend on the affected arterial distribution.

Clinical Correlate

Strokes frequently occur in the middle cerebral artery territory.

Table 20-3. Gross and Microscopic Changes Associated with Cerebral Infarction

Time	Gross Changes	Microscopic Changes
0–12 h	No changes	Minimal or no changes
12–24 h	Minimal changes	Red (hypereosinophilic) neurons with pyknotic nuclei
24–48 h	Indistinct gray-white matter junction	Neutrophilic infiltration
2–10 d	Friable tissue with marked edema	Histiocytic infiltration; neurons disappear
2–3 wk	Tissue liquefies	Liquefactive necrosis; histiocytes filled with products of myelin breakdown
3 wk–mo	Fluid-filled cavity demarcated by gliotic scar	Fluid-filled cavity; reactive astrocytes and lipid-laden macrophages
Years	Old cyst surrounded by gliotic scar	Astrogliosis surrounding a cyst

Note: Hemorrhagic infarct leads to erythrocyte degradation and hemosiderin deposition.

Hemorrhage causes 15% of strokes.

- **Intracerebral (intraparenchymal) hemorrhage** causes severe headache, frequent nausea/vomiting, steady progression of symptoms over 15–20 minutes, and coma. It is most frequently due to hypertension, and in those instances, it most commonly involves the basal ganglia, cerebellum, pons, and centrum semiovale.

Other causes include vascular malformations (especially arteriovenous malformations), cerebral amyloid angiopathy, neoplasms, vasculitides, abnormal hemostasis, hematological malignancies, infections, and diabetes mellitus.

- **Subarachnoid hemorrhage** is most frequently caused by ruptured berry aneurysm. Less frequent causes include extension of an intracerebral or subdural hematoma, vascular malformations, trauma, abnormal hemostasis, and tumors. Subarachnoid hemorrhage causes sudden headache ("worst headache of my life"), nuchal rigidity, neurological deficits on one side, and stupor.

  ○ **Berry aneurysms** are thin-walled saccular outpouchings, consisting of intima and adventitia only. They are the most frequent cause of subarachnoid hemorrhage. The most frequent sites are the anterior circle of Willis at branching points. Rupture is precipitated by a sudden increase in blood pressure; the prognosis after rupture is that one-third die, one-third recover, and one-third rebleed. The pathogenesis involves a congenital focal weakness of vessel media that is not identifiable at birth. Associated disorders include Marfan syndrome, Ehlers-Danlos type 4, and adult polycystic kidney disease. Hypertension and cigarette smoking predispose to formation.

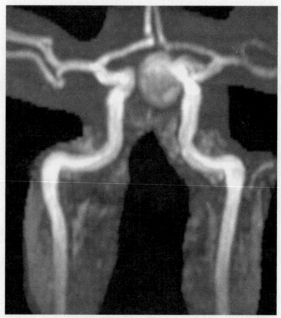

© Charles Gould, National Capital Consortium.
Used with permission.

Figure 20-2. Large Berry Aneurysm Seen on Angiography of Circle of Willis

CNS TRAUMA AND HERNIATIONS

Cranial Cavity and Brain

Concussion is mild traumatic brain injury with a transient loss of brain function. The trauma is commonly due to a change in the momentum of the head (impact against a rigid surface). Concussion causes loss of consciousness and reflexes, temporary respiratory arrest, and amnesia for the event. The pathogenesis is uncertain. Parenchymal injuries may or may not be evident at autopsy.

Contusions are bruises of the brain tissue. Common sites of injury include crests of orbital gyri in frontal and temporal poles, in addition to *coup* (site of injury) and *contrecoup* (site diametrically opposite) injuries. Coup and contrecoup develop when the head is mobile at the time of impact.

- **Acute contusion** is characterized by hemorrhage of brain tissue in a wedge-shaped area.

- **Subacute contusion** shows necrosis and liquefaction of brain.

- **Remote contusion** causes a depressed area of cortex with yellow discoloration ("*plaque jaune*").

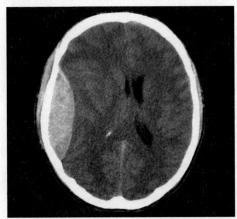

© Andrew Mullins, National Naval Medical Center.
Used with permission.

Figure 20-3. Epidural Hematoma

Epidural hematoma (*See* Anatomy Lecture Notes.)

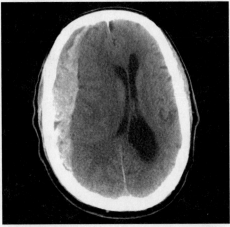

© Brendan T. Doherty, National Capital Consortium.
Used with permission.

Figure 20-4. Subdural Hematoma

Subdural hematoma is caused by the rupture of bridging veins (from the cerebral convexities to the sagittal sinus); it is usually traumatic in older individuals. Predisposing conditions include brain atrophy (due simply to aging) and abnormal hemostatis. Symptoms include headache, drowsiness, focal neurological deficits, and sometimes dementia. It recurs frequently.

Diffuse axonal injury refers to damage to axons at nodes of Ranvier with impairment of axoplasmic flow. It causes coma after trauma without evidence of direct parenchymal injuries. There is a poor prognosis, related to duration of coma. The injury to the white matter is due to acceleration/deceleration forces with shearing of axons.

The histopathology shows axonal swellings appreciable in the white matter. It is diffuse, but with a predilection for the corpus callosum, periventricular white matter, and hippocampus, as well as cerebral and cerebellar peduncles.

Spinal cord injuries are usually traumatic, due to vertebral displacement. Symptomatology depends on the interruption of ascending and descending tracts.

- Lesions to thoracic segments or below cause paraplegia.

- Lesions to cervical segments cause tetraplegia.

- Lesions above C4 cause respiratory arrest due to paralysis of the diaphragm.

Chronic traumatic encephalopathy is a neurodegenerative disorder that occurs years or decades after a sports career with repetitive brain trauma. Neuropathological changes include neurofibrillary tangles, cerebellar atrophy and gliosis, hypopigmentation of the substantia nigra, and cavum septum pellucidum.

Cerebral Herniations

Subfalcine (cingulate gyrus) herniation occurs when the cingulate gyrus is displaced underneath the falx to the opposite side. Compression of the anterior cerebral artery can occur.

Transtentorial (uncal) herniation occurs when the uncus of the temporal lobe is displaced over the free edge of the tentorium. Clinical features include compression of the third nerve, ipsilateral pupillary dilatation, and infarction of the tissue supplied by the posterior cerebral artery. Advanced stages of transtentorial herniation can cause Duret hemorrhages within the central pons and midbrain.

Cerebellar tonsillar herniation occurs when there is displacement of cerebellar tonsils through the foramen magnum. Compression of the medulla may lead to cardiorespiratory arrest.

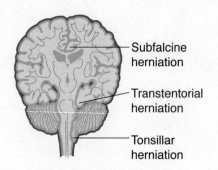

Subfalcine herniation

Transtentorial herniation

Tonsillar herniation

Cerebral Herniations

DEVELOPMENTAL ABNORMALITIES AND PERINATAL BRAIN INJURY

Neural tube defects are the most common developmental central nervous system abnormalities. They result from defective closure of the neural tube, and they tend to occur at the 2 extremities of the neuraxis. Folate deficiency is involved in the pathogenesis.

- **Anencephaly** is the absence of cranial vault. It is incompatible with life; babies die soon after birth.

- **Neural tube defects of the spinal cord** may take a variety of forms. Significant defects lead to paraplegia and urinary incontinence from birth.

- **Spina bifida occulta** is a bony defect of the vertebral arch.
- **Meningocele** is a bony defect with outpouching of meninges.
- **Meningomyelocele** is a defective formation of the bony arch with cystic outpouching of meninges, spinal cord, and spinal roots.
- **Myelocele** is a defective bony arch with complete exposure of the spinal cord.

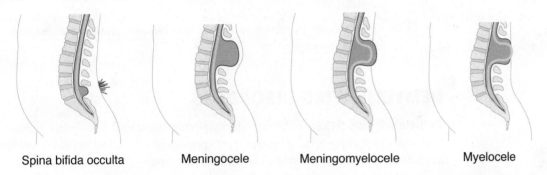

Spina bifida occulta   Meningocele   Meningomyelocele   Myelocele

Figure 20-5. Neural Tube Defects of the Spinal Cord

Syringomyelia is an ependymal-lined, CSF-filled channel parallel to and connected with the central canal in the spinal cord. (*Hydromyelia* means the central canal is dilated with CSF.) About 90% of cases are associated with Arnold-Chiari type 2; the remaining 10% are posttraumatic or associated with intraspinal tumors. *Syrinx* (the cyst) enlarges progressively and destroys the spinal parenchyma. Symptoms include paralysis and loss of sensory functions. (*See* Anatomy Lecture Notes.)

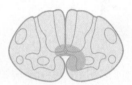

Syringomyelia

Perinatal brain injury is injury to the brain during prenatal or immediately postnatal period. This is the most common cause of cerebral palsy, and it occurs most frequently in premature babies.

- **Germinal matrix hemorrhage** is hemorrhage localized in the germinal matrix due to its fragile vessels.
- **Periventricular leukomalacia** causes infarcts in watershed areas (periventricular white matter in the fetus).
- **Multicystic encephalopathy** refers to multiple brain infarcts occurring early in pregnancy.

Fetal alcohol syndrome is characterized by structural abnormalities (microcephaly, agenesis of the corpus callosum, cerebellar hypoplasia), functional impairments including learning disabilities, and neurological impairments including epilepsy.

Cerebellar Malformations

Cerebellar malformations have chromosomal, single-gene and complex inheritance. *FOXCI* deletions and duplications are associated with cerebellar vermis hypoplasia, mega-cisterna magna and Dandy-Walker malformation, the most common human cerebellar malformation.

- **Dandy-Walker malformation** is a non-communicating hydrocephalus with dilation of the fourth ventricle and hypoplasia of the cerebellar vermis.

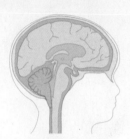

**Arnold-Chiari
Malformation**

- **Arnold-Chiari malformations**
  - **Type 1** (common) is a downward displacement of cerebellar tonsils and the medulla through the foramen magnum. This lesion is mostly asymptomatic.
  - **Type 2** is due to a faulty craniospinal junction, resulting in a small posterior fossa, with abnormal development of the cerebellar vermis and medulla leading to downward displacement. It is mostly symptomatic because of compression of the fourth ventricle with obstructive hydrocephalus.
  - Other frequently related manifestations include syringomelia and lumbar meningomyelocele.

DEMYELINATING DISORDERS

Multiple sclerosis (MS) is a chronic relapsing-remitting disorder of probable autoimmune origin characterized by recurrent episodes of demyelination in the brain (including optic nerves) and spinal cord; it results in progressive neurological deficits.

- The overall prevalence of MS is 1/1,000, with higher prevalence in northern countries.
- Those who emigrate age >15 from areas of high prevalence to areas of low prevalence maintain their original risk.
- Women have 2x the risk of men.

Genetic and environmental factors contribute to the pathogenesis. HLA DR 15 confers genetic susceptibility. Environmental factors include viral infection, vitamin D deficiency, and smoking.

- **Acute lesions** on gross examination show well-circumscribed gray lesions (plaques), with bilateral distribution that is frequently periventricular. Histology shows chronic inflammation with phagocytosis of myelin by macrophages; axons are initially preserved.
- **Chronic lesions** have no inflammation, with axons showing remyelination. Remyelination is defective because myelin sheaths are thinner with shorter internodes.

During an acute attack, nerve conduction is entirely blocked, leading to acute neurological deficits. Chronic plaques are associated with slower nerve conduction, allowing for partial recovery. Recurrent attacks cause progressive neurological deterioration.

Clinical onset is typically in decades 3–4. About 85% of cases show a relapsing-remitting course; a minority of cases show primary progressive (slow deterioration) or progressive-relapsing (slow progression punctuated by acute exacerbations) course. Recovery from each episode of demyelination occurs in weeks or months.

Early symptoms include sensory problems, paresis, and visual dysfunction. As the disease progresses, other symptoms include fatigue, bladder dysfunction, spasticity and ataxia. Neuropsychological symptoms affect 40–60% of patients.

Diagnosis of MS requires the demonstration of the dissemination of disease in space and time. Clinical history, MRI, CSF studies and electrophysiological studies are important. Treatment is immunomodulatory drugs (e.g., interferon beta), immunosuppressive therapies (e.g., mitoxantrone), and monoclonal antibodies (e.g., natalizumab). The latter is used as monotherapy in cases of relapsing MS; its use is linked to PML.

Central pontine myelinolysis (CPM) is a focal demyelination of the central area of the basis pontis. It probably derives from rapid correction of hyponatremia, and the condition is very often fatal. Patients at risk include the severely malnourished and alcoholics with liver disease.

DEGENERATIVE AND DEMENTING DISORDERS

Parkinson disease (PD) is a progressive neurodegenerative disease that involves genetic and environmental factors. The *SNCA* gene (alpha-synuclein) has been identified as a risk factor, and gene mutations and multiplications are associated with familial PD, but the majority of cases are sporadic. PD is due to loss of dopaminergic neurons in the substantia nigra, leading to tremor, rigidity, and akinesia.

- **Parkinson disease** is the idiopathic form.
- **Parkinson syndrome** is secondary to known injuries to the substantia nigra (e.g., infection, vascular condition, toxic insult).

Parkinson disease is common, affecting 2% of the population. Clinical onset is typically in decades 5–8. Loss of dopaminergic neurons is still unexplained, though theories emphasize oxidative stress. Pesticides and meperidine have been associated with increased risk, while smoking and caffeine are protective.

On gross examination there is pallor of the substantia nigra. Histology shows loss of pigmented (dopaminergic) neurons in the substantia nigra. Residual neurons show Lewy bodies, which are intracytoplasmic round eosinophilic inclusions that contain α-synuclein. Electron microscopy shows filaments most likely of cytoskeletal origin. There is also a secondary degeneration of dopaminergic axons in the striatum.

Loss of the extrapyramidal nigrostriatal pathway leads to inhibition of movement of proximal muscles and disruption of fine regulation of distal muscles. Involvement of the amygdala, cingulate gyrus and higher cortical regions causes dementia and psychosis.

About 60% of patients experience dementia 12 years after diagnosis; 50% also experience depression and psychosis. Those treated with medication (combination carbidopa and levodopa) and surgery (deep brain stimulation) will become refractory to therapy.

A clinical diagnosis is difficult to make early in disease because symptoms overlap with other conditions. Early symptoms include hyposmia, constipation, and fatigue. Key features are bradykinesia, rigidity, tremor and postural instability. Early in the disease course, a response to levodopa can help confirm the diagnosis. Imaging studies are not useful in most cases.

Huntington disease (HD) is an autosomal dominant disorder. It is characterized pathologically by the degeneration of GABAergic neurons of the caudate nucleus, and clinically by involuntary movements, cognitive decline, and behavioral changes.

- Affects those of northwestern European descent
- Has an incidence in high-prevalence regions of 1/12,000–20,000
- Gene (*HTT*), located on chromosome 4, codes for a protein called huntingtin

- Mutations due to expansion of unstable cytosine-adenine-guanine (CAG) repeats

- Shows features of anticipation and genomic imprinting

The pathophysiology is that loss of caudate nucleus GABAergic neurons removes inhibitory influences on extrapyramidal circuits, thus leading to chorea.

Clinical onset is typically in decades 3–5. The chorea is characterized by sudden, unexpected, and purposeless contractions of proximal muscles while awake. Psychiatric symptoms may predate motor symptoms. Disease progression leads to dependency and death.

Gross examination shows atrophy of the caudate nucleus with secondary ventricular dilatation. Histology shows loss of small neurons in the caudate nucleus followed by loss of the larger neurons.

A definitive diagnosis can be based on clinical symptoms with an affected parent. Otherwise, DNA determination is the gold standard. Prenatal diagnosis and pre-implantation diagnostics are available. Treatment is medical therapeutics for chorea (dopamine receptor blocking or depleting agents).

Alzheimer disease (AD) causes 60% of all cases of dementia. It is the most common cause of dementia in people age >65.

- Incidence is 2% at age 65 and doubles every 5 years

- Risk factors include aging and significant head trauma

    ○ Aluminum is an epiphenomenon, not a risk factor

- Protective factors include high level of education and smoking

About 5–10% of AD cases are hereditary, early onset, and transmitted as an autosomal dominant trait. There are 3 genes that cause autosomal dominant AD:

- *APP* (amyloid precursor protein)

- Presenilin 1 and 2 (*PSEN1* and *2*)

Carriers of *APP* and *PSEN1* mutations develop early-onset AD. Other AD susceptibility genes have been identified. *APOE* is the largest effect locus for late-onset AD.

Table 20-4. Genetics of AD

Genes causing autosomal dominant AD	• *APP* • *PSEN1* • *PSEN2* All can cause early onset disease but *PSEN2* is associated with a broad range of onset ages.

Susceptibility genes	• Apolipoprotein E gene (*APOE*)
	  • ε2 allele: associated with decreased risk
	  • ε3 allele: neutral
	  • ε4 allele: high-risk
	• *SORL1*

AD is characterized by amyloid-β deposition, neurofibrillary tangle formation, and neuronal degeneration.

- **Abnormal proteins**. Aβ amyloid is a 42-residue peptide derived from a normal transmembrane protein, the amyloid precursor protein (APP). There is also an abnormal tau (a microtubule-associated protein).

- **Neuritic plaques** have a core of Aβ amyloid and are surrounded by abnormal neurites.

- **Neurofibrillary tangles** are intraneuronal aggregates of insoluble cytoskeletal elements, mainly composed of abnormally phosphorylated tau forming paired helical filaments.

- **Cerebral amyloid angiopathy** is accumulation of Aβ amyloid within the media of small and medium-size intracortical and leptomeningeal arteries; it may occur by itself and cause intracerebral hemorrhage.

- Additional changes include granulovacuolar degeneration and Hirano bodies, which develop in the hippocampus and are less significant diagnostically.

Affected areas are involved in learning and memory. Lesions involve the neocortex, hippocampus, and several subcortical nuclei including forebrain cholinergic nuclei (i.e., basal nucleus of Meynert). The earliest and most severely affected are the hippocampus and temporal lobe. Small numbers of neuritic plaques and neurofibrillary tangles also form in intellectually normal aging persons.

Macroscopic changes include atrophy of affected regions, producing brains that are smaller (atrophic), with thinner gyri and wider sulci. Hippocampi and temporal lobes are markedly atrophic.

Clinical manifestations have insidious onset, typically beginning in decades 7–8. They include progressive memory impairment, especially related to recent events; alterations in mood and behavior; progressive disorientation; and aphasia (loss of language skills) and apraxia (loss of learned motor skills). Within 5–10 years patients become mute and bedridden.

No effective treatment is available for AD but there is mild improvement with inhibitors of acetylcholinesterase (e.g., tacrine).

Lewy body dementia is a progressive brain disease associated with the formation of Lewy bodies in neurons involving neocortex and subcortical nuclei. The etiopathogenesis is obscure, with no known risk factors; it is the second leading cause of degenerative dementia in the elderly.

The histopathological hallmark is the Lewy body. Neuron loss accompanies Lewy body formation. Sites involved include the neocortex (especially the limbic system and cingulate gyrus), and subcortical nuclei, including basal nucleus of Meynert, amygdala, and substantia nigra.

The involvement of the neocortex and substantia nigra is responsible for cognitive deterioration and parkinsonism. Clinical manifestations include memory loss, parkinsonism, and visual hallucinations. There is a possible treatment benefit from cholinesterase inhibitors.

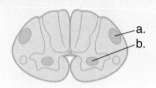

ALS
a. Primary lateral sclerosis (corticospinal tract)
b. Progressive spinal muscular atrophy (ventral horn)

Amyotrophic lateral sclerosis (ALS) is the most common adult-onset, progressive motor neuron disease.

The clinical diagnosis is supported by a biopsy of muscles. The etiopathogenesis is obscure; 5–10% of cases are hereditary, and a small number are caused by mutation of the gene encoding zinc-copper superoxide dismutase on chromosome 21.

- **Loss of upper motor neurons** produces hyperreflexia and spasticity. In some cases, involvement of cranial nerve nuclei also occurs.

- **Loss of lower motor neurons** produces weakness, atrophy, and fasciculations.

There is no cure for ALS. Ultimately, involvement of respiratory muscles will lead to death.

Friedreich ataxia is an autosomal recessive disorder which leads to degeneration of nerve tissue in the spinal cord, especially those sensory neurons connected to the cerebellum affecting muscle movement of the arms and legs. Onset is early childhood.

Friedreich ataxia is caused by the expansion of an unstable triplet nucleotide repeat (GAA repeats in the first intron) in the frataxin gene on chromosome 9. The frataxin protein is essential for mitochondrial function by helping in mitochondrial iron regulation; in the absence of frataxin, mitochondrial iron builds up, leading to free radical damage and mitochondrial dysfunction.

Clinical manifestations include gait ataxia, dysarthria, hand clumsiness, loss of sense of position, impaired vibratory sensation, and loss of tendon reflexes. There is an increased incidence of heart disorders and diabetes. Patients become wheelchair-bound by age 5.

Wilson disease (*See* Liver Pathology chapter.)

Acute intermittent porphyria is an autosomal dominant defect in porphyrin metabolism with deficient uroporphyrinogen synthase. Both porphobilinogen and aminolevulinic acid are increased. Urine is initially colorless but on exposure to light turns dark red. Patients may develop recurrent severe abdominal pain, psychosis, neuropathy, and dementia.

Vitamin B12 deficiency causes megaloblastic anemia, demyelination of the spinal cord posterior columns and lateral corticospinal tracts (subacute combined degeneration of the spinal tract). It also causes dementia and peripheral neuropathy.

Alcohol abuse causes generalized cortical and cerebellar atrophy, as well as Wernicke-Korsakoff syndrome. The neurologic disease is usually related to thiamine deficiency. There can be hemorrhages in the mamillary bodies and the walls of the third and fourth ventricles. Neuronal loss and gliosis may be prominent.

- **Wernicke encephalopathy** has reversible confusion, ataxia, and nystagmus.

- **Korsakoff psychosis** is more severe and has irreversible anterograde and retrograde amnesia.

- **Central pontine myelinolysis** may cause death.

CNS TUMORS

CNS tumors account for 20% of all pediatric tumors. Most pediatric tumors mainly arise in the posterior fossa, while adult tumors arise in the supratentorial region. Factors determining prognosis and response to therapy include the following:

- Age
- Tumor location
- Grade
- Extent of surgical resection
- Molecular subgroupings

The World Health Organization (WHO) grading system assigns grades I–IV, with grade IV tumors the most aggressive. While grade IV glioblastoma patients usually succumb to disease within a year, other patients with treatable grade IV tumors may survive 5 years. Metastasis of CNS tumors is rare.

Table 20-5. Primary Versus Metastatic (CNS) Tumors

Primary	Metastatic
Poorly circumscribed	Well circumscribed
Usually single	Often multiple
Location varies according to specific type	Location typically at the junction between gray and white matter

Tumors of Neuroepithelial Tissue

Tumors of neuroepithelial tissue are categorized as **astrocytic** tumors, **oligodendroglial** tumors, **ependymal** tumors, and **embryonal** tumors (further broken down as **medulloblastoma** or **CNS primitive neuroectodermal tumor**).

Astrocytoma originates from astrocytes and exhibits fibrillary background, immunoreactivity for glial fibrillary acidic protein (GFAP), and diffuse (ill-demarcated) pattern of growth.

- **Pilocytic astrocytoma** is a well-differentiated, benign astrocytic tumor that arises throughout the neuraxis; it is common in children and young adults. It is the most common benign CNS tumor in children.
- Sites of involvement include posterior fossa (cerebellum) and diencephalon
    - Radiographically, most show cystic lesion with a mural nodule
    - Histology shows spindly neoplastic astrocytes with long bipolar processes
    - Rosenthal fibers are thick, corkscrew-like eosinophilic structures that derive from hypertrophic processes of astrocytes
    - Posterior fossa tumors have favorable prognosis
    - Activating mutations in *BRAF* are common

- **Fibrillary (diffuse) astrocytoma** is a low-grade tumor that arises in the cerebral hemisphere of young to middle-aged adults and the brainstem of children.

    ◦ IDH1 (immunostain) is positive.

- **Anaplastic astrocytoma** is cellular, pleomorphic and mitotically active.

- **Glioblastoma** is the most common CNS primary malignancy in adults.

    ◦ Histology shows necrosis and/or vascular proliferation in addition to features seen in anaplastic astrocytoma.

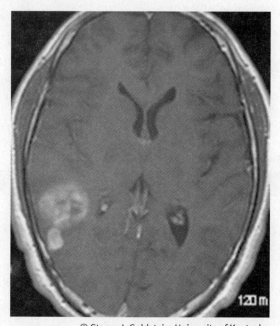

© Steven J. Goldstein, University of Kentucky.
Used with permission.

Figure 20-6. White Mass in the Cerebral Cortex Showing a Glioblastoma Multiforme

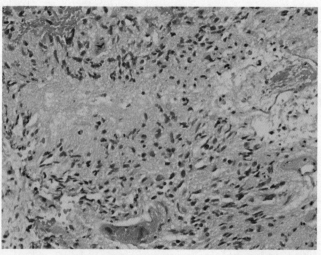

© Gregg Barré, M.D.
Used with permission.

Figure 20-7. Glioblastoma with Necrosis

The prognosis of astrocytomas varies.

- Well-differentiated astrocytomas grow slowly; affect younger patients.

- Anaplastic astrocytomas and glioblastoma are aggressive; affect older patients; median survival for glioblastoma is 15 months.

Oligodendroglioma occurs more often in adults than in children. Its cortical location may cause seizures. Histologically, perinuclear halos are a fixation artifact that is not seen on frozen section. This tumor is slow-growing. Tumors with deletions of 1p and 19q respond well to therapy.

Ependymoma is typically located in the fourth ventricle in children, where it presents with obstructive hydrocephalus. In adults the spinal cord is the most common site. Pseudorosettes are a helpful diagnostic feature on microscopic study. Multifocality in the spinal cord is associated with NF2. The prognosis depends on tumor location and adequacy of resection.

Embryonal (primitive) tumors are a group of small round cell tumors that occur predominantly in children. In the cerebellum, they are called medulloblastoma.

- Medulloblastoma is the most common malignant brain tumor in children.

- Molecular subgroupings are proving useful for prognosis; Wnt subgroup has the best prognosis.

Tumors of Cranial and Paraspinal Nerves

Schwannoma originates from Schwann cells of cranial or spinal nerves. The most frequent location is on CN 8 at the cerebellopontine angle (CPA). Schwannoma manifests characteristically with unilateral loss of hearing and tinnitus. The prognosis is good after surgical resection.

- Has spindly cells arranged in hypercellular Antoni A areas; alternating hypocellular Antoni B areas; and *Verocay bodies*, parallel rows of neoplastic Schwann cells.

- Neoplastic cells are immunoreactive for S-100.

Tumors of the Meninges

Meningioma is a tumor that originates from meningothelial cells of the arachnoid. It is common in adults (women > men) and rare in children. It is a dura-based mass that can recur if the brain has been invaded, but invasion is unusual. It has varied clinical features but commonly presents with headache, seizures, and neurological deficits.

- Histology shows cellular whorls and psammoma bodies. Many patterns are seen; the syncytial pattern is common.

- Abnormalities of chromosome 22 are sometimes present.

- Multiple meningiomas occur in NF2 patients.

The prognosis of meningioma is good, though tumors in some locations may not be amenable to complete resection.

Note

Glioblastoma multiforme has a tendency to cross the midline by involving the corpus callosum ("butterfly glioma").

Note

Bilateral acoustic schwannoma is pathognomonic of neurofibromatosis type 2.

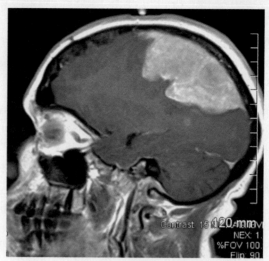

Figure 20-8. Large Meningioma Pushing into the Cerebral Cortex.

> Note the thin dark shadow around the lesion which occurs because the tumor is not actually invading the brain.

Tumors of the Sellar Region

Craniopharyngioma arises from rests of odontogenic epithelium within the suprasellar/diencephalic region. It most commonly affects children and young adults. The most common presenting symptoms are headache, hypopituitarism, and visual field disturbances.

- Contains deposits of calcium, evident on x-ray

- Histology shows squamous cells and resembles **adamantinoma**, a bone tumor of unknown histological origin that is the most common tumor of the tooth

- Is benign but tends to recur after resection

- Beta-catenin (*CTNNB1*) gene mutations have been reported

Other Neoplasms

- **Lymphomas** are the most common CNS tumors in the immunosuppressed. Primary CNS lymphomas may be multiple, unlike other histologic types. They do not respond well to chemotherapy.

- **Germ cell tumors** are more common in children than adults. The germinoma is the most common histologic type. It resembles the seminoma of the testis and the dysgerminoma of the ovary; the cells are large with a prominent nucleolus. These tumors are radiosensitive.

Metastatic Tumors

About 25–50% of all CNS tumors are metastatic tumors from sources outside the CNS. **Carcinomas** are the most common.

Chapter Summary

- Acute aseptic meningitis (usually viral, enteroviruses are the most common cause) is less severe than bacterial meningitis. The CSF shows lymphocytosis and a normal glucose level.

- *S. pneumoniae* is the most common cause of community-acquired bacterial meningitis in infants, young children and adults. The CSF shows decreased glucose; PMNs predominate.

- Mycobacterial (either *M. tuberculosis* or atypicals such as MAI, particularly in AIDS patients) meningoencephalitis causes tuberculomas of the basal surface of the brain and dura mater.

- Viral encephalitides are commonly caused by mosquito viruses (St. Louis), Herpes simplex viruses (HSV-1), and enteroviruses (poliovirus).

- Fungal meningoencephalitis can be caused by *Candida*, *Aspergillus*, *Mucor*, and *Cryptococcus* ("soap bubble lesions"). Toxoplasmosis occurs in AIDS patients (ring-enhancing lesions).

- Cerebral abscess (usually bacterial) can complicate a variety of systemic medical conditions (acute bacterial endocarditis) or local predisposing conditions (mastoiditis), and causes increased intracranial pressure, focal neurologic defects, and a ring-enhancing lesion on CT/MRI.

- HIV-associated neurocognitive disorder (HAND) presents as cognitive decline with behavioral changes and motor symptoms in HIV patients.

- Subacute sclerosing panencephalitis is a potentially fatal slow-virus encephalitis which can follow measles infection.

- Creutzfeldt-Jakob is a prion disease that causes a spongiform encephalopathy.

- Cerebrovascular disease can occur in several clinicopathological forms, including global cerebral ischemia, transient ischemic attack, infarction, and hemorrhage. Infarctions can be due to atherosclerosis with superimposed thrombosis (anemic: white infarct), thromboemboli (hemorrhagic: red infarct), or small vessel disease (tiny lacunar infarcts).

- Berry aneurysms of the circle of Willis are the most frequent cause of subarachnoid hemorrhage, which can present as "the worst headache of my life."

- CNS trauma can take several forms:

  - Concussion (transient loss of consciousness after impact against a rigid surface)

  - Contusions (brain bruises, sometimes in a coup and contrecoup pattern, can cause local infarction)

  - Subdural hematoma (injury of the bridging veins) and epidural hematoma (middle meningeal artery)

  - Diffuse axonal injury (acceleration/deceleration with subsequent axonal swelling)

  - CNS trauma to the spinal cord

  - Chronic traumatic encephalopathy (repetitive brain trauma associated with sports)

(continued)

Chapter Summary (cont'd)

- Acute aseptic meningitis (usually viral, enteroviruses are the most common cause) is less severe than bacterial meningitis. The CSF shows lymphocytosis and a normal glucose level.

- *S. pneumoniae* is the most common cause of community-acquired bacterial meningitis in infants, young children and adults. The CSF shows decreased glucose; PMNs predominate.

- Mycobacterial (either *M. tuberculosis* or atypicals such as MAI, particularly in AIDS patients) meningoencephalitis causes tuberculomas of the basal surface of the brain and dura mater.

- Viral encephalitides are commonly caused by mosquito viruses (St. Louis), Herpes simplex viruses (HSV-1), and enteroviruses (poliovirus).

- Fungal meningoencephalitis can be caused by *Candida*, *Aspergillus*, *Mucor*, and *Cryptococcus* ("soap bubble lesions").

- Toxoplasmosis occurs in AIDS patients (ring-enhancing lesions).

- Cerebral abscess (usually bacterial) can complicate a variety of systemic medical conditions (acute bacterial endocarditis) or local predisposing conditions (mastoiditis), and causes increased intracranial pressure, focal neurologic defects, and a ring-enhancing lesion on CT/MRI.

- HIV-associated neurocognitive disorder presents as cognitive decline with behavioral changes and motor symptoms in HIV patients.

- Subacute sclerosing panencephalitis is a potentially fatal slow-virus encephalitis which can follow measles infection.

- Creutzfeldt-Jakob is a prion disease that causes a spongiform encephalopathy.

- Cerebrovascular disease can occur in several clinicopathological forms, including global cerebral ischemia, transient ischemic attack, infarction, and hemorrhage. Infarctions can be due to atherosclerosis with superimposed thrombosis (anemic: white infarct), thromboemboli (hemorrhagic: red infarct), or small vessel disease (tiny lacunar infarcts).

- Berry aneurysms of the circle of Willis are the most frequent cause of subarachnoid hemorrhage, which can present as "the worst headache of my life."

- CNS trauma can take several forms: concussion, contusions, subdural hematoma, epidural hematoma, diffuse axonal injury (acceleration/deceleration with subsequent axonal swelling), CNS trauma to the spinal cord, or chronic traumatic encephalopathy

- Herniation can take several forms, including subfalcine, transtentorial, and tonsillar.

- Neural tube defects (risk factor: folate deficiency) include anencephaly, spina bifida occulta (bony defect of the vertebral arch), meningocele (bony defect with outpouching of meninges), meningomyelocele (with outpouching meninges, spinal cord, and spinal roots), and myelocele (complete exposure of spinal cord).

(continued)

Chapter Summary (cont'd)

- Posterior fossa defects include Arnold-Chiari malformation type I (often asymptomatic downward displacement of the cerebellar tonsils), type 2 (small posterior fossa, downward displacement of cerebellar vermis and medulla, compressed fourth ventricle with obstructive hydrocephalus, and lumbar meningomyelocele) and Dandy-Walker malformation (noncommunicating hydrocephalus characterized by cerebellar vermis hypoplasia and enlarged fourth ventricle).

- Perinatal brain injury (risk factor prematurity) can manifest as germinal matrix hemorrhage, periventricular leukomalacia, and multicystic encephalopathy.

- Fetal alcohol syndrome is characterized by structural abnormalities, functional impairments, and neurological impairments.

- Demyelinating diseases include multiple sclerosis (chronic relapsing-remitting autoimmune disorder with progressive neurological deficits including visual changes, sensation changes, motor changes, neuropsychiatric disturbances) and central pontine myelinolysis (a rare, potentially fatal, focal demyelination of the basis pontis possibly related to rapid correction of hyponatremia).

- Neurodegenerative diseases include:

  - Parkinson disease (loss of substantia nigra dopaminergic neurons with Lewy body formation, tremor, rigidity, and akinesia)

  - Huntington disease (autosomal dominant disorder with degeneration of GABAergic neurons of the caudate nucleus causing chorea and dementia)

  - Alzheimer disease (cortical atrophy, neuritic plaques, neurofibrillary tangles, and cerebral amyloid angiopathy)

  - Lewy body dementia (cognitive deterioration coupled with parkinsonism)

  - Amyotrophic lateral sclerosis (upper motor neuron and lower motor neuron loss)

  - Friedreich ataxia (autosomal recessive disorder with degeneration in the cerebellum, brain stem, and spinal cord producing gait ataxia)

- Metabolic and toxic disorders include Wilson disease, acute intermittent porphyria, vitamin B12 deficiency, and alcohol abuse.

- CNS tumors mainly arise in the posterior fossa in children and in the supratentorial region in adults. Neuroepithelial tumors include astrocytic tumors, oligodendrogliomas, ependymomas, and embryonal (primitive) tumors, of which the cerebellar medulloblastoma is the most common malignant brain tumor in childhood. Tumors may also derive from the meninges, nerves, and the sellar region. Other neoplasms include lymphomas (resistant to chemotherapy) and germinoma (radiosensitive).

Hematopoetic Pathology–White Blood Cell Disorders & Lymphoid and Myeloid Neoplasms

21

Learning Objectives

❏ Explain information related to reactive changes in white blood cells

❏ Describe lymphoid, mature B-cell, peripheral T-cell, and natural killer cell neoplasms

❏ Solve problems concerning Hodgkin lymphoma, acute leukemias, B and T lymphoblastic lymphoma/leukemia, and myeloid neoplasms

❏ Solve problems concerning diseases of histiocytes and dendritic cells

❏ Demonstrate understanding of mast cell diseases

❏ Answer questions about diseases of the spleen and thymus

REACTIVE CHANGES IN WHITE BLOOD CELLS

Leukocytosis

Leukocytosis is characterized by an elevated white blood cell count. It has the following features:

- **Increased neutrophils** (neutrophilia)

  ◦ Increased bone marrow production is seen with acute inflammation associated with pyogenic bacterial infection or tissue necrosis

  ◦ Increased release from bone marrow storage pool may be caused by corticosteroids, stress, or endotoxin

  ◦ Increased bands ("left shift") noted in peripheral circulation

  ◦ Reactive changes include Döhle bodies (aggregates of rough endoplasmic reticulum), toxic granulations (prominent granules), and cytoplasmic vacuoles of neutrophils

- **Increased eosinophils** (eosinophilia) occurs with allergies and asthma (type I hypersensitivity reaction), parasites, drugs (especially in hospitals), and certain skin diseases and cancers (adenocarcinomas, Hodgkin disease).

- **Increased monocytes** (monocytosis) occurs with certain chronic diseases such as some collagen vascular diseases and inflammatory bowel disease, and with certain infections, especially TB.

- **Increased lymphocytes** (lymphocytosis) occurs with acute (viral) diseases and chronic inflammatory processes.

  ◦ **Infectious mononucleosis**, an acute, self-limited disease, which usually resolves in 4–6 weeks, is an example of a viral disease that causes lymphocytosis. The most common cause is Epstein-Barr virus (a herpesvirus) though other viruses can cause it as well (heterophile-negative infectious mononucleosis is most likely due to cytomegalovirus).

- Age groups include adolescents and young adults ("kissing disease").

- The "classic triad" includes fever, sore throat with gray-white membrane on tonsils, and lymphadenitis involving the posterior auricular nodes. Another sign is hepatosplenomegaly.

- Complications include hepatic dysfunction, splenic rupture, and rash if treated with ampicillin.

- Diagnosis is often made based on symptoms. Lymphocytosis and a rising titer of EBV antibodies are suggestive of the infection. Atypical lymphocytes may be present in peripheral blood. Monospot test is often negative early in infection.

- **Increased basophils** are seen with chronic myeloproliferative disorders such as polycythemia vera.

Leukopenia

Leukopenia is characterized by a decreased white blood cell count. It has the following features:

- **Decreased neutrophils** can be due to decreased production (aplastic anemia, chemotherapy), increased destruction (infections, autoimmune disease such as systemic lupus erythematosus), and activation of neutrophil adhesion molecules on endothelium (as by endotoxins in septic shock).

- **Decreased eosinophils** are seen with increased cortisol, which causes sequestering of eosinophils in lymph nodes; examples include Cushing syndrome and exogenous corticosteroids.

- **Decreased lymphocytes** are seen with immunodeficiency syndromes such as HIV, DiGeorge syndrome (T-cell deficiency), and severe combined immunodeficiency (B- and T-cell deficiency); also seen secondary to immune destruction (systemic lupus erythematosus), corticosteroids, and radiation (lymphocytes are the most sensitive cells to radiation).

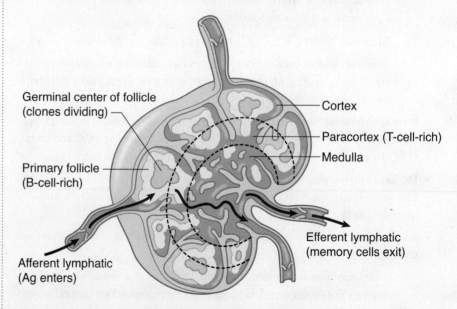

Figure 21-1. Lymph Node

Lymphadenopathy

Lymphadenopathy is lymph node enlargement due to reactive conditions or neoplasia.

- **Acute nonspecific lymphadenitis** produces tender enlargement of lymph nodes; focal involvement is seen with bacterial lymphadenitis. Microscopically, there may be neutrophils within the lymph node. Cat scratch fever (due to *Bartonella henselae*) causes stellate microabscesses. Generalized involvement of lymph nodes is seen with viral infections.

- **Chronic nonspecific lymphadenitis** causes nontender enlargement of lymph nodes. Follicular hyperplasia involves B lymphocytes and may be seen with rheumatoid arthritis, toxoplasmosis, and early HIV infections. Paracortical lymphoid hyperplasia involves T cells and may be seen with viruses, drugs (Dilantin), and systemic lupus erythematosus. Sinus histiocytosis involves macrophages and, in most cases, is nonspecific; an example is lymph nodes draining cancers.

- **Neoplasia** usually causes nontender enlargement of lymph nodes. The most common tumor to involve lymph nodes is metastatic cancer (e.g., breast, lung, malignant melanoma, stomach and colon carcinoma), which is initially seen under the lymph node capsule. Other important causes of lymphadenopathy are malignant lymphoma and infiltration by leukemias.

LYMPHOID NEOPLASMS

Lymphoid neoplasia is grouped according to the 2008 WHO classification as follows (note that B and T lymphoblastic lymphoma/leukemia is grouped by the WHO with myeloid neoplasia):

- Mature B-cell neoplasms

- Mature T-cell and NK-cell neoplasms

- Hodgkin lymphoma

- Histiocytic and dendritic cell neoplasms

- Posttransplantation lymphoproliferative disorders

MATURE B-CELL NEOPLASMS

Chronic lymphocytic leukemia (CLL) and **small lymphocytic lymphoma (SLL)** are very similar; they both represent an abnormal proliferation of B cells. Patients who present with **lymph node findings** are classified as having SLL. Patients who present with **blood findings** are classified as having CLL; 50% of CLL patients also have lymph node involvement.

- CLL is the most indolent of all of the leukemias.

- Mean age at time of diagnosis is age 60.

- The malignant cells are nonfunctional, so patients develop hypogammaglobulinemia, leading to an increased risk of infections.

- CLL is associated with warm autoimmune hemolytic anemia (AIHA) (10% of cases), which will cause spherocytes to be observed in peripheral blood.

- CLL rarely transforms into a worse disease such as prolymphocytic leukemia or large cell lymphoma (Richter syndrome).

CLL and SLL can be categorized by the markers present on the B cells:

- **B-chronic lymphocytic leukemia cells** (95% of cases) have B-cell markers, such as CD19 and CD20. One T-cell marker, CD5, is also present. Also important is that the cells are CD23 positive and CD10 negative.

  ○ SLL occurs only as this type.

- **T-chronic lymphocytic leukemia cells** (5% of cases) have T-cell markers. The histology of affected lymph nodes reveals only a diffuse pattern (not nodular), but proliferation centers may also be present.

- Peripheral blood findings show increased numbers of normal-appearing lymphocytes. Numerous smudge cells ("parachute cells") are also present; the smudge cells result from the fact that the neoplastic lymphocytes are unusually fragile.

- Bone marrow shows numerous normal-appearing neoplastic lymphocytes.

Hairy cell leukemia is a rare B-cell neoplasm that causes indolent disease in middle-aged Caucasian men. There can be a "dry tap" with bone marrow aspiration. Lymphocytes have "hairlike" cytoplasmic projections; the diagnostic stain is positive tartrate-resistant acid phosphatase (TRAP).

Physical examination shows a markedly enlarged spleen (splenomegaly) due to infiltration of red pulp by malignant cells.

Treatment is 2-chloro-deoxyadenosine (2-CdA), which inhibits adenosine deaminase (ADA) and increases levels of toxic deoxyadenosine.

Follicular lymphoma is a well-differentiated B-cell lymphoma with follicular architecture. All follicular lymphomas are derived from B lymphocytes.

- Most common form of non-Hodgkin lymphoma in the United States

- Characteristic translocation is t(14;18), involving the immunoglobulin heavy chain gene and *BCL2* gene (activation of bcl-2 inhibits apoptosis by blocking the bax channel)

- Frequently presents with disseminated disease (more advanced stage)

- Prognosis is better than diffuse lymphoma, but it doesn't respond to therapy (unlike the more aggressive diffuse non-Hodgkin lymphomas)

Diffuse large B-cell lymphoma is a high grade large B-cell lymphoma with a diffuse growth pattern. It is an aggressive, rapidly proliferating tumor which may respond to therapy. Special subtypes include immunodeficiency-associated B-cell lymphomas (often infected with Epstein-Barr virus) and body-cavity large B-cell lymphomas (sometimes associated with human herpes virus [HHV]-8).

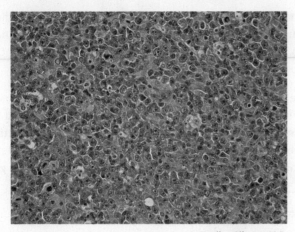

Bradley Gibson, M.D.
Used with permission.

Figure 21-2. Diffuse Large B-Cell Lymphoma

Small noncleaved lymphoma (Burkitt lymphoma) is a high grade B-cell lymphoma. It is composed of intermediate-sized lymphoid cells with a "starry sky" appearance due to numerous reactive tingible-body macrophages (phagocytosis of apoptotic tumor cells). There is a characteristic t(8;14) translocation juxtaposing MYC to the immunoglobulin heavy chain locus in most cases.

- **African type:** endemic form
  - Involvement of mandible or maxilla is characteristic; is associated with Epstein-Barr virus
- **American type**: nonendemic, sporadic form
  - Involvement of the abdomen (such as bowel, retroperitoneum, or ovaries); has a high incidence in AIDS patients

Both endemic and sporadic forms of Burkitt lymphoma are seen most often in children and young adults.

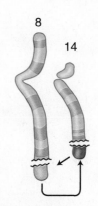

Normal Chromosome

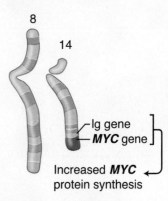

Burkitt Lymphoma

Bradley Gibson, M.D.
Used with permission.

Figure 21-3. "Starry Sky" Appearance of Burkitt Lymphoma

Mantle cell lymphoma (MCL) is a rare B-cell lymphoma in which the tumor cells arise from mantle zone B lymphocytes (positive for CD19, CD20, and CD5; negative for CD23). The characteristic translocation is t(11;14), involving *CCD1* and the heavy chain locus.

Marginal zone lymphoma (MALToma) is a diverse group of B-cell neoplasms that arise within lymph nodes, spleen, or extranodal tissue. It is associated with mucosa-associated lymphoid tissue (MALTomas). The lesion begins as a reactive polyclonal reaction and may be associated with previous autoimmune disorders or infectious disease (e.g., Sjögren disease, Hashimoto thyroiditis, *Helicobacter* gastritis). The lymphoma remains localized for long periods of time.

Multiple myeloma is a malignant neoplasm of plasma cells.

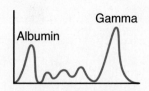

Serum electrophoresis pattern of IgG myeloma with γ spike and reduced albumin

- Most common primary tumor arising in the bone marrow of adults

- Lab studies show increased serum protein with normal serum albumin; an M spike in serum electrophoresis is a monoclonal immunoglobulin spike—most commonly IgG (60%) and next most commonly IgA (20%)

- Bence Jones proteins are light chains that are small and can be filtered into urine.

Histologically, bone marrow shows increased plasma cells (>20% is characteristic). Peripheral blood may show rouleaux formation ("stack of coins"). Multiple lytic bone lesions are due to the osteoclastic activating factor. Lytic bone lesions cause hypercalcemia, bone pain, and increased risk of fracture.

Increased risk of infection is the most common cause of death. Other complications include renal disease (such as myeloma nephrosis) and primary amyloidosis (10% of patients) due to amyloid light (AL) chains. Increased amounts of IL-6 are associated with a poorer prognosis because survival of myeloma cells is dependent on IL-6.

Plasmacytoma is a solitary myeloma within bone or soft tissue.

- **Within bone**: precursor lesion that can later develop into myeloma

- **Outside bone** (extramedullary): usually found within upper respiratory tract

Monoclonal gammopathy of undetermined significance (MGUS) (an old name was benign monoclonal gammopathy). Serum M protein is found in 1–3% of asymptomatic individuals age >50; the incidence increases with increasing age. The annual risk of developing a plasma cell dyscrasia, usually multiple myeloma, is 1–2% per year. MGUS may also evolve into Waldenström macroglobulinemia, primary amyloidosis, B-cell lymphoma, or CLL.

Lymphoplasmacytic lymphoma (Waldenström macroglobulinemia) is a small lymphocytic lymphoma with plasmacytic differentiation. It is a cross between multiple myeloma and SLL.

Like myeloma, it has an M spike (IgM). Like SLL (and unlike myeloma), the neoplastic cells infiltrate many organs (e.g., lymph nodes, spleen, bone marrow). Also unlike multiple myeloma, there are no lytic bone lesions and there is no increase in serum calcium. Russell bodies (cytoplasmic immunoglobulin) and Dutcher bodies (intranuclear immunoglobulin) may be present.

- May have hyperviscosity syndrome, because IgM is a large pentamer

- Visual abnormalities may be due to vascular dilatations and hemorrhages in the retina

- Neurologic symptoms include headaches and confusion

- Bleeding and cryoglobulinemia can be due to abnormal globulins, which precipitate at low temperature and may cause Raynaud phenomenon

PERIPHERAL T-CELL AND NATURAL KILLER CELL NEOPLASMS

Peripheral T-cell lymphoma, unspecified is a "wastebasket" diagnostic category.

Adult T-cell leukemia/lymphoma (ATLL) is a malignant T-cell disorder (CD4-T cells) due to HTLV-1 infection. It is often seen in Japan and the Caribbean. Clinical symptoms include skin lesions, hypercalcemia, enlarged lymph nodes, heptomegaly, and splenomegaly. Microscopically, characteristic hyperlobated "4-leaf clover" lymphocytes can be found in the peripheral blood.

Mycosis fungoides is a malignant T-cell disorder (CD4+ cells) that has a better prognosis than ATLL. It can present with a generalized pruritic erythematous rash (no hypercalcemia), which develops as a sequence of skin changes:

inflammatory eczematous stage → plaque stage → tumor nodule stage

Microscopically, atypical PAS-positive lymphocytes are present in the epidermis (epidermotropism); aggregates of these cells are called Pautrier microabscesses. If there is erythroderma and cerebriform Sézary cells are present in peripheral blood, the condition is called **Sézary syndrome**.

HODGKIN LYMPHOMA

Hodgkin lymphoma has some characteristics that are different from non-Hodgkin lymphoma.

- May present similar to infection (with fever)

- Spread is contiguous to adjacent node groups

- No leukemic state

- Extranodal spread is uncommon

The malignant cells are the diagnostic **Reed-Sternberg cells**; these malignant cells are intermixed with reactive inflammatory cells. The Reed-Sternberg cell is a large malignant tumor cell that has a bilobed nucleus with a prominent large inclusion-like nucleolus in each lobe.

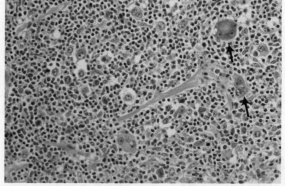

© Katsumi M. Miyai, M.D., Ph.D.; Regents of the University of California.
Used with permission.

Figure 21-4. Reed-Sternberg Cells (arrows) of Hodgkin Lymphoma
Appear as Large Binucleate Cells with Macronucleoli

Hodgkin lymphoma classification:

- **Lymphocyte-rich** type (rare): composed primarily of reactive lymphocytes; associated with Epstein-Barr virus (40% of cases)

- **Lymphocyte-predominant** type: has lymphohistocytic variants (L&H cells, called "popcorn cells") and a unique phenotype (CD45+, CD15-, CD30-, CD20+)

- **Mixed cellularity** type: occurs in middle-aged and older males; the increased number of eosinophils is related to IL-5 secretion

- **Lymphocyte-depleted** type: presents with abdominal adenopathy; Reed-Sternberg cells predominate

- **Nodular sclerosis** type (most common subtype (65–70% of cases)): is only type in which females > males

  - Lymph node has broad collagen bands

  - Reed-Sternberg cell has clear space in the cytoplasm (lacunar cell)

Hodgkin lymphoma has a bimodal age group distribution (age late 20s and >50). Patients usually present with painless enlargement of lymph nodes.

Poor prognosis is directly proportional to the number of Reed-Sternberg cells present. Survivors of chemotherapy and radiotherapy have increased risk for secondary non-Hodgkin lymphoma or acute leukemia.

ACUTE LEUKEMIAS

In acute leukemias, the peripheral blood has decreased mature forms and increased immature forms called **blasts**, which have immature chromatin with nucleoli. The bone marrow has increased immature cells (blasts). Acute symptoms are secondary to marrow failure, which can produce decreased erythrocytes (causing anemia and fatigue), decreased leukocytes (permitting infections and fever), and decreased platelets (inducing bleeding).

In a Nutshell

The classical Hodgkin lymphomas (nodular sclerosis, mixed cellularity, lymphocyte-rich, lymphocyte-depleted) share the immunophenotype CD45-, CD15+, CD30+.

Note

Hodgkin lymphoma patients who have symptoms (fever, night sweats, unexplained weight loss > 10%) have a worse prognosis.

B AND T LYMPHOBLASTIC LYMPHOMA/LEUKEMIA

Acute Lymphoblastic Leukemia (ALL)

- **Karyotypic abnormalities:** Most pre-B-cell tumors are hyperdiploid. Translocations are common in both B-ALL and T-ALL.

- **Immunophenotyping.** Most tumors are positive for terminal deoxytransferase (TdT).

  ◦ **B-cell lineage** classification is based on presence or absence of cytoplasmic or surface markers, including surface immunoglobulin (sIg) presence (mature B-ALL) and cytoplasmic μ presence (pre-BALL). The B-cell tumors almost always express B-cell molecules CD19 and CD10.

  ◦ **T-cell lineage:** The majority of T-ALLs stain with CD2, CD3, CD5, and CD7.

- **B-ALL** is more common in children; symptoms include fever, anemia, and bleeding

- **T-ALL** often presents as a mediastinal mass in an adolescent male

Lymphoblastic Lymphoma

Most cases of lymphoblastic lymphoma are T-cell neoplasms that are aggressive and rapidly progressive. Most patients are young males with a mediastinal mass (think thymus). The leukemic phase of lymphoblastic lymphoma is similar to T-ALL and some consider them the same entity. Most cells are CD1+, CD2+, CD5+, and CD7+.

MYELOID NEOPLASMS

Acute Myelogenous Leukemia

Acute myelogenous leukemia is a cancer of the myeloid line of blood cells. Median age at diagnosis is age 50. Symptoms include fatigue, unusual bleeding, and infections.

Lab findings: Myeloid blasts or promyelocytes represent at least 20% of the marrow cells. **Auer rods** (linear condensations of cytoplasmic granules) are characteristic of AML and are not found in normal myeloid precursors.

The WHO classification of AML (2008) is as follows:

- AML with recurrent genetic abnormalities (for some of these entities, the karyotype is diagnostic regardless of the blast percentage)

  ◦ Promyelocytic leukemia has t(15;17)(q22;q12) with fusion gene PML/RARA and responds to all-transretinoic acid (ATRA); DIC is common

  ◦ AML with either t(8;21)(q22;q22) or inv(16)(p13.1;q22)

- AML with myelodysplasia-related changes

- Therapy-related myeloid neoplasms

- AML, not otherwise specified

Note

With some exceptions, lymphoblasts stain with PAS; myeloblasts are myeloperoxidase (MPO) positive.

Clinical Correlate

ALL is associated with infiltration of the CNS and testes (**sanctuary sites**). Thus, prophylactic radiation and/or chemotherapy to the CNS is used because malignant cells in the brain are protected from chemotherapy by the blood–brain barrier.

Clinical Correlate

Tumor lysis syndrome is a group of metabolic complications that can occur after treatment of neoplastic disorders. These complications, which include hyperkalemia, hyperphosphatemia, hyperuricemia, hypocalcemia, and acute renal failure, are caused by the breakdown products of dying cancer cells. Treatment is hydration and allopurinol.

Myelodysplastic Syndromes (MDS)

MDS are classified according to the number of blasts in the marrow. Dysplastic changes include Pelger-Huët cells ("aviator glasses" nuclei), ring sideroblasts, nuclear budding, and "pawn ball" megakaryocytes. MDS are considered preleukemias, so patients are at increased risk for developing acute leukemia.

MDS mainly affect older adults (age 50–70); they also predispose to infection, hemorrhage and anemia. Transformation to AML is common.

Myeloproliferative Neoplasms (MPN)

MPN are clonal neoplastic proliferations of multipotent myeloid stem cells. The bone marrow is usually markedly hypercellular (hence the name *myeloproliferative*). All cell lines are increased in number (erythroid, myeloid, and megakaryocytes).

- **Chronic myelogenous leukemia (CML)** is a clonal proliferation of pluripotent granulocytic precursor stem cells. In most cases it is associated with a *BCR-ABL* fusion gene due to a balanced (9;22) translocation; however, this Philadelphia chromosome is not specific to CML.

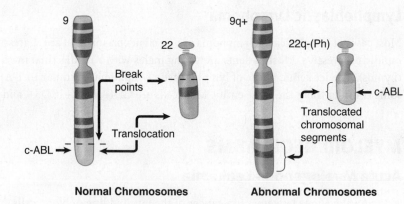

Figure 21-5. Translocation of Chromosomal Segments between Chromosomes 9 and 22

- CML has an insidious onset (i.e., chronic) and causes massive splenomegaly. Progression is typically slow (50% develop accelerated phase <5 years), unless blast crisis develops (very poor prognosis; doesn't respond to chemotherapy). In blast crisis, 70% of cases show myeloid blasts and 30% show lymphoid blasts.

- Microscopically, the bone marrow is hypercellular, with all cell lines increased in number. Peripheral leukocytosis is present, including markedly increased neutrophils (and bands and metamyelocytes), as well as increased eosinophils and basophils (as in the other MPS).

- Treatment is imatinib mesylate, which blocks the P210 tyrosine kinase protein produced by the translocation. Hematopoietic stem cell transplantation is also used.

- **Polycythemia vera** is a stem cell disorder with trilineage (erythroid, granulocytic, megakaryocytic) proliferation. It may develop into a "spent phase" with myelofibrosis. It causes an increased risk for acute leukemia. Phlebotomy is therapeutic.

Polycythemia vera characteristically shows the following:

- Increased erythroid precursors with increased red cell mass

- Increased hematocrit

- Increased blood viscosity, which can cause deep vein thrombosis and infarcts

- Decreased erythropoietin, but erythrocytes have increased sensitivity to erythropoietin and overproliferate

- Increased basophils. Histamine release from basophils can cause intense pruritus and gastric ulcer (bleeding may cause iron deficiency).

- Increased eosinophils (like all of the MPS)

- High cell turnover can cause hyperuricemia, resulting in gout. Other clinical characteristics include plethora (redness) and cyanosis (blue).

- **Essential thrombocythemia** is characterized by increased megakaryocytes (and other cell lines) in bone marrow. Peripheral blood smear shows increased platelets, some with abnormal shapes. There are also increased leukocytes. Clinical signs include excessive bleeding and occlusion of small vessels.

- **Myelofibrosis (MF) with myeloid metaplasia** has unknown etiology (agnogenic).

    - Marrow fibrosis is secondary to factors released from megakaryocytes, such as platelet-derived growth factor (PDGF).

    - Bone marrow aspiration may be a "dry tap." The biopsy specimen shows hypocellular marrow with fibrosis (increased reticulin). The fibroblasts are a polyclonal proliferation and are not neoplastic.

    - There is an enlarged spleen due to extramedullary hematopoiesis (myeloid metaplasia). Peripheral smear shows leukoerythroblastosis (immature white cells and nucleated red cells) with teardrop RBCs. High cell turnover causes hyperuricemia and gout.

Note

The most common site for extramedullary hematopoiesis is the spleen.

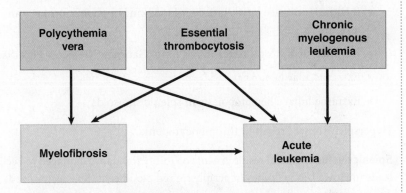

Figure 21-6. Natural History of the Myeloproliferative Syndromes

DISEASES OF HISTIOCYTES AND DENDRITIC CELLS

Langerhans histiocytosis is common in children. It can affect many sites, including skin, bone, CNS (diabetes insipidus), and lungs. Biopsy is required for diagnosis. The Langerhans cells are CD1a positive and on electron microscopy show cytoplasmic Birbeck granules (tennis racket–shaped organelles).

- Multisystem variant: Letterer-Siwe disease (marrow involvement can be fatal)
- Hand-Schuller-Christian triad is calvarial involvement, diabetes insipidus, and exophthalmos
- Unisystem variant: eosinophilic granuloma (most often found in bone)

MAST CELL DISEASES

Mastocytosis occurs from birth to adulthood; adult-onset cases are more severe. The WHO separates mastocytosis into 3 categories:

- **Cutaneous mastocytosis**, seen in children, regresses over time. Mast cell degranulation enzymes (histamine and tryptase) cause pruritus.
- **Systemic mastocytosis** is a clonal proliferation of mast cells associated with a KIT mutation; ≥1 organs are involved, as are the skin and bone marrow. The WHO now classifies systemic mastocytosis as one of the myeloproliferative neoplasms.
    - Variants include some rare leukemias.
    - Diagnosis is made with bone marrow biopsy and molecular analysis.
- **Localized extracutaneous mast cell neoplasms** can be benign (mastocytoma) or malignant (sarcoma).

DISEASES OF THE SPLEEN AND THYMUS

Splenomegaly (splenic enlargement) can be caused by multiple things:

- Vascular congestion (portal hypertension)
- Reactive hyperplasia of white pulp (autoimmune disorder, infectious mononucleosis, malaria)
- Infiltrative disease (metastatic non-Hodgkin lymphoma, primary amyloidosis, leukemia)
- Accumulated macrophages in red pulp (Gaucher, Niemann-Pick disease)
- Extravascular hemolysis
- Extramedullary hematopoiesis in splenic sinusoids

Hypersplenism will result in thrombocytopenia.

Splenic dysfunction will result in a loss of ability to remove damaged red cells, which leads to Howell-Jolly bodies in peripheral red blood cells. Splenectomized, asplenic, and hyposplenic individuals are at risk for infection (sepsis, peritonitis), particularly due to *Streptococcus*, *Haemophilus*, and *Salmonella*.

Thymomas are low-grade tumors of the thymic epithelium with many histologic patterns. Recent large case series have shown that tumor behavior does not always correlate with histopathological features.

True thymic hyperplasia is enlargement of a histologically normal thymus; it can occur as a complication of chemotherapy.

Thymic lymphoid hyperplasia shows germinal center hyperplasia.

Chapter Summary

- Leukocytosis and leukopenia are common reactive patterns of white cells; determining whether the leukocytosis is related to neutrophilia, eosinophilia, monocytosis, or lymphocytosis may be helpful in narrowing the diagnostic possibilities.

- Infectious mononucleosis is a common viral disease which can cause lymphocytosis, fever, sore throat, lymphadenitis, and hepatosplenomegaly.

- Acute nonspecific lymphadenitis tends to cause tender lymph nodes and can be seen with bacterial or viral infections. Chronic nonspecific lymphadenitis tends to cause non-tender lymph nodes and can be seen with chronic inflammatory conditions, viral infections, medicines, and in nodes draining cancers.

- Acute lymphoblastic leukemia (ALL) is a leukemia of precursor lymphoid cells of either B-cell or T-cell lineage. Early pre-B-ALL is usually seen in children and is the most common type of ALL.

- T-ALL typically causes a mediastinal mass in adolescent or young adult men. A similar presentation to T-ALL is seen in lymphoblastic lymphoma, which is usually of T-cell lineage.

- Non-Hodgkin lymphomas were most recently classified by the WHO Classification of Lymphoid Neoplasia.

- Mature B-cell lymphomas include the following:

- Chronic lymphocytic leukemia (CLL)/small lymphocytic lymphoma (SLL) occurs in the elderly and has an indolent course.

- Hairy cell leukemia is an indolent disease of older men with characteristic lymphocytes with "hair-like" cytoplasmic projections that stain positive for TRAP.

- Follicular lymphomas are the most common form of non-Hodgkin lymphoma in the United States and are all derived from B cells. They tend to present with diffuse disease and have a better prognosis than diffuse lymphomas.

- Diffuse large B-cell lymphoma is an aggressive, rapidly proliferating tumor that may be present at extranodal sites and may be associated with EBV or HHV-8 infection.

- Small noncleaved lymphoma (Burkitt lymphoma) occurs in African type with jaw involvement and American type with involvement of the abdomen. It has a characteristic "starry-sky" microscopic appearance and is related to a characteristic t(8;14) translocation.

- Mantle cell lymphoma arises from mantle zone B lymphocytes and has a characteristic t(11;14) translocation.

- Marginal zone lymphomas often involve mucosa-associated lymphoid tissue and appear to often begin as reactive polyclonal disorders.

- Multiple myeloma, a tumor of plasma cells, is the most common primary tumor arising in the bone marrow of adults. It can be associated with production of a monoclonal immunoglobulin spike (M protein) in serum or urine.

- *Monoclonal gammopathy of undetermined significance* is the term used when an M protein is found in an asymptomatic individual.

(continued)

Chapter Summary (cont'd)

- Lymphoplasmacytic lymphoma (Waldenström macroglobulinemia) is a cross between multiple myeloma and small lymphocytic lymphoma with M spike, but with neoplastic cells that tend to infiltrate many organs and do not cause lytic bone lesions.

- Adult T-cell leukemia/lymphoma is a malignant T-cell disorder due to HTLV-1 infection; it is seen in Japan and the Caribbean.

- Mycosis fungoides is a malignant T-cell disorder with a predilection for involving skin. The term *Sézary syndrome* is used if the abnormal lymphocytes are found in the blood and erythroderma is present.

- In Hodgkin disease, the malignant cell is the Reed-Sternberg cell. There is a bimodal age group distribution (late 20s and ›50).

- In acute myelogenous leukemia, myeloid blasts or promyelocytes represent at least 20% of the marrow cells. Karyotype is the most important prognostic factor.

- Myelodysplastic syndromes are proliferations of dysplastic myeloid precursors and are associated with an increased risk of developing acute leukemias.

- Myeloproliferative neoplasms are clonal neoplastic proliferations of multipotent myeloid stem cells. The diseases in this category include CML, polycythemia vera, essential thrombocytopenia, and myelofibrosis with myeloid metaplasia.

- Langerhans cell histiocytosis has several clinical forms and can behave in a malignant or benign fashion.

- Splenomegaly can have many causes; splenic dysfunction manifests with erythrocyte abnormalities and predisposes to serious infections.

- Thymomas are tumors of thymic epithelium.

- Mastocytosis has myriad clinical presentations; adult-onset mastocytosis has a worse prognosis.

Female Genital Pathology 22

Learning Objectives

❑ Demonstrate understanding of the pathology of the vulva, vagina, cervix, uterus, and ovary

❑ Solve problems concerning the placenta

VULVA

Non-Neoplastic Disorders

- **Lichen sclerosis** is caused by epidermal thinning and dermal changes which cause pale skin in postmenopausal women. There is a small risk of progression to squamous cell carcinoma (SCC).

- In **lichen simplex chronicus**, a chronic scratch/itch cycle produces the white plaques seen clinically. These plaques are characterized microscopically by squamous cell hyperplasia and dermal inflammation.

Infections

- **Human papillomavirus (HPV)** causes warty lesions (condylomata acuminata) and precursor dysplastic lesions of squamous cell carcinoma called vulvar intraepithelial neoplasia (VIN). Vulvar HPV is commonly subtype 6 and 11 and therefore has low oncogenic potential.

- **Herpes simplex virus (HSV)**. Most cases of vulvar herpes are caused by HSV-2. Painless vesicles progress to pustules and painful ulcers.

- **Syphilis** is a sexually transmitted disease caused by *Treponema pallidum*. The primary lesion is a chancre, a painless ulcer that does not scar after healing.

- **Molluscum contagiosum** is a viral disease caused by a DNA poxvirus. It presents as smooth papules and has characteristic cytoplasmic viral inclusions.

- **Bartholin gland abscess** is a polymicrobial infection requiring drainage or excision.

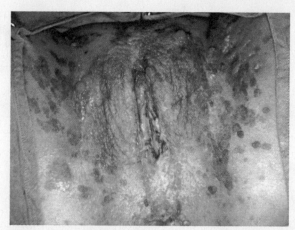

© Katsumi M. Miyai, M.D., Ph.D.; Regents of the University of California.
Used with permission.

Figure 22-1. Severe Case of Condyloma Acuminata

Tumors

- **Papillary hidradenoma** is a benign tumor of modified apocrine sweat glands of the labia majora or interlabial folds. It occurs along the milk line and may ulcerate, mimicking carcinoma. Papillary hidradenoma is histologically similar to an intraductal papilloma of the breast.

- **Extramammary Paget disease of the vulva** usually involves the labia majora, and it causes an erythematous, crusted rash that is characterized microscopically by intraepidermal malignant cells with pagetoid spread. This form of Paget disease is not usually associated with underlying tumor.

- **Squamous cell carcinoma** is the most common malignancy of the vulva. The most common form occurs in women age >60. The less common form occurs in younger women with HPV serotypes 16 and 18.

- **Melanoma** can occur on the vulva, and must be differentiated from lentigo simplex which is more common.

VAGINA

- **Vaginal adenosis and clear cell adenocarcinoma** are rare conditions with increased risk in females exposed to diethylstilbestrol (DES) *in utero*.

- **Embryonal rhabdomyosarcoma** (sarcoma botryoides) affects infants and young children (age <5), in whom it can cause a polypoid, "grapelike," soft tissue mass that protrudes from the vagina. Microscopically, the mass is characterized by polypoid epithelial growth with an underlying immature (cambium) proliferation of spindle-shaped tumor cells with rare cross-striations. Tumor cells are positive for desmin.

- **Primary forms of vaginal squamous cell carcinoma** are usually related to HPV infection; secondary forms are more common and are usually due to extension from a cervical cancer. Treatment is radiotherapy.

- **Rhabdomyoma** is a benign skeletal muscle tumor that can involve the vagina. It occurs in middle-aged women.

Clinical Correlate

DES was used in high-risk pregnancies from 1940–1970, after which time vaginal adenosis and clear cell carcinoma were discovered in the female offspring. Vaginal adenosis is a benign condition that is presumed to be a precursor of clear cell carcinoma.

- **Gartner duct cyst** is a cyst of the lateral wall of the vagina that is due to persistence of a mesonephric (Wolffian) duct remnant. Urinary tract abnormalities may exist.

- **Mayer-Rokitansky-Kuster-Hauser (MRKH) syndrome** is congenital absence of the upper part of the vagina and uterus. Patients present with primary amenorrhea.

- **Vaginitis/vaginosis:** All of the following conditions require vaginal swab for definitive diagnosis; molecular diagnostic tests may be indicated in certain situations.

  - **Vulvovaginal candidiasis** can occur spontaneously or from antibiotic therapy; it is not usually sexually transmitted. Symptoms include discharge and pruritis. Yeast cells and pseudohyphae are seen on microscopy. Antimycotics are therapeutic.

  - **Bacterial vaginosis (BV)** is implicated in preterm labor and pelvic inflammatory disease. Some patients are asymptomatic. BV is a sexually transmitted bacterial infection of polymicrobial origin (although it used to be attributed only to *Gardnerella vaginalis*); recurrence rate is high after treatment with antibiotics. "Clue cells" are squamous cells coated with coccobacilli that may be seen microscopically in swab material.

  - ***Trichomonis vaginalis*** is a sexually transmitted motile protozoan. Most infected people are asymptomatic. It can also cause cervicitis, but "strawberry cervix" is not a consistent diagnostic feature. Antibiotics are therapeutic.

CERVIX

Pelvic inflammatory disease (PID) is an ascending infection (sexually transmitted disease) from the cervix to the endometrium, fallopian tubes, and pelvic cavity. The infecting organisms are most frequently nongonococcal organisms, including *Chlamydia*, *Mycoplasma hominis* and endogenous flora. Broad-spectrum antibiotics are therapeutic.

The distribution of disease includes the endometrium (endometritis), fallopian tubes (salpingitis), and pelvic cavity (peritonitis and pelvic abscesses). **Fitz-Hugh–Curtis syndrome** (perihepatitis) can occur, characterized by "violin-string" adhesions between the fallopian tube and liver capsule. Symptoms include the following:

- Vaginal discharge (cervicitis)
- Vaginal bleeding and midline abdominal pain (endometritis)
- Bilateral lower abdominal and pelvic pain (salpingitis)
- Abdominal tenderness and peritoneal signs (peritonitis)
- Pleuritic right upper quadrant pain (perihepatitis)

Complications of PID include tubo-ovarian abscess; tubal scarring (increasing risk of infertility and ectopic tubal pregnancies), and intestinal obstruction secondary to fibrous adhesions.

Clinical Correlate

Tubal ectopic pregnancies usually occur in the ampulla of the fallopian tube. Tubal rupture will cause severe, acute lower abdominal pain.

Table 22-1. Malignant Tumors of the Lower Female Genital Tract in the U.S.

Order of Incidence	Order of Greatest Mortality
1. Endometrial cancer	1. Ovarian cancer
2. Ovarian cancer	2. Endometrial cancer
3. Cervical cancer	3. Cervical cancer

Cervical carcinoma is most commonly squamous cell carcinoma but can also be adenocarcinoma or small cell neuroendocrine carcinoma. It is the third most common malignant tumor of the lower female genital tract in the United States, with peak incidence at ages 35–44. Risk factors include the following:

- Early age of first intercourse
- Multiple sexual partners
- Multiple pregnancies
- Oral contraceptive use
- Smoking
- STDs (including human papilloma virus)
- Immunosuppression

Human papilloma virus infection is the most important risk factor, with high-risk types being 16, 18, 31, and 33, and having viral oncoproteins E6 (binds to p53) and E7 (binds to Rb).

The precursor lesion is **cervical intraepithelial neoplasia (CIN)**, which is increasing in incidence and occurs commonly at the squamocolumnar junction (transformation zone). Cervical intraepithelial lesions show a progression of changes on histologic examination:

- Low grade SIL (squamous intraepithelial lesion)
- High grade SIL
- Carcinoma in situ
- Superficially invasive squamous cell carcinoma
- Invasive squamous cell carcinoma

Squamous cell carcinoma of the cervix may be asymptomatic or may present with postcoital vaginal bleeding, dyspareunia, and/or malodorous discharge. To establish the diagnosis, the Papanicolaou (**Pap**) test is useful for early detection, and colposcopy with biopsy for microscopic evaluation.

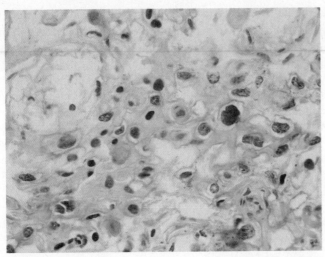

© Gregg Barré, M.D.
Used with permission.

Figure 22-2. Cervix Biopsy Showing Squamous Cells with Nuclear Hyperchromasia and Perinuclear Vacuoles, Characteristic of HPV Cytopathic Effect

Acute cervicitis and chronic cervicitis are common and usually nonspecific inflammatory conditions.

- Acute cervicitis is often caused by *C. trachomatis, N. gonorrhoeae, T. vaginalis, Candida*, and herpes simplex type 2.

- A specific, severe form of chronic cervicitis (**follicular cervicitis**) can be caused by *C. trachomatis*; it can result in neonatal conjunctivitis and pneumonia in infants delivered vaginally through an infected cervix.

Cervical polyp is a common non-neoplastic polyp that can be covered with columnar or stratified squamous epithelium.

UTERUS

Endometritis is inflammation of the endometrial lining in the uterus. It can be acute or chronic.

- **Acute endometritis** is an ascending infection from the cervix; it is associated with pregnancy and abortion.

- **Chronic endometritis** is associated with PID and intrauterine devices; plasma cells are seen in the endometrium.

Endometriosis is the presence of endometrial glands and stroma outside the uterus. It most commonly affects women of reproductive age. Common sites of involvement are the ovaries, ovarian and uterine ligaments, pouch of Douglas, serosa of bowel and urinary bladder, and peritoneal cavity. It can present with chronic pelvic pain, dysmenorrhea and dyspareunia, rectal pain and constipation, abnormal uterine bleeding, or infertility.

Grossly, endometriosis causes red-brown serosal nodules (an *endometrioma* is an ovarian "chocolate" (hemolyzed blood) cyst).

Leiomyoma (fibroid), the most common tumor of the female genital tract, is a benign, smooth muscle tumor of the myometrium. Leiomyomas have a high incidence in African Americans, though they are common across all populations. Their growth is estrogen-dependent.

Leiomyomas may present with menorrhagia, abdominal mass, pelvic/back pain, suprapubic discomfort, or infertility and spontaneous abortion.

Grossly, leiomyomas form well-circumscribed, rubbery, white-tan masses with a whorled, trabeculated appearance on cut section. Leiomyomas are commonly multiple, and may have subserosal, intramural, and submucosal location. The malignant variant is leiomyosarcoma.

Endometrial hyperplasia refers to a histological proliferation of endometrial glands with 2 important histopathologic categories:

- **Benign endometrial hyperplasia** shows uniform remodeling of glands with cyst formation.

- **Endometrial intraepithelial neoplasia** shows crowded architecture and cytologic alteration on biopsy.

    ◦ Patients are at high risk for endometrial adenocarcinoma.

    ◦ Treatment options include total hysterectomy or progestin therapy with biopsy surveillance.

Endometrial adenocarcinoma is the most common malignant tumor of the lower female genital tract. It most commonly affects postmenopausal women who present with abnormal uterine bleeding. Risk factors are mostly related to estrogen:

- Early menarche and late menopause
- Nulliparity
- Hypertension and diabetes
- Obesity
- Chronic anovulation
- Estrogen-producing ovarian tumors (granulosa cell tumors)
- ERT and tamoxifen
- Endometrial hyperplasia (complex atypical hyperplasia)
- Lynch syndrome (colorectal, endometrial, and ovarian cancers)

Endometrial adenocarcinoma typically forms a tan polypoid endometrial mass; invasion of myometrium is prognostically important.

- Endometroid adenocarcinoma (most common histological type): associated with *PTEN* mutations

- Serous tumors: associated with *TP53* mutations

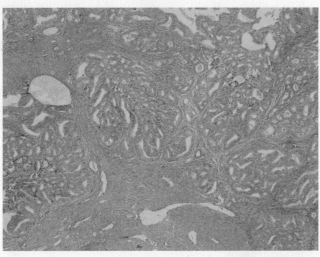

© Gregg Barré, M.D.
Used with permission.

Figure 22-3. Endometrial Carcinoma Invading the Myometrium

Less common types of uterine malignancy include **leiomyosarcoma**, a malignant, smooth muscle tumor, and **carcinosarcoma**, which contains both malignant stromal cells and endometrial adenocarcinoma.

Adenomyosis is an invagination of the deeper layers of the endometrium into the myometrium, which causes menorrhagia and dysmenorrhea.

Anovulation can cause abnormal uterine bleeding, especially in women near menarche and menopause. Biopsy shows glandular and stromal breakdown in a background of proliferative phase endometrium.

OVARY

Polycystic ovarian disease (Stein-Leventhal syndrome) is an endocrine disorder of unknown etiology showing signs of androgen excess (clinical or biochemical), oligoovulation and/or anovulation, and polycystic ovaries.

Accurate diagnosis requires exclusion of other endocrine disorders that might affect reproduction. Patients are usually young women of reproductive age who present with oligomenorrhea or secondary amenorrhea, hirsutism, infertility, or obesity. Treatment is lifestyle change and hormone therapy.

Lab studies show elevated luteinizing hormone (LH), low follicle-stimulating hormone (FSH), and elevated testosterone. Gross examination is notable for bilaterally enlarged ovaries with multiple cysts; microscopic examination shows multiple cystic follicles.

Epithelial Ovarian Tumors

Epithelial ovarian tumors are the most common form of ovarian tumor. Risk factors include nulliparity, family history, and germline mutations.

Previously, epithelial tumors were characterized by histology into the categories cystadenoma (benign), borderline, and cystadenocarcinoma. Now, **serous tumors** are classified as **low grade** and **high grade** for prognostic significance.

- Low grade serous tumors are associated with *KRAS*, *BRAF*, or *ERB2* mutations.
- Most high grade serous tumors have *TP53* mutations.

The most common malignant ovarian tumor is **serous cystadenocarcinoma**. Hereditary risk factors include *BRCA1* (breast and ovarian cancers) and Lynch syndrome.

- Well-differentiated serous tumors show psammoma bodies and a lining similar to that of the fallopian tube.

Mucinous tumors commonly have goblet cells like intestinal mucosal cells.

CA 125 can be used to follow treatment.

Ovarian Germ Cell Tumors

- **Teratoma** (dermoid cyst)
  - Vast majority (>95%) of ovarian (but not testicular) teratomas are benign; commonly occurs in early reproductive years
  - Include elements from all 3 germ cell layers: ectoderm (skin, hair, adnexa, neural tissue), mesoderm (bone, cartilage), and endoderm (thyroid, bronchial tissue)
  - Complications include torsion, rupture, and malignant transformation
  - Can contain hair, teeth, and sebaceous material
  - The term *struma ovarii* is used when there is a preponderance of thyroid tissue
  - Immature teratoma is characterized by histologically immature tissue
- **Dysgerminoma**
  - Malignant; commonly occurs in children and young adults
  - Risk factors include Turner syndrome and disorders of sexual development
  - Gross and microscopic features are similar to seminomas
  - Are radiosensitive; prognosis is good

Ovarian Sex Cord–Stromal Tumors

- **Ovarian fibroma**
  - Most common stromal tumor; forms a firm, white mass
  - **Meigs syndrome** refers to the combination of fibroma, ascites, and pleural effusion.

Note
- The Pap test has reduced the incidence of cervical cancer in the United States.
- There is no screening test for ovarian cancer.

- **Granulosa cell tumor**

  - Potentially malignant, **estrogen-producing** tumor

  - Presentation depends on age:

    - Prepuberal patients with juvenile granulosa cell tumor present with precocious puberty

    - Reproductive age patients present with irregular menses

    - Postmenopausal patients present with vaginal bleeding

  - Complications include endometrial hyperplasia and cancer

  - Tumor forms a yellow-white mass that microscopically shows polygonal tumor cells and formation of follicle-like structures (Call-Exner bodies)

- **Sertoli-Leydig cell tumor** (androblastoma) is an **androgen-producing tumor** that presents with virilization, usually in young women.

Primary sites for **metastatic tumor** to the ovary include breast cancer, colon cancer, endometrial cancer, and gastric "signet-ring cell" cancer (Krukenberg tumor).

Table 22-2. Origins of Common Ovarian Neoplasms

	Surface Epithelial Cells	Germ Cell	Sex Cord–Stroma	Metastasis to Ovaries
Age group affected	20+ years	0–25+ years	All ages	Variable
Types	• Serous tumor • Mucinous tumor • Endometrioid tumor • Clear cell tumor • Brenner tumor	• Teratoma • Dysgerminoma • Endodermal sinus tumor • Choriocarcinoma	• Fibroma • Granulosa–theca cell tumor • Sertoli-Leydig cell tumor	
Overall frequency	65–70%	15–20%	5–10%	5%
Percentage of malignant ovarian tumors	90%	3–5%	2–3%	5%

PLACENTA

Hydatidiform mole (molar pregnancy) is a tumor of placental trophoblastic tissue. Incidence in the United States is 1 per 1,000 pregnancies, with an even higher incidence in Asia. Women ages <15 and >40 are at increased risk.

- **Complete mole** results from fertilization of an ovum that *lost* all of its chromosomal material, so that all chromosomal material is derived from sperm.

  - 90% of the time, the molar karyotype is 46,XX

  - 10% of the time, the molar karyotype includes a Y chromosome

  - The embryo does not develop

- **Partial mole** results from fertilization of an ovum (that has not lost its chromosomal material) by 2 sperms, one 23,X and one 23,Y.

    ◦ Results in a triploid cell 69, XXY (23,X [maternal] + 23,X [one sperm] + 23,Y [the other sperm])

    ◦ The embryo may develop for a few weeks

Patients with hydatidiform mole typically present with the following:

- Excessive uterine enlargement ("size greater than dates")

- Vaginal bleeding

- Passage of edematous, grape-like soft tissue

- Elevated beta-human chorionic gonadotropin (β-hCG)

Microscopically, molar tissue will show edematous chorionic villi, trophoblast proliferation, and fetal tissue (only in partial mole). Diagnosis is by U/S. Treatment is endometrial curettage and following of β-hCG levels.

Table 22-3. Partial Mole Versus a Complete Mole

	Partial Mole	Complete Mole
Ploidy	Triploid	Diploid
Number of chromosomes	69	46 (All paternal)
β-hCG	Elevated (+)	Elevated (+++)
Chorionic villi	Some are hydropic	All are hydropic
Trophoblast proliferation	Focal	Marked
Fetal tissue	Present	Absent
Invasive mole	2%	10%
Choriocarcinoma	Rare	2%

Invasive mole is a mole that invades the myometrium of the uterine wall.

Choriocarcinoma is a malignant germ cell tumor derived from the trophoblast that forms a necrotic and hemorrhagic mass. Almost 50% arise from complete moles. The most common presentation is a rising or plateaued titer of hCG after a molar pregnancy, abortion, or ectopic pregnancy.

Microscopically, choriocarcinoma shows proliferation of cytotrophoblasts, intermediate trophoblasts, and syncytiotrophoblasts. Hematogenous spread can occur, with seeding of tumor to lungs, brain, liver, etc. Treatment is chemotherapy.

Placental site trophoblastic tumor is a tumor of intermediate trophoblast which usually presents <2 years after pregnancy with bleeding and an enlarged uterus. Treatment is surgical; it does not respond well to chemotherapy.

In **ectopic pregnancy**, the fetus implants outside the normal location, most often in the fallopian tube, and less often in the ovaries or abdominal cavity. The fetus almost never survives. The mother is at risk for potentially fatal intra-abdominal hemorrhage. Risk factors include scarring of fallopian tubes from PID, endometriosis, and decreased tubal motility.

Enlarged placenta is common with maternal diabetes mellitus, Rh hemolytic disease, and congenital syphilis.

Succenturiate lobes are accessory lobes of the placenta which may cause hemorrhage if torn away from the main part of the placenta during delivery.

Placental abruption is partial premature separation of the placenta away from the endometrium, with resulting hemorrhage and clot formation. Risk factors include hypertension, cigarette use, cocaine, and older maternal age.

Placenta previa describes when the placenta overlies the cervical os. Vaginal delivery can cause the placenta to tear, with potentially fatal maternal or fetal hemorrhage.

In **placenta accreta**, the placenta implants directly in the myometrium rather than in endometrium. Hysterectomy is required after delivery to remove the rest of the placenta.

Twin placentation

- **Fraternal twins** always have 2 amnions and 2 chorions; placental discs are usually separate, but can grow together to appear to be a single placental disc.

- **Identical twins** have a variable pattern in the number of membranes and discs due to variations in the specific point in embryonic development at which the twins separated. Twin-twin transfusion syndrome can occur if (a) there is only one placental disc and (b) one twin's placental vessels connect to the other twin's placental vessels.

- **Conjoined twins** are always identical twins with one amnion, one chorion, and one disc, though there are rare reports of diamniotic placentation.

Preeclampsia is a condition of new onset hypertension and either proteinuria or end-organ dysfunction after 20 weeks gestation in a previously normotensive woman. It is linked to abnormal uteroplacental blood flow.

- The term **eclampsia** is used when the patient has seizures not attributable to other causes.

- **HELLP syndrome** is a rare complication of preeclampsia characterized by hemolysis, elevated liver enzymes, and low platelets.

Chapter Summary

- Lesions of the vulva include condyloma acuminatum, papillary hidradenoma, extramammary Paget disease, squamous cell carcinoma (SCC), melanoma, Bartholin gland abscess, lichen sclerosis, and lichen simplex chronicus.

- Lesions of the vagina include vaginal adenosis, clear cell adenocarcinoma, embryonal rhabdomyosarcoma, squamous cell carcinoma, rhabdomyoma, Gartner duct cyst, and Rokitansky-Kuster-Hauser syndrome.

- Pelvic inflammatory disease is an ascending infection of polymicrobial origin, from the cervix to the endometrium, fallopian tubes, and pelvic cavity; it is an important cause of infertility.

- Cervical carcinoma is the third most common malignant tumor of the female genital tract and typically arises from HPV-types 16, 18, 31, and 33. Cervical polyps and cervicitis can also affect the cervix.

- Acute endometritis is usually due to an ascending infection of the cervix, sometimes associated with pregnancy or abortions; chronic endometritis is associated with PID and intrauterine devices.

- Endometriosis is the presence of endometrial glands and stroma outside the uterus.

- Leiomyomas are benign smooth muscle tumors that are the most common tumors of the female tract.

- Endometrial adenocarcinoma is the most common malignant tumor of the female genital tract and usually presents as postmenopausal bleeding.

- Polycystic ovarian disease is a cause of infertility and hirsutism in young women.

- Ovarian tumors are subclassified as epithelial, germ cell, or sex cord–stromal origin.

- The most common **epithelial** tumors are serous tumors, classified as low grade (*KRAS*, *BRAF*, *ERB2* mutations) or high grade (*TP53*).

- Ovarian **germ cell** tumors include teratoma, dysgerminoma and yolk sac tumor.

- Ovarian **sex cord**–stromal tumors include ovarian fibroma, granulosa cell tumor, and Sertoli-Leydig cell tumor.

- Gestational trophoblastic disease includes benign and malignant tumors derived from trophoblast, including hydatidiform mole, invasive mole, choriocarcinoma, and placental site trophoblastic tumor.

- Abnormalities of the placenta include ectopic pregnancy, enlarged placentas, succenturiate lobes, placental abruption, placenta previa, and placenta accreta.

- Preeclampsia is a maternal hypertensive condition linked to uteroplacental vascular abnormalities.

Learning Objectives

❏ Explain information related to mastitis

❏ Demonstrate understanding of fibrocystic changes

❏ Solve problems concerning benign and malignant neoplasms

❏ Answer questions about gynecomastia

MASTITIS

Mastitis is an infection of the breast tissue.

Acute mastitis causes an area of erythema and firmness in the breast, commonly during lactation. The most common infecting organism is *S. aureus*. The breast is often biopsied to differentiate the condition from inflammatory carcinoma, another painful breast condition. Microscopically there is acute and chronic inflammation with abscess formation in some cases.

Fat necrosis is often related to trauma or prior surgery, and it may produce a palpable mass or a discrete lesion with calcifications on mammography. Microscopic changes include fat necrosis, chronic inflammation, hemosiderin deposits and fibrosis with calcification.

FIBROCYSTIC CHANGES

Fibrocystic changes (formerly called *fibrocystic disease*) are a group of very common, benign changes that can be classified as **proliferative** (having an increase in the glandular elements or epithelial cells) or **nonproliferative**. Because they carry varying degrees of risk for breast cancer, it is important to identify each type histologically.

Fibrocystic changes primarily affect women in their reproductive years. The changes most often involve the upper outer quadrant and may produce a palpable mass or nodularity.

- **Fibrosis** may mimic a tumor on clinical exam and U/S.

- **Cysts** can usually be diagnosed by U/S.

- **Apocrine metaplasia** is often seen in cyst walls.

- **Microcalcifications** occur in benign and malignant processes.

- **Ductal hyperplasia** is classified as usual or atypical on the basis of cytology and microlumen architecture; **atypical ductal hyperplasia** is differentiated from DCIS on the basis of microscopic extent.

- **Atypical lobular hyperplasia** is differentiated from LCIS histologically on the basis of the percentage of acini involved.
- **Sclerosing adenosis** is distinguished from carcinoma histologically by the preservation of the myoepithelial layer.

Table 23-1. Nonproliferative Versus Proliferative Fibrocystic Changes

Nonproliferative	Proliferative Changes
Fibrosis	Ductal hyperplasia ± atypia
Cysts (blue-domed)	Sclerosing adenosis
Apocrine metaplasia	Atypical lobular hyperplasia
Microcalcifications	

Table 23-2. Relative Risk of Developing Breast Cancer with Fibrocystic Change

Relative Risk	Fibrocystic Change
No increase	Fibrosis, cysts, apocrine metaplasia, adenosis
1.5–2×	Sclerosing ductal hyperplasia, papillomas
4–5×	Atypical ductal or lobular hyperplasia

Table 23-3. Features That Distinguish Fibrocystic Change from Breast Cancer

Fibrocystic Change	Breast Cancer
Often bilateral	Often unilateral
May have multiple nodules	Usually single
Menstrual variation	No menstrual variation
May regress during pregnancy	Does not regress during pregnancy

BENIGN NEOPLASMS

Fibroadenoma is the most common benign breast tumor in women age <35. It causes a palpable, round, movable, rubbery mass, which on cross-section shows small, cleft-like spaces. Microscopically, the mass shows proliferation of benign stroma, ducts, and lobules.

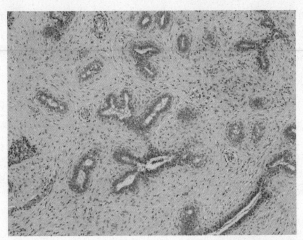

© Gregg Barré, M.D.
Used with permission.

Figure 23-1. Fibroadenoma

Phyllodes tumor (cystosarcoma phyllodes) usually involves an older patient population (age 50s) and can be benign or malignant. Local recurrence is common but the incidence of metastasis is low. Microscopically, the mass shows increased stromal cellularity, clefts lined by epithelium, stromal overgrowth, and irregular margins.

Intraductal papilloma commonly presents as a bloody nipple discharge. Microscopically, papilloma causes benign papillary growth within lactiferous ducts or sinuses; the myoepithelial layer is preserved.

MALIGNANT NEOPLASMS

Carcinoma of the breast is the most common cancer in women and affects 1 in 9 women in the United States. It is also the second most common cause of cancer death. The incidence is increasing and is higher in the United States than in Japan. Many risk factors have been identified.

The incidence increases with the following factors:

- Age
- Unusually long/intense exposure to estrogens (long length of reproductive life, nulliparity, obesity, exogenous estrogens)
- Presence of proliferative fibrocystic changes, especially **atypical hyperplasia**
- First-degree relative with breast cancer

Hereditary influences are thought to be involved in 5–10% of breast cancers, with important genes as follows:

- *BRCA1* (error-free repair of DNA double-strand breaks) chromosome 17q21
- *BRCA2* (error-free repair of DNA double-strand breaks) chromosome 13q12.3
- *TP53* germline mutation (Li-Fraumeni syndrome)

Carcinoma in situ and risk of invasive carcinoma. About 35% of women with untreated DCIS will develop invasive cancer, usually in the same quadrant of the breast. About 35% of women with LCIS will develop invasive lobular or ductal carcinoma, in either breast.

Breast cancer is most common in the upper outer quadrant. Gross examination of a breast cancer typically shows a stellate, white-tan, gritty mass. Clinically, it can cause:

- Mammographic calcifications or architectural distortion
- Palpable solitary painless mass
- Nipple retraction or skin dimpling
- Fixation of breast tissue to the chest wall

Paget disease of the nipple is an intra-epidermal spread of tumor cells from an underlying ductal carcinoma in situ or invasive ductal carcinoma. The tumor cells often lie in lacunae, and there can be a dermal lymphocytic infiltrate.

Histologic variants of breast cancer are as follows:

- **Preinvasive lesions** include ductal carcinoma in situ (**DCIS**) and lobular carcinoma in situ (**LCIS**). Preservation of the myoepithelial cell layer distinguishes them from their invasive counterparts.
- **Invasive (infiltrating) ductal carcinoma** is the most common form (>80% of cases). Microscopically, it shows tumor cells forming ducts within a desmoplastic stroma. About 70% of cases are ER/PR positive and 30% overexpress HER2.

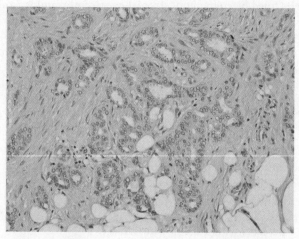

© Gregg Barré, M.D.
Used with permission.

Figure 23-2. Invasive Ductal Carcinoma

- **Invasive (infiltrating) lobular carcinoma** (5–10% of cases) is characterized by small, bland tumor cells forming a single-file pattern.
- Multifocal and bilateral disease occurs commonly.
  - About 50% are ER/PR-positive; these tumors do not overexpress HER2.
- **Mucinous (colloid) carcinoma** is characterized microscopically by clusters of bland tumor cells floating within pools of mucin. It has a better prognosis.
  - Hormone receptors are positive; these tumors do not overexpress HER2.
- **Tubular carcinoma** rarely metastasizes and has an excellent prognosis.
  - Hormone receptors are positive; these tumors do not overexpress HER2.
- **Medullary carcinoma** is characterized microscopically by pleomorphic tumor cells forming syncytial groups surrounded by a dense lymphocytic host response. It has a better prognosis.

○ Hormone receptors are negative; the tumors do not overexpress HER2.

- **Inflammatory carcinoma** is related to tumor invasion into the dermal lymphatics with resulting lymphatic edema; it presents with red, warm, edematous skin. The prognosis is poor.

  ○ The term *peau d'orange* is used when the thickened skin resembles an orange peel. This is caused by the accentuation of the attachments of the suspensory ligaments of Cooper to the dermis.

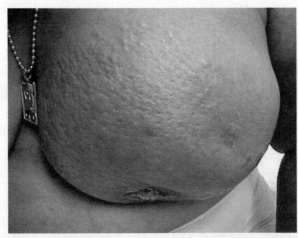

© Richard P. Usatine, M.D.
Used with permission.

Figure 23-3. Advanced Breast Cancer with Peau d'Orange Skin Involvement

Mammary Paget disease (Paget disease of the nipple) is commonly associated with an underlying invasive or in situ ductal carcinoma. It may present with ulceration, oozing, crusting, and fissuring of the nipple and areola. Microscopic examination shows intraepidermal spread of tumor cells (Paget cells), with the cells occurring singly or in groups within the epidermis; there is often a clear halo surrounding the nucleus.

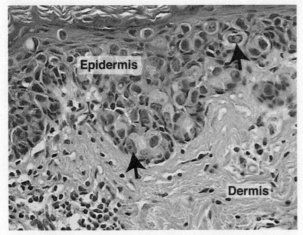

© Giovannini, D'Atri, et al. *World Journal of Surgical Oncology.* 2006.
Used with permission.

Figure 23-4. Paget Disease of the Nipple

Note the intraepidermal tumor cells (arrows) with prominent nucleoli and dermal lymphocytic infiltrate.

The prognosis of breast cancer depends on the following:

- Axillary lymph node status as determined by sentinel node biopsy (SNB) or axillary dissection. In most cases, SNB is recommended to evaluate clinically tumor-free regional nodes.

- Size of tumor

- Histological type and grade of tumor

- ER/PR receptor status is used to select patients for endocrine forms of therapy.

- Overexpression of HER2/neu is associated with more aggressive behavior than other types of breast cancer; patients may respond to therapy with trastuzumab.

Treatment of breast cancer depends on the stage and other tests.

- Urokinase plasminogen activator (uPA) and plasminogen activator inhibitor (PAI-1) as measured by ELISA are used to guide treatment decisions with node-negative breast cancer, along with multiparameter gene expression analysis.

- Cancer antigen 15-3 (CA 15-3), cancer antigen 27.29 (CA 27.29), and carcinoembryonic antigen (CEA) are used to monitor patients with metastatic disease undergoing therapy.

Although the majority of cancers in the breast are primaries, **cancer from other organs can spread to the breast**. Lung cancer may spread by contiguity or via the lymphatics.

GYNECOMASTIA

Gynecomastia is a unilateral or bilateral benign breast enlargement in a male. It is usually caused by an altered androgen-estrogen balance that favors estrogen effect. Microscopically, it is characterized by:

- Ductal epithelial hyperplasia

- Ductal elongation and branching

- Proliferation of periductal fibroblasts

- Increase in vascularity in the involved tissue

Clinical Correlate

Causes of gynecomastia can be:

- Physiologic (newborn infants, pubescent adolescents, and elderly)

- Pathologic (cirrhosis, Klinefelter syndrome, pituitary tumors such as prolactinomas)

- Side effect of drugs (spironolactone and ketoconazole)

Chapter Summary

- Acute mastitis commonly occurs during lactation and is usually due to *S. aureus*.

- Fibrocystic change is an extremely common condition of women age 20–50. It can produce fibrosis, cyst formation, apocrine metaplasia, microcalcifications, ductal hyperplasia with or without atypia, sclerosing adenosis, and atypical lobular hyperplasia.

- Fibroadenoma is the most common benign breast tumor of women age ‹35. It produces a palpable, rubbery, movable mass.

- Cystosarcoma phyllodes is a large tumor involving both stroma and glands. It behaves malignantly in 10–20% of cases.

- Carcinoma of the breast is the most common cancer in women, with a 1 in 9 incidence in the United States.

- Preinvasive lesions which may progress to breast cancer include DCIS and LCIS.

- Invasive cancer occurs in several histologic variants:
  - Ductal carcinoma
  - Lobular carcinoma
  - Mucinous carcinoma
  - Tubular carcinoma
  - Medullary carcinoma
  - Inflammatory carcinoma

- Paget disease of the nipple is an intraepidermal spread of tumor cells. It is commonly associated with an underlying invasive or in situ ductal carcinoma.

- Gynecomastia is benign breast enlargement in a male, usually caused by an increased estrogen to androgen ratio.

Male Pathology 24

Learning Objectives

❑ Explain information related to the pathology of the penis and testes

❑ Solve problems concerning testicular cancer

❑ Solve problems concerning prostate disease

PENIS

Malformations of the penis include epispadias and hypospadias. Both may be associated with undescended testes. **Epispadias** is a urethral opening on the dorsal surface of the penis, while **hypospadias** is a urethral opening on the ventral surface. Both have an increased risk of urinary tract infection and infertility.

Balanitis/balanoposthitis is inflammation of the glans penis, and the glans and foreskin, respectively. Causes include poor hygiene and lack of circumcision.

Peyronie disease is penile fibromatosis resulting in curvature of the penis during erection.

Condyloma acuminatum is a warty, cauliflower-like growth, with the causative agents most frequently being HPV serotypes 6 and 11.

Squamous cell carcinoma (SCC) is uncommon in the United States, and is often related to infection with HPV serotypes 16 and 18. There is an increased risk in uncircumcised males (multicentric carcinoma in situ). Precursor lesions include Bowen disease, bowenoid papulosis, and erythroplasia of Queyrat (a red plaque with carcinoma in situ histology).

Priapism is a persistent painful erection that can be caused by sickle cell anemia (causes blood sludging in penis), trauma, and drugs (e.g., trazodone).

Erectile dysfunction (ED). Causes of impotence include psychological factors, decreased testosterone, vascular insufficiency (most common cause age >50), neurologic disease (multiple sclerosis, diabetic neuropathy, radical prostatectomy), some medications (leuprolide, methyldopa, finasteride, psychotropic medications), hypothyroidism, prolactinoma, and penile disorders.

TESTES

Varicocele is a dilated pampiniform venous plexus and internal spermatic vein, usually on the left side. It may cause infertility. Clinically, it resembles a "bag of worms" superior to the testicle.

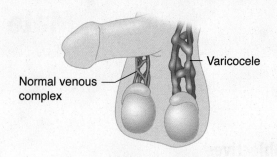

Figure 24-1. Varicocele

Hydrocele refers to fluid within the tunica vaginalis.

Spermatocele is an epididymal cyst containing sperm. On physical examination it transilluminates.

Epididymitis presents with fever and gradual onset of scrotal pain.

- Acute epididymitis that affects men age <35 is often caused by *N. gonorrhoeae* or *C. trachomatis.*

- Acute epididymitis that affects men age >35 is often caused by *E. coli* or *Pseudomonas.*

- Chronic epididymitis can be caused by TB.

Orchitis presents with sudden onset of testicular pain and fever. It is frequently viral, particularly due to the mumps virus.

Testicular torsion is twisting of the spermatic cord; may be associated with physical activity or trauma; and is a clinical emergency that can cause painful hemorrhagic infarction leading to gangrene.

Cryptorchidism is a failure of one or both testes to descend; the undescended testes are most commonly found in the inguinal canal. The undescended testes have an increased risk for developing seminoma.

Male infertility

- Decreased sperm count due to **primary testicular dysfunction** can be caused by Leydig cell dysfunction or seminiferous tubule dysfunction.

- Decreased sperm count due to **secondary hypogonadism** can be caused by pituitary and hypothalamic dysfunction.

- Inability of sperm to exit the body in sufficient numbers may be caused by **obstruction of the vas deferens** or **disordered ejaculation**.

TESTICULAR CANCER

Testicular cancer typically presents with a firm, painless testicular mass; nonseminomatous tumors may present with widespread metastasis. Caucasians have a higher incidence than African Americans.

Clinical Correlate

The most common regional metastatic lymph nodes for testicular cancer are the **para-aortic lymph nodes,** with lymphatic drainage following the gonadal vessels to the retroperitoneum.

Risk factors include:

- Cryptorchidism (3–5 times increased risk)

- Testicular dysgenesis (testicular feminization and Klinefelter syndrome)

- Positive family history

Clinically, U/S typically shows a hypoechoic intratesticular mass. Serum tumor marker studies can be helpful in confirming the diagnosis. Treatment is radical orchiectomy and possible chemotherapy/radiotherapy. Staging includes examination of the surgically resected specimen, including a lymph node dissection, along with imaging studies and lab tests.

Serum markers are used to monitor disease.

- AFP is produced by yolk sac tumors.

- β-hCG is produced by choriocarcinoma and any tumor with syncytiotrophoblastic giant cells.

- LDH is used to measure tumor burden.

Germ Cell Tumors

Germ cell tumors are usually hyperdiploid.

Seminoma is the most common germ cell tumor in adults, with mean age 40. It is characteristically sensitive to both chemotherapy and radiation, and has an excellent prognosis (early stage seminoma has 95% cure rate). A variant is spermatocytic seminoma, a disease of older men, also with an excellent prognosis.

On gross examination the tumor has a pale tan, bulging cut surface. Microscopic exam shows sheets of monotonous cells (with clear cytoplasm and round nuclei) separated by fibrous septae. Lymphocytes, granulomas, and giant cells may be seen.

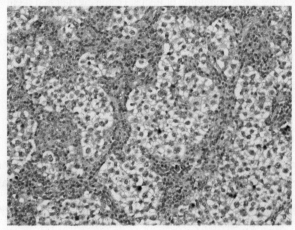

© Gregg Barré, M.D.
Used with permission.

Figure 24-2. Seminoma

Embryonal carcinoma is more aggressive than seminoma and affects adults ages 20–40. It causes bulky masses with hemorrhage and necrosis. Microscopy shows large primitive cells.

Choriocarcinoma is a highly malignant tumor that often has widespread metastasis at the time of diagnosis; hematogenous spread to lungs and liver is particularly common. The often small tumor has extensive hemorrhage and necrosis. Microscopically, syncytiotrophoblasts and cytotrophoblasts are seen.

Yolk sac tumor (endodermal sinus tumor) is the most common germ cell tumor in children; in pediatric cases, the prognosis is good. In adults, the prognosis may depend on the other histologic types that are admixed. Microscopically, yolk sac tumors show numerous patterns. Schiller-Duval bodies are glomeruloid structures.

Teratoma often causes cystic masses which may contain cartilage and bone. Microscopically, mature teratoma usually contains ectodermal, endodermal, and mesodermal tissue in a haphazard arrangement. Immature elements contain embryonic tissue. Prepubertal cases are benign regardless of immature elements; teratomas in adults have malignant potential.

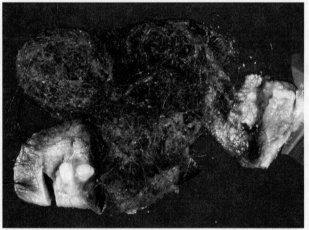

© Katsumi M. Miyai, M.D., Ph.D.; Regents of the University of California.
Used with permission.

Figure 24-3. Teratoma of Testes, Producing Hair and Teeth

Mixed germ cell tumors. As many as 60% of germ cell tumors contain >1 component. When both teratoma and embryonal carcinoma are present, the name *teratocarcinoma* is used.

Sex Cord–Stromal Tumors

Sex cord–stromal tumors include Leydig cell and Sertoli cell tumors.

- **Leydig cell tumors** cause painless testicular masses, and have a bimodal distribution (prepubertal and age >50). They may produce androgens and estrogens.

  ◦ In adults, the hormonal secretion can produce gynecomastia; in children, it can produce precocious puberty.

  ◦ Benign tumors (90%) have an excellent prognosis; malignant tumors (10%) can be refractory to chemotherapy and radiation therapy.

  ◦ Tumor cells have abundant pink cytoplasm.

- **Sertoli cell tumors** are rare and usually benign. Microscopically, they show tubule formation.

Other Tumors

- **Testicular lymphoma** is the most common testicular tumor in men >age 60. It is most commonly non-Hodgkin lymphoma, diffuse large cell type.

- **Scrotal squamous cell carcinoma** is associated with exposure to soot (chimney sweeps).

PROSTATE

Benign prostatic hyperplasia (BPH) (also called nodular hyperplasia; glandular and stromal hyperplasia) is extremely common. Androgens (dihydrotestosterone) play an important role in the pathogenesis, and the lesion is not premalignant. The incidence increases with age (age 60 is 70%; age 70 is 80%). BPH typically presents with the following:

- Decreased caliber and force of stream

- Trouble starting (hesitancy)/stopping the stream

- Postvoid dribbling

- Urinary retention

- Incontinence

- Urgency/frequency

- Nocturia/dysuria

- Possible elevation in prostate specific antigen (PSA) but usually <10 ng/mL

Complications include urinary tract infection, urinary bladder trabeculation and diverticula formation, and hydronephrosis and renal failure (rare). Treatment varies, with available modalities including transurethral resection of prostate (TURP); the 5-alpha reductase inhibitor, finasteride (Proscar); and the selective alpaha-1 receptor blockers, terazosin and prazosin.

Grossly, BPH causes an enlarged prostate with well-demarcated nodules in the transition and central (periurethral) zones, which often results in slit-like compression of the prostatic urethra. Microscopically, the lesion shows glandular and stromal hyperplasia resulting in the characteristic prostate enlargement.

Prostate adenocarcinoma is the most common cancer in men in the United States and the second most common cause of cancer death in men. The incidence increases with age, and the highest rate is in African Americans.

- Often clinically silent but may present with lower back pain secondary to metastasis

- Advanced localized disease may present with urinary tract obstruction or UTI (rare)

- Tumor can be detected with digital rectal exam (induration), serum PSA level, and transrectal U/S and biopsy

- Metastases most commonly involve obturator and pelvic lymph nodes

- Osteoblastic bone metastasis to lumbar spine can occur, and can be associated with elevated alkaline phosphatase

Bridge to Anatomy

- Prostatic hyperplasia → transitional/periurethral zone
- Prostatic carcinoma → peripheral zone

Treatment of local disease is prostatectomy and/or external beam radiation. Metastatic disease is treated with orchiectomy, estrogens, or LHRH agonists and antiandrogens. The disease course can be monitored with PSA levels.

Pathologically, an ill-defined, firm, yellow mass commonly arises in the posterior aspect of the peripheral zone. Microscopically, adenocarcinoma is graded with the **Gleason system**, which scores glandular differentiation. *TMPRSS2-ETS* fusion genes are present in nearly 50% of all prostatic carcinomas.

Prostatitis

- Acute prostatitis is usually caused by intraprostatic reflux of urinary tract pathogens.

- Chronic prostatitis may develop following recurrent acute prostatitis, and bacterial pathogens may not be detectable. Chronic nonbacterial prostatitis (**chronic pelvic pain syndrome**) is more common than bacterial prostatitis.

- Clinical findings can include fever (acute prostatitis), pain (lower back, perineal, or suprapubic), painful prostate on rectal exam, and dysuria (with possible hematuria).

Chapter Summary

- Malformations of the penis related to aberrant opening of the urethra include epispadias (opening on dorsal surface) and hypospadias (opening on ventral surface).

- Balanitis is inflammation of the glans penis, often related to poor hygiene and lack of circumcision.

- Peyronie disease is penile fibromatosis resulting in curvature of the erect penis.

- Condyloma acuminatum is a warty growth of HPV infection.

- Squamous cell carcinoma (SCC) of the penis is uncommon in the United States and is caused by HPV infection.

- Priapism is a persistent painful erection.

- Erectile dysfunction has many causes.

- Varicocele is a dilated pampiniform venous plexus and internal spermatic vein. Hydrocele is fluid within the tunica vaginalis. Spermatocele is an epididymal cyst containing sperm.

- Acute epididymitis is usually caused by *N. gonorrhoeae* and/or *C. trachomatis*. Chronic epididymitis is usually caused by TB. Orchitis or testicular inflammation can be caused by mumps.

- Testicular torsion is a twisting of the spermatic cord that may lead to gangrene.

- Cryptorchidism is a failure of descent of one or both testes, and is associated with an increased risk of developing seminoma.

- Seminoma is a chemotherapy- and radiation therapy–sensitive cancer of young adult men that causes bulky testicular masses. Spermatocytic seminoma is a variant affecting older men.

- Embryonal carcinoma also affects young men and behaves more aggressively than seminoma.

- Choriocarcinoma is a highly malignant testicular carcinoma.

- Pure yolk sac tumor is the most common germ cell tumor in children and carries a good prognosis.

- Testicular teratoma (as opposed to ovarian teratoma) is almost always malignant and aggressive in adults.

- Mixed germ cell tumors are common and usually behave aggressively.

- Most sex cord tumors of the testes are Leydig cell tumors, of which 10% are malignant.

- Testicular lymphoma is the most common testicular tumor in men age >60.

- Male infertility has many causes including conditions that cause low sperm counts or poor sperm mobility.

- Benign prostatic hyperplasia (nodular hyperplasia) may alter the function of the urinary tract by compressing the urethra.

- Prostate cancer is the most common cancer in men in the United States; it frequently arises in the posterior aspect of the peripheral zone of the prostate.

- Prostatitis can be acute or chronic, and causes dysuria and back pain.

Learning Objectives

❑ Demonstrate understanding of disease of the thyroid, parathyroid, adrenal, pituitary, and pineal gland

❑ Describe the relationship between the hypothalamus and pituitary gland

❑ Solve problems concerning multiple endocrine neoplasia syndromes

❑ Explain information related to diabetes mellitus

THYROID GLAND

Multinodular goiter (nontoxic goiter) refers to an enlarged thyroid gland with multiple colloid nodules. Females are affected more often than males. It is frequently asymptomatic, and the patient is typically euthyroid, with normal T4, T3, and TSH. **Plummer syndrome** is the development of hyperthyroidism (toxic multinodular goiter) late in the course.

Microscopically, the tissue shows nodules of varying sizes composed of colloid follicles. Calcification, hemorrhage, cystic degeneration, and fibrosis can also be present.

Hyperthyroidism

The term *hyperthyroidism* is used when the mean metabolic rate of all cells is increased due to increased T4 or T3. Clinical features include tachycardia and palpitations; nervousness and diaphoresis; heat intolerance; weakness and tremors; diarrhea; and weight loss despite a good appetite. Lab studies show elevated free T4.

- In primary hyperthyroidism, TSH is decreased.

- In secondary and tertiary hyperthyroidism, TSH is elevated.

Graves disease is an autoimmune disease characterized by production of IgG autoantibodies to the TSH receptor. Females are affected more frequently than males, with peak age 20–40. Clinical features include hyperthyroidism, diffuse goiter, ophthalmopathy (exophthalmus), and dermopathy (pretibial myxedema). Microscopically, the thyroid has hyperplastic follicles with scalloped colloid.

Other causes of hyperthyroidism include toxic multinodular goiter, toxic adenoma (functioning adenoma producing thyroid hormone), and Hashimoto and subacute thyroiditis (transient hyperthyroidism).

Clinical Correlate

TSH is the most sensitive test in thyroid disease. If it is normal, the patient is euthyroid.

Hypothyroidism

The term *hypothyroidism* is used when the mean metabolic rate of all cells is decreased due to decreased T4 or T3. Clinical features include fatigue and lethargy; sensitivity to cold temperatures; decreased cardiac output; myxedema (accumulation of proteoglycans and water); facial and periorbital edema; peripheral edema of the hands and feet; deep voice; macroglossia; constipation; and anovulatory cycles. Lab studies show decreased free T4.

- In primary hypothyroidism, TSH is elevated.

- In secondary and tertiary hypothyroidism, TSH is decreased.

Iatrogenic hypothyroidism is the most common cause of hypothyroidism in the United States, and is secondary to thyroidectomy or radioactive iodine treatment. Treatment is thyroid hormone replacement.

Congenital hypothyroidism (cretinism) in endemic regions is due to iodine deficiency during intrauterine and neonatal life, and in nonendemic regions is due to thyroid dysgenesis. Patients present with failure to thrive, stunted bone growth and dwarfism, spasticity and motor incoordination, and mental retardation. Goiter is seen in endemic cretinism.

Endemic goiter is due to dietary deficiency of iodine; it is uncommon in the United States.

Thyroiditis

Hashimoto thyroiditis is a chronic autoimmune disease characterized by immune destruction of the thyroid gland and hypothyroidism. It is the most common noniatrogenic/nonidiopathic cause of hypothyroidism in the United States; it most commonly causes painless goiter in females more than males, with peak age 40–65.

Hashimoto thyroiditis is the most common cause of hypothyroidism (due to destruction of thyroid tissue), though the initial inflammation may cause transient hyperthyroidism (hashitoxicosis). Hashimoto may be associated with other autoimmune diseases (SLE, rheumatoid arthritis, Sjögren syndrome, etc.), and it has an increased risk of non-Hodgkin B-cell lymphoma. Grossly, Hashimoto produces a pale, enlarged thyroid gland; microscopically, it shows lymphocytic inflammation with germinal centers and epithelial "Hürthle cell" changes.

Subacute thyroiditis (also called de Quervain thyroiditis and granulomatous thyroiditis) is the second most common form of thyroiditis; it affects females more than males, with peak age 30–50. Patients may complain of odynophagia (pain on swallowing).

- Typically preceded by a viral illness

- Produces a tender, firm, enlarged thyroid gland

- May be accompanied by transient hyperthyroidism

Microscopy shows granulomatous thyroiditis. The disease typically follows a self-limited course.

Note

The original name for the autoantibodies of Graves disease was long-acting thyroid stimulator (LATS). The current name is **thyroid-stimulating immunoglobulin (TSI)**.

Riedel thyroiditis is a rare disease of unknown etiology, characterized by destruction of the thyroid gland by dense fibrosis and fibrosis of surrounding structures (trachea and esophagus). It affects females more than males, and most patients are middle-aged.

- Causes an irregular, hard thyroid that is adherent to adjacent structures
- May clinically mimic carcinoma and present with stridor, dyspnea, or dysphagia

Microscopic exam shows dense fibrous replacement of the thyroid gland with chronic inflammation. Reidel thyroiditis is associated with retroperitoneal and mediastinal fibrosis.

Thyroid Neoplasia

Thyroglossal duct cyst presents as a midline neck mass in a young patient. Its epithelium varies with location (squamous/respiratory). It may become infected and painful. Treatment is surgical.

Adenomas: follicular adenoma is the most common. Clinically, adenomas are usually painless, solitary, encapsulated nodules that appear "cold" on thyroid scans. They may be functional and cause hyperthyroidism (toxic adenoma).

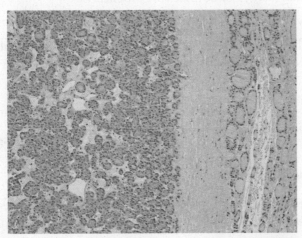

© Gregg Barré, M.D.
Used with permission.

Figure 25-1. Follicular Adenoma *(left)*, Separated from Normal Thyroid Parenchyma *(right)*, by the Capsule *(center)*

Papillary carcinoma accounts for 80% of malignant thyroid tumors. It affects females more than males, with peak age 20–50. Radiation exposure is a risk factor. Resection is curative in most cases. Radiotherapy with iodine 131 is effective for metastases. The prognosis is excellent, with 20-year survival 90% due to slow growth and metastasis to regional cervical lymph nodes. There are chromosomal rearrangements of the *RET* oncogene.

Microscopically, the tumor typically exhibits a papillary pattern. Occasional psammoma bodies may be seen. Characteristic nuclear features include clear "Orphan Annie eye" nuclei, nuclear grooves, and intranuclear cytoplasmic inclusions. Lymphatic spread to cervical nodes is common.

Follicular carcinoma accounts for 15% of malignant thyroid tumors. It affects females more than males, with peak age 40–60. Hematogenous metastasis to the bones or lungs is common. These cancers are microscopically distinguished from follicular adenoma by the presence of capsular invasion.

Medullary carcinoma accounts for 5% of malignant thyroid tumors. It arises from C cells (parafollicular cells) and secretes calcitonin. Microscopic exam shows nests of polygonal cells in an amyloid stroma. A minority of cases (25%) is associated with MEN 2 and MEN 3 syndromes, and those cases tend to be multicentric. Activating *RET* mutations are present in familial and sporadic types.

Anaplastic carcinoma affects females more than males, with peak age >60. It can present with a firm, enlarging, and bulky mass, or with dyspnea and dysphagia. The tumor has a tendency for early widespread metastasis and invasion of the trachea and esophagus. Microscopically, the tumor is composed of undifferentiated, anaplastic, and pleomorphic cells. This very aggressive tumor is often rapidly fatal.

PARATHYROID GLANDS

Primary hyperparathyroidism can be caused by the following:

- Adenomas (80%); may be associated with MEN 1
- Parathyroid hyperplasia (15%)
  - Characterized by diffuse enlargement of all 4 glands; the enlarged glands are usually composed of chief cells
  - Parathyroid carcinoma is very rare
- Hyperparathyroidism can also occur as a paraneoplastic syndrome of lung and renal cell carcinomas.

The excess production of parathyroid hormone (PTH) leads to hypercalcemia, with lab studies showing elevated serum calcium and PTH.

Primary hyperparathyroidism is often asymptomatic, but may cause kidney stones, osteoporosis and osteitis fibrosa cystica, metastatic calcifications, or neurologic changes.

Secondary hyperparathyroidism is caused by any disease that results in hypocalcemia, leading to increased secretion of PTH by the parathyroid glands; it can result from chronic renal failure, vitamin D deficiency, or malabsorption.

Hypoparathyroidism can result from the surgical removal of glands during thyroidectomy, DiGeorge syndrome, or a hereditary autoimmune syndrome caused by mutations in the autoimmune regulator gene *AIRE*. Patients present with muscle spasm and tingling of toes and lips. The hypocalcemia may also cause psychiatric disturbances and cardiac conduction defects (ECG: prolonged QT interval).

Treatment of hypoparathyroidism is vitamin D and calcium.

In a Nutshell

Osteitis fibrosa cystica (von Recklinghausen disease) is seen when excessive parathyroid hormone (hyperparathyroidism) causes osteoclast activation and generalized bone resorption (causing possible bone pain, deformities, and fractures). It is common in primary hyperparathyroidism.

- Excess parathyroid hormone may be produced by parathyroid adenoma or parathyroid hyperplasia
- "Brown tumors" are masses produced by cystic enlargement of bones with areas of fibrosis and organized hemorrhage

PITUITARY GLAND, HYPOTHALAMUS, AND PINEAL GLAND

Pituitary adenomas are categorized as follows:

- **Microadenoma** if <1 cm

- **Macroadenoma** if >1 cm

Macroadenomas cause visual field defects.

GNAS1 mutations are common. Pathologically, adenomas are monomorphic compared with normal pituitary.

- **Prolactinoma** is the most common type of pituitary adenoma. Lactotroph cells secrete prolactin, which results in hyperprolactinemia. Clinical features include galactorrhea, amenorrhea, and infertility, or decreased libido and impotence.

- **Nonfunctional adenoma** may produce hypopituitarism.

- **Growth-hormone–producing adenoma** is characterized by elevated growth hormone (GH) and elevated somatomedin C (insulin-like growth factor 1 [IGF-1]). It causes gigantism in children and acromegaly in adults.

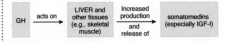

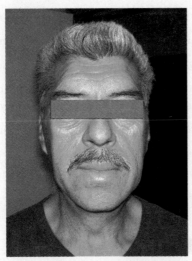

© Richard P. Usatine, M.D.
Used with permission.

Figure 25-2. Coarse Facial Features and Protruding Jaw Seen with Acromegaly

Sheehan syndrome is ischemic necrosis of the pituitary secondary to hypotension from postpartum hemorrhage resulting in panhypopituitarism.

Clinical Correlate

Any pituitary tumor that destroys >75% of the pituitary may result in panhypopituitarism, which is characterized by abnormalities of the thyroid, adrenal gland, and reproductive organs. Common causes are:

- Pituitary adenomas
- Sheehan syndrome
- Craniopharyngiomas

Clinical Correlate

The most common cause of ectopic ADH secretion is cancer (especially small cell lung cancer, though any lung lesion can lead to this manifestation). For this reason, SIADH may be a marker for occult malignancy. Drugs that may also lead to SIADH include chlorpropamide, carbamazepine, cyclophosphamide, tricyclic antidepressants, and SSRIs.

Posterior pituitary syndromes include the following:

- **Diabetes insipidus**
    - Central diabetes insipidus is caused by ADH deficiency, which results in hypotonic polyuria, polydipsia, hypernatremia, and dehydration. Causes include head trauma and tumors.
    - Nephrogenic diabetes insipidus is caused by a lack of renal response to ADH.

- **Syndrome of inappropriate ADH secretion (SIADH)** is caused by excessive production of antidiuretic hormone (ADH), resulting in oliguria, water retention, hyponatremia, and cerebral edema. Causes include paraneoplastic syndrome and head trauma.

Craniopharyngioma is a benign pituitary tumor derived from Rathke pouch remnants that is usually located above the sella turcica, but can extend downward to destroy the pituitary. It is the most common cause of hypopituitarism in children.

Hypothalamic disorders can cause a variety of problems:

- **Hypopituitarism** (including dwarfism) can be due to a lack of releasing hormones from the hypothalamus.

- **Central diabetes insipidus** is due to lack of ADH synthesis.

- **Precocious puberty** is usually due to a midline hamartoma in boys.

- The hypothalamus can also be affected in **hydrocephalus**.

- **Visual field changes** can complicate hypothalmic disorders.

- Masses can affect the hypothalamus, i.e., pituitary adenoma, craniopharyngioma, midline hamartoma, and Langerhans histiocytosis.

- Inflammatory processes can affect the hypothalamus, i.e., sarcoidosis and meningitis.

Pineal diseases include dystrophic calcification (a useful landmark for radiologists) and rarely tumors, with most being germ cell tumors.

ADRENAL GLAND

Cushing syndrome is characterized by increased levels of glucocorticoids. It is investigated with lab and imaging studies (*see* Physiology Lecture Notes). The most common cause is exogenous glucocorticoid administration.

Endogenous causes include:

- Cushing disease (hypersecretion of ACTH, usually due to a pituitary microadenoma)

- Secretion of ACTH from nonpituitary tumors (e.g., small cell lung cancer)

- ACTH-independent Cushing syndrome due to adrenal neoplasia

Clinical manifestations include hypertension, weight gain (truncal obesity, "buffalo hump" and moon facies), cutaneous striae, hirsutism and mental disturbances.

Note

Administration of **dexamethasone** (a cortisol analog) will typically suppress pituitary ACTH production, resulting in suppression of adrenal cortisol production and a decrease in urinary free cortisol.

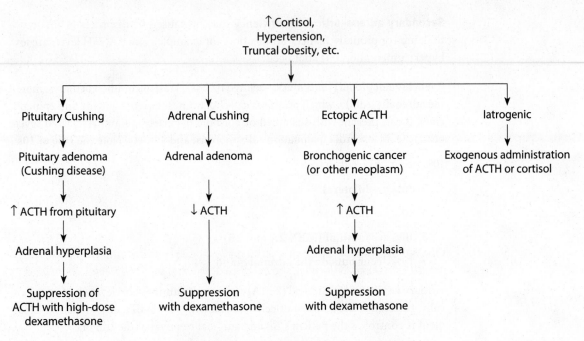

Figure 25-3. Cushing Syndrome and Its Effects

Hyperaldosteronism may cause hypertension and hypokalemia.

- **Primary** (decreased plasma renin)
    - Adrenocortical neoplasm: adenoma (Conn syndrome)
        - Circumscribed yellow nodule with vacuolated cells
        - Carcinoma: poorly demarcated lesion with cystic change and pleomorphic cells
    - Bilateral nodular hyperplasia of the adrenal
- **Secondary** (increased plasma renin) (e.g., renal artery stenosis)

Adrenogenital syndromes are adrenal disorders characterized by excess production of androgens and virilization. They are caused either by adrenocortical adenoma/ carcinoma, which produces androgens, or by congenital adrenal hyperplasia, a cluster of autosomal recessive enzyme defects (most common is 21-hydroxylase deficiency).

Waterhouse-Friderichsen syndrome (acute adrenal insufficiency) is a potentially fatal, bilateral hemorrhagic infarction of the adrenal glands associated with sepsis, often due to a *N. meningitidis* infection in children. It is clinically characterized by disseminated intravascular coagulation (DIC), acute respiratory distress syndrome, hypotension and shock, and acute adrenal insufficiency. Treatment is antibiotics and steroid replacement.

Addison's disease (chronic adrenocortical insufficiency) is caused by destruction of the adrenal cortex, leading to a deficiency of glucocorticoids, mineralocorticoids, and androgens. The most common cause is autoimmune adrenalitis, though adrenal involvement by TB or metastatic cancer are other possible causes. Patients present with gradual onset of weakness, skin hyperpigmentation, hypotension, hypoglycemia, poor response to stress, and loss of libido. Treatment is steroid replacement.

Bridge to Embryology

- The cells of the **adrenal medulla** are derived from neural crest cells.
- The cells of the **adrenal cortex** are derived from mesoderm.

Secondary adrenocortical insufficiency may be caused by disorders of the hypothalamus or pituitary (cancer or infection, for example). Since ACTH levels are low, hyperpigmentation does not occur.

Pheochromocytoma ("dark/dusky-colored tumor") is an uncommon benign tumor of the adrenal medulla, which produces catecholamines (norepinephrine and epinephrine). It can present with sustained or episodic hypertension and associated severe headache, tachycardia, palpitations, diaphoresis, and anxiety. Note the **rule of 10s:**

10% occur in **children**

- 10% are **bilateral**

- 10% are **malignant**

- 10% are **familial (MEN 2A and 2B)**

- 10% occur **outside the adrenal gland**

Urinary vanillylmandelic acid (VMA) and catecholamines are elevated. Microscopically, the tumor shows nests of cells (Zellballen) with abundant cytoplasm. Treatment is control of the patient's BP and surgical removal of the tumor.

MULTIPLE ENDOCRINE NEOPLASIA SYNDROMES

Multiple endocrine neoplasia (MEN) syndromes are autosomal dominant conditions with incomplete penetrance that are characterized by hyperplasia and tumors of endocrine glands occurring at a young age.

- **MEN 1** (Werner syndrome) features tumors of the pituitary gland, parathyroids, and pancreas.

- Associated with peptic ulcers and Zollinger-Ellison syndrome

  ◦ Affected gene is *MEN1*, a tumor suppressor gene which encodes a nuclear protein called menin

- **MEN 2A** (Sipple syndrome) features medullary carcinoma of the thyroid, pheochromocytoma, and parathyroid hyperplasia or adenoma.

  ◦ Mutation of *RET* proto-oncogene

- **MEN 2B** features medullary carcinoma of the thyroid, pheochromocytoma, and mucocutaneous neuromas.

- Mutation of *RET* proto-oncogene

DIABETES MELLITUS

Diabetes mellitus (DM) is a chronic systemic disease characterized by insulin deficiency or peripheral resistance, resulting in hyperglycemia and nonenzymatic glycosylation of proteins. Diagnosis is established by demonstrating **either** of the following:

- Fasting glucose >126 mg/dL on at least 2 separate occasions

- Positive glucose tolerance test

A glycated hemoglobin (HbA1c) assay is used for certain patient populations. The diagnostic cutoff is 6.5%.

Type 1 diabetes (T1D) represents 10% of cases of diabetes.

- Affects children and adolescents, usually age <20

- Risk factors include Northern European ancestry and specific HLA types (DR3, DR4, and DQ)

- Pathogenesis is a lack of insulin due to autoimmune destruction of β cells (type IV hypersensitivity reaction)

- Patients are absolutely dependent on insulin to prevent ketoacidosis and coma

- Thought to be caused by autoimmune reaction triggered by an infection (Coxsackie B virus) in a genetically susceptible individual

T1D can present with polydipsia, polyuria, and polyphagia; dehydration and electrolyte imbalance; metabolic ketoacidosis; and coma and potentially death. Microscopically, lymphocytic inflammation involves the islets of Langerhans (insulitis), leading to loss of β cells and fibrosis of the islets. Treatment is insulin.

Type 2 diabetes (T2D) represents 90% of cases.

- Affects obese individuals, both children and adults

- Approximately 10 million people in the United States are affected (half are undiagnosed), and incidence increases with age

- Risk factors include obesity, increasing age, and genetic predisposition

- Pathogenesis involves relatively reduced insulin secretion; *peripheral insulin resistance* is the term used for reduced tissue sensitivity to insulin due to decreased numbers of insulin receptors on the cell membranes.

T2D is often asymptomatic, but it can present with either polydipsia, polyuria, and polyphagia, or with hyperosmolar nonketotic diabetic coma. Microscopically, the changes are nonspecific, and can include focal atrophy and amyloid deposition in islets (hyalinization). Treatment is diet/weight loss, oral antidiabetic drugs, and insulin as needed (more common in long-standing cases).

Vascular pathology. Diabetes is a major risk factor for atherosclerosis and its complications, including myocardial infarction (most common cause of death), stroke (CVA), and peripheral vascular disease. The vascular disease can lead to atrophy of skin and loss of hair of the lower extremities, claudication, nonhealing ulcers, and gangrene of lower extremities.

Diabetic nephropathy includes glomerular lesions, arteriolosclerosis, and pyelonephritis (*see* Renal chapter).

Diabetic retinopathy. Nonproliferative retinopathy is characterized by microaneurysms, retinal hemorrhages, and retinal exudates. Proliferative retinopathy is characterized by neovascularization and fibrosis. Diabetics also have an increased incidence of cataracts and glaucoma.

Diabetic neuropathy can cause peripheral neuropathy, neurogenic bladder, and sexual impotence.

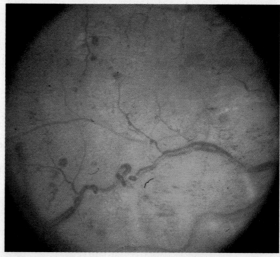

© Richard P. Usatine, M.D. / Paul D. Comeau, M.D.
Used with permission.

Figure 25-4. Diabetic Retinopathy with Hemorrhages, Venous Beading, and Looping of Vessels

Chapter Summary

- Multinodular goiter is an enlarged thyroid gland with multiple colloid nodules that is frequently asymptomatic and euthyroid.

- General features of hyperthyroidism include tachycardia, nervousness, diaphoresis, heat intolerance, weakness, tremors, diarrhea, and weight loss. Free T4 is elevated and TSH is decreased in primary hyperthyroidism and increased in secondary and tertiary hyperthyroidism. Hyperthyroidism can be caused by Graves disease, toxic multinodular goiter, toxic adenoma, and (transiently during) Hashimoto disease and subacute thyroiditis.

- Graves disease is an autoimmune disease characterized by production of IgG autoantibodies to the TSH receptor. Clinical features include hyperthyroidism, goiter, exophthalmos, and pretibial myxedema.

- General features of hypothyroidism include fatigue, lethargy, sensitivity to cold temperatures, decreased cardiac output, myxedema, and constipation. Free T4 is decreased and TSH is elevated in primary hypothyroidism and decreased in secondary and tertiary hypothyroidism.

- Hashimoto thyroiditis is a chronic autoimmune disease characterized by immune destruction of the thyroid gland and hypothyroidism.

- Subacute thyroiditis is a cause of transient hyperthyroidism following a viral illness.

- Riedel thyroiditis is a rare disease of unknown etiology characterized by destruction of the gland by dense fibrosis.

- Thyroid adenomas are usually painless, solitary nodules.

- Thyroid carcinomas occur in a number of histologic types, including papillary (most common with excellent prognosis), follicular (tends to spread hematogenously), medullary (secretes calcitonin, makes amyloid, and may be associated with MEN-2A or 2B), and anaplastic (rapidly fatal).

(continued)

Chapter Summary *(cont'd)*

- Primary hyperparathyroidism is most often due to a parathyroid adenoma or to parathyroid hyperplasia. Secondary hyperparathyroidism may occur secondary to any disease causing hypocalcemia.

- Hypoparathyroidism presents as hypocalcemia. Causes include surgical removal of the glands, DiGeorge syndrome, and *AIRE* mutations.

- Pituitary adenomas can produce prolactin (causing galactorrhea, amenorrhea, and infertility), growth hormone (causing gigantism and acromegaly), or other pituitary hormones.

- Diabetes insipidus is ADH deficiency resulting in hypotonic polyuria, hypernatremia and dehydration.

- SIADH is excessive production of ADH, resulting in oliguria, water retention, hyponatremia, and cerebral edema.

- Cushing syndrome is characterized by increased levels of glucocorticoids, whose origin may be iatrogenic, pituitary corticotroph adenoma, adrenocortical adenoma, or paraneoplastic syndrome.

- Primary hyperaldosteronism causes hypertension, hypokalemia, elevated aldosterone, and decreased renin. Causes include neoplasia and hyperplasia.

- Adrenogenital syndromes are adrenal disorders characterized by excess production of androgens and virilization and can be due to either an adrenocortical adenoma/carcinoma or congenital adrenal hyperplasia.

- Waterhouse-Friderichsen syndrome (acute adrenal insufficiency) is a potentially fatal, bilateral hemorrhagic infarction of the adrenal glands, usually in a patient with sepsis.

- Addison's disease (chronic adrenocortical insufficiency) is caused by destruction of the adrenal cortex; the most common cause is autoimmune adrenalitis.

- Pheochromocytoma is an uncommon tumor of the adrenal medulla that produces catecholamines and may present with severe headache, tachycardia, diaphoresis, and hypertensive episodes.

- MEN 1, 2A and 2B are inherited disorders of endocrine glands.

- DM is a chronic systemic disease characterized by insulin deficiency or peripheral resistance, resulting in hyperglycemia and non-enzymatic glycosylation of proteins.

  - Type 1 usually develops in children and adolescents and is related to lack of insulin secondary to autoimmune destruction of beta cells.

  - Type 2 usually develops in obese adults; it is much more common than type 1.

  - Both types of diabetes may lead to long-term complications including atherosclerosis, myocardial infarction, stroke, peripheral vascular disease, nephropathy, retinopathy, and neuropathy.

Learning Objectives

❏ Describe normal bone

❏ Explain information related to hereditary bone disorders

❏ Answer questions about Paget disease

❏ Differentiate osteoporosis, osteomalacia, and rickets

❏ Solve problems concerning osteomyelitis, benign tumors of bone, and malignant tumors of bone

NORMAL BONE

Normal bone is composed of organic matrix and inorganic matrix.

- The **organic matrix** includes cells, type I collagen (90% of bone protein), osteocalcin, glycoproteins, and proteoglycans.

- The **inorganic matrix** includes calcium hydroxyapatite $Ca_{10}(PO_4)_6(OH)_2$, magnesium, potassium, chloride, sodium, and fluoride.

There are 3 cell types.

- **Osteoblasts** are responsible for the production of osteoid (unmineralized bone); they contain high amounts of alkaline phosphatase, have receptors for parathyroid hormone (PTH), and modulate osteoclast function.

- **Osteocytes** are responsible for bone maintenance; they are osteoblasts that have become incorporated in the matrix.

- **Osteoclasts** are responsible for bone resorption; they contain high amounts of acid phosphatase and collagenase, and resorb bone within Howship's lacunae.

Bone remodeling occurs throughout life and is necessary to maintain healthy bones. Bone resorption by osteoclasts is tightly balanced with bone formation by osteoblasts.

Important hormones involved in bone physiology include parathyroid hormone (PTH), calcitonin, vitamin D, estrogen, thyroid hormone, cortisol, and growth hormone.

Formation of bones is as follows:

- **Intramembranous bone** occurs as direct bone formation without a "cartilage model." Intramembranous bones include flat bones such as the cranium, clavicle, vertebrae, wrist, and ankle bones. Intramembranous growth is also involved in appositional bone growth.

- **Endochondral bone** is indirect bone formation from a "cartilage model" at the epiphyseal growth plates; this type of bone formation occurs in long bones such as the femur, humerus, tibia, fibula, etc.

HEREDITARY BONE DISORDERS

Achondroplasia is the most common form of inherited dwarfism. It is caused by an autosomal dominant mutation in fibroblast growth factor receptor 3 (*FGFR3*). Activation of *FGFR3* inhibits cartilage synthesis at the epiphyseal growth plate, resulting in decreased enchondral bone formation and premature ossification of the growth plates.

- Long bones are short and thick, leading to dwarfism with short extremities.

- Cranial and vertebral bones are spared, leading to relatively large head and trunk.

- Intelligence, life span, and reproductive ability are normal.

Osteogenesis imperfecta (OI) ("brittle bone disease") is a hereditary defect leading to abnormal synthesis of type I collagen.

- Patients have generalized osteopenia (brittle bones), resulting in recurrent fractures and skeletal deformity

- Abnormally thin sclera with blue hue is common

- Laxity of joint ligaments leads to hypermobility

- Involvement of inner and middle ear bones produces deafness

- Occasional dentinogenesis imperfecta, characterized by small, fragile, and discolored teeth due to a deficiency of dentin

- Dermis may be abnormally thin, and skin is susceptible to easy bruising

- Treatment is supportive

Osteopetrosis (or marble bone disease) is a hereditary defect leading to decreased osteoclast function, with resulting decreased resorption and thick sclerotic bones. X-ray shows symmetrical generalized osteosclerosis. Long bones may have broadened metaphyses, causing an "Erlenmeyer flask"-shaped deformity. Treatment is hematopoietic stem cell transplantation.

- **Autosomal recessive** type (**malignant**):

  ○ Affects infants and children (causes multiple fractures and early death due to anemia, infection, and hemorrhage)

- **Autosomal dominant** type (**benign**):

  ○ Affects adults (causes fractures, mild anemia, and cranial nerve impingement)

Pathology shows increased bone density and thickening of bone cortex. Myelophthisic anemia may result from marrow crowding. Cranial nerve compression due to narrowing of cranial foramina may result in blindness, deafness, and facial nerve palsies. Hydrocephalus may develop due to obstruction of CSF.

PAGET DISEASE

Paget disease (osteitis deformans) is a localized disorder of bone remodeling, resulting in excessive bone resorption followed by disorganized bone replacement, producing thickened but weak bone that is susceptible to deformity and fracture. There is an association with paramyxovirus and mutations of *SQSTM1*.

- Seen in those age >40
- Common in those of European ancestry
- Common sites of involvement include the skull, pelvis, femur, and vertebrae
- Majority of cases are polyostotic and mild

Paget disease develops in 3 stages:

- **Osteolytic stage** (osteoclastic activity predominates)
- **Mixed osteolytic-osteoblastic stage**
- **Osteosclerotic stage** (osteoblastic activity predominates in this "burnout stage")

Paget disease can cause bone pain and deformity, fractures, and warmth of the overlying skin due to bone hypervascularity. X-rays show bone enlargement with lytic and sclerotic areas. Lab studies show highly elevated serum alkaline phosphatase and increased levels of urinary hydroxyproline. Complications include arteriovenous shunts within marrow, which may result in high-output cardiac failure and an increased incidence of osteosarcoma and other sarcomas.

Microscopically, there is a haphazard arrangement of cement lines, creating a "mosaic pattern" of lamellar bone. Involved bones are thick but weak and fracture easily. Skull involvement leads to increased head size and foraminal narrowing that can impinge on cranial nerves, often leading to deafness. Involvement of facial bones may produce a lion-like facies.

OSTEOPOROSIS

Osteoporosis is decreased bone mass (osteopenia), resulting in thin, fragile bones susceptible to fracture. It is the most common bone disorder in the United States. It most commonly occurs in postmenopausal Caucasian women and the elderly.

Note

In osteoporosis, bone is formed normally but in decreased amounts.

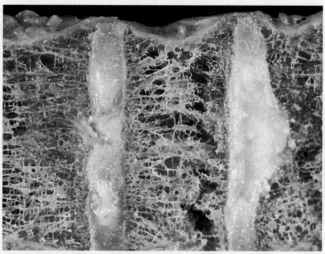

© Katsumi M. Miyai, M.D., Ph.D.; Regents of the University of California.
Used with permission.

Figure 26-1. Marked Thinning of Bony Trabeculae in Osteoporosis

Primary causes of osteoporosis include the following:

- Estrogen deficiency (postmenopausal, Turner syndrome)
- Genetic factors (low density of original bone)
- Lack of exercise
- Old age
- Nutritional factors

Secondary causes include immobilization, endocrinopathies (e.g., Cushing disease, thyrotoxicosis), malnutrition (e.g., deficiencies of calcium, vitamins C and D, protein), corticosteroids, smoking/alcohol consumption, genetic disease (e.g., Gaucher disease).

- Patients may experience bone pain and fractures; weight-bearing bones are predisposed to fractures.
- Common fracture sites include vertebrae (compression fracture); femoral neck (hip fracture); and distal radius (Colles fracture).
- Kyphosis and loss of height may result.
- X-rays show generalized radiolucency of bone (osteopenia).

Dual-energy x-ray absorptiometry (DEXA) can measure bone mineral density to predict fracture risk. Lab studies may show normal serum calcium, phosphorus, and alkaline phosphatase, but the diagnosis is not based on labs. Microscopically, the bone has thinned cortical and trabecular bone.

Treatment can include estrogen replacement therapy (controversial; not recommended currently); weight-bearing exercise; calcium and vitamin D; bisphosphonate (alendronate); and calcitonin.

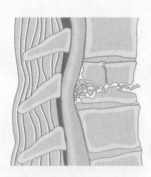

Compression Fracture

OSTEOMALACIA AND RICKETS

Osteomalacia and **rickets** are both characterized by decreased mineralization of newly formed bone. They are usually caused by deficiency or abnormal metabolism of vitamin D. Specific causes include dietary deficiency of vitamin D, intestinal malabsorption, lack of sunlight, and renal and liver disease. Treatment is vitamin D and calcium supplementation.

Osteomalacia (adults) is due to impaired mineralization of the osteoid matrix resulting in thin, fragile bones susceptible to fracture. The patient may present clinically with bone pain or fractures (vertebrae, hips, and wrist). X-rays show transverse lucencies called Looser zones. Lab studies show low serum calcium, low serum phosphorus, and high alkaline phosphatase.

Rickets (children) occurs in children prior to closure of the epiphyses. Both remodeled bone and bone formed at the epiphyseal growth plate are undermineralized. Enchondral bone formation is affected, leading to skeletal deformities. Skull deformities include craniotabes (softening, seen in early infancy) and frontal bossing (hardening, later in childhood). The "rachitic rosary" is a deformity of the chest wall as a result of an overgrowth of cartilage at the costochondral junction. Pectus carinatum, lumbar lordosis, bowing of the legs, and fractures also occur.

OSTEOMYELITIS

Pyogenic osteomyelitis is bone inflammation due to bacterial infection. The most common route of infection is **hematogenous spread** (leading to seeding of bone after bacteremia); this type of spread often affects the metaphysis. Other routes of spread include direct inoculation (e.g., trauma) and spread from an adjacent site of infection (e.g., prosthetic joint).

The most common infecting organism is *S. aureus*; other important pathogens include *E. coli*, streptococci, gonococci, *H. influenzae*, *Salmonella* (common in sickle cell disease), and *Pseudomonas* (common in IV drug abusers and diabetics).

Clinically, osteomyelitis is characterized by fever and leukocytosis; and localized pain, erythema, and swelling. X-ray studies may be normal for up to 2 weeks, and then initially show periosteal elevation followed by a possible lytic focus with surrounding sclerosis. MRI and nuclear medicine studies are more sensitive and specific.

Microscopic examination shows suppurative inflammation. Vascular insufficiency can lead to ischemic necrosis of bone; a sequestrum is an area of necrotic bone, while an involucrum is the new bone formation that surrounds the sequestrum. The diagnosis is established with blood cultures or with bone biopsy and culture.

Patients are treated with antibiotics and some may require surgical drainage. Complications include fracture, intraosseous (Brodie) abscess, secondary amyloidosis, sinus tract formation, squamous cell carcinoma of the skin at the site of a persistent draining sinus tract, and, rarely, osteogenic sarcoma.

Note

Rickets and osteomalacia are disorders of osteoid mineralization; osteoid is produced in normal amounts but is not calcified properly.

Clinical Correlate

Lab findings help to distinguish osteomalacia from osteoporosis.

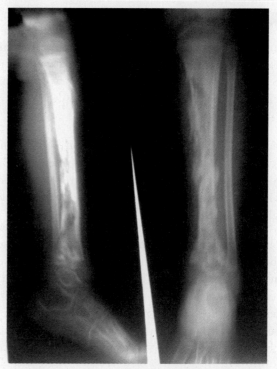

Source: commons.wikimedia.org

Figure 26-2. Tibial Radiolucencies Representing Osteomyelitis.

Tuberculous osteomyelitis is seen in 1% of cases of TB. It presents with pain or tenderness, fever, night sweats, and weight loss. Biopsy shows caseating granulomas with extensive destruction of the bones. Common sites of involvement include thoracic and lumbar vertebrae ("Pott disease"). Complications include vertebral compression fracture, psoas abscesses, and secondary amyloidosis.

MISCELLANEOUS BONE DISORDERS

Avascular necrosis (or aseptic necrosis and osteonecrosis) is the term used for ischemic necrosis of bone and bone marrow. Causes include trauma and/or fracture (most common); idiopathic; steroid use; sickle cell anemia; Gaucher disease; and caisson disease. Avascular necrosis can be complicated by osteoarthritis and fractures.

Osteitis fibrosa cystica (or von Recklinghausen disease of bone) is seen when excessive parathyroid hormone (hyperparathyroidism) causes osteoclast activation and generalized bone resorption, resulting in possible bone pain, bone deformities, and fractures.

- Seen commonly in primary hyperparathyroidism
- Excess parathyroid hormone may be produced by parathyroid adenoma or parathyroid hyperplasia
- Can be resolved if hyperparathyroidism is treated

Microscopic exam shows excess bone resorption with increased number of osteoclasts, fibrous replacement of marrow, and cystic spaces in trabecular bone (dissecting osteitis). "Brown tumors" are brown bone masses produced by cystic enlargement of bones with areas of fibrosis and organized hemorrhage.

Hypertrophic osteoarthropathy presents with painful swelling of wrists, fingers, ankles, knees, or elbows.

- Seen in the setting of bronchogenic carcinoma (a paraneoplastic syndrome), chronic lung diseases, cyanotic congenital heart disease, and inflammatory bowel disease

- Can regress if underlying disease is treated

Pathologically, the ends of long bones show periosteal new bone formation, which can produce digital clubbing and often arthritis of adjacent joints.

Osgood-Schlatter disease is a common cause of knee pain in adolescents. It develops when stress from the quadriceps during rapid growth causes inflammation of the proximal tibial apophysis at the insertion of the patellar tendon. Permanent changes to the knees (knobby knees) may develop. The lesion is not usually biopsied.

Fibrous dysplasia presents with painful swelling, deformity, or pathologic fracture of involved bone (typically ribs, femur, or cranial bones), usually in children and young adults. *GNAS* gene mutations cause osteoblasts to produce fibrous tissue (microscopically, irregularly scattered trabelculae) rather than bone.

BENIGN TUMORS OF BONE

Osteoma is a benign neoplasm that frequently involves the skull and facial bones. Osteoma can be associated with Gardner syndrome. Malignant transformation doesn't occur.

Osteoid osteoma is a benign, painful growth of the diaphysis of a long bone, often the tibia or femur. Males are affected more than females, with peak age 5–25. Pain tends to be worse at night and relieved by aspirin. X-rays show central radiolucency surrounded by a sclerotic rim. Microscopically, ostoblasts line randomly connected trabeculae.

Osteoblastoma is similar to an osteoid osteoma but larger (>2 cm) and often involves vertebrae.

Osteochondroma (exostosis) is a benign bony metaphyseal growth capped with cartilage, which originates from epiphyseal growth plate. It typically presents in adolescent males who have firm, solitary growths at the ends of long bones. It may be asymptomatic, cause pain, produce deformity, or undergo malignant transformation (rare). *Osteochondromatosis* (multiple hereditary exostoses) produces multiple, often symmetric, osteochondromas. Excision is usually curative.

In a Nutshell

McCune-Albright syndrome presents with café au lait spots, precocious puberty (and other endocrine abnormalities), and polyostotic fibrous dysplasia.

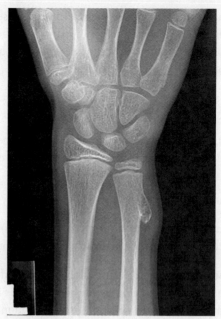

© Roger Boodoo, National Naval Medical Center.
Used with permission.

Figure 26-3. Osteochondroma Seen on Bony Protuberance on Distal Ulna

Enchondroma is a benign cartilaginous growth within the medullary cavity of bone, usually involving the hands and feet. It is typically solitary, asymptomatic, and requires no treatment. Multiple enchondromas (*enchondromatosis*) can occur as part of both Ollier disease (multiple and unilateral) and Maffucci syndrome (with hemangiomas), and carry a risk of malignant transformation.

Giant cell tumor of bone ("osteoclastoma") is a benign neoplasm containing multi-nucleated giant cells admixed with stromal cells. It is uncommon but occurs more often in females than in males, with peak age 20–50. Clinically, the tumor produces a bulky mass with pain and fractures. X-rays show an expanding lytic lesion surrounded by a thin rim of bone, with a possible "soap bubble" appearance. Treatment is surgery (curettage or *en bloc* resection). Osteoclastoma is locally aggressive with a high rate of recurrence (40–60%). In spite of being considered benign, approximately 2% will metastasize to the lungs.

Grossly, the tumor causes a red-brown mass with cystic degeneration that often involves the epiphyses of long bones, usually around the knee (distal femur and proximal tibia). Microscopically, multiple osteoclast-like giant cells are distributed within a background of mononuclear stromal cells.

MALIGNANT TUMORS OF BONE

Osteosarcoma (osteogenic sarcoma) is the most common primary malignant tumor of bone. It occurs more frequently in males than in females, with most cases in teenage years (ages 10–25). Patients with familial retinoblastoma have a high risk.

Osteosarcoma presents with localized pain and swelling. The classic x-ray findings are Codman triangle (periosteal elevation), "sun burst" pattern, and bone destruction. Treatment is surgery and chemotherapy. The prognosis is poor, but is improved with aggressive management such as resection of single pulmonary metastases (hematogenous metastasis to the lungs is common). **Secondary osteosarcoma** is seen in the elderly; these highly aggressive tumors are associated with Paget disease, irradiation, and chronic osteomyelitis.

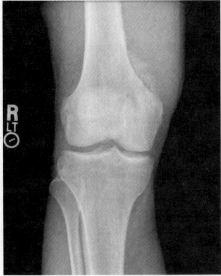

© James W. Graham, National Naval Medical Center.
Used with permission.

Figure 26-4. Osteosarcoma Seen in
Fuzzy Calcifications Adjacent to Distal Femur

Grossly, osteosarcoma often involves the metaphyses of long bones, usually around the knee (distal femur and proximal tibia). It produces a large, firm, white-tan mass with necrosis and hemorrhage. Microscopically, anaplastic cells producing osteoid and bone are seen.

Chondrosarcoma is a malignant tumor of chondroblasts which may arise *de novo* or secondary to a preexisting enchondroma, exostosis, or Paget disease. Males are affected more frequently than females, with peak ages 30–60. It presents with enlarging mass with pain and swelling, and it typically involves the pelvic bones, spine, and shoulder girdle. Microscopically, there is cartilaginous matrix production. Radiographs show osteolytic destruction and "popcorn" calcification. The 5-year survival is predicted by histologic differentiation.

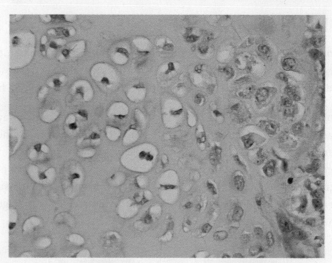

© Gregg Barré, M.D.
Used with permission.

Figure 26-5. Chondrosarcoma

Ewing sarcoma is a malignant neoplasm of undifferentiated cells arising within the marrow cavity. Males are affected slightly more often than females, with most cases in teenage years (ages 5–20). The classic translocation for Ewing sarcoma is t(11;22), which produces the EWS-FLI1 fusion protein.

Clinically, patients present with pain, swelling, and tenderness. X-ray studies show concentric "onion-skin" layering of new periosteal bone with soft tissue extension. Treatment is chemotherapy, surgery, and/or radiation; the 5-year survival rate is 75%.

Grossly, Ewing sarcoma often affects the diaphyses of long bones, with the most common sites being the femur, pelvis, and tibia. The tumor characteristically produces a white-tan mass with necrosis and hemorrhage. Microscopically, Ewing sarcoma is characterized by sheets of undifferentiated small, round, blue cells resembling lymphocytes, which may form Homer Wright pseudorosettes. The tumor cells erode through the cortex and periosteum and invade surrounding tissues.

Metastasis to bone is much more common than primary bone tumor. Common primary sites include prostate (often osteoblastic), breast, lung, thyroid, and kidney.

Chapter Summary

- Normal bone is composed of an **organic matrix** (containing collagen, osteocalcin, glycoproteins, and cells) and an **inorganic matrix** (containing calcium hydroxyapatite and other minerals). Osteoblasts and osteocytes form bone; osteoclasts resorb bone.

- Bone remodeling occurs throughout life and is under complex hormonal control by PTH, calcitonin, vitamin D, estrogen, cortisol, growth hormone, and thyroid hormone.

- **Autosomal dominant achondroplasia** is the most common form of inherited dwarfism. It is clinically characterized by short extremities, normal head and trunk, and normal life span and intelligence.

- **Osteogenesis imperfecta** has variable genetics and severity. Clinical manifestations may include brittle bones, blue sclera, joint hypermobility, deafness, and teeth abnormalities.

- **Osteopetrosis**, or marble bone disease, is a hereditary disease (variable genetics) characterized by thick sclerotic bones that fracture easily. Secondarily, it may compromise marrow cavities (leading to pancytopenia), foramina (leading to nerve palsies, blindness, or deafness), and CSF flow (leading to hydrocephalus).

- **Paget disease of bone** is an acquired, localized disorder of bone remodeling, resulting in excessive bone resorption followed by disorganized bone replacement (in a characteristic "mosaic" microscopic pattern), producing thickened bone that fractures easily and may impinge on nerves.

- **Osteoporosis** is a common disease in which bone mass decreases, resulting in thin, fragile bones that are susceptible to fracture. Predisposing factors include:

  - Estrogen deficiency
  - Genetically low density of original bone
  - Lack of exercise (or immobilization)
  - Old age
  - Nutritional deficiencies
  - Corticosteroid use

- **Osteomalacia** (adults) and **rickets** (children) are both characterized by decreased mineralization of newly formed bone, often secondary to vitamin D deficiency or abnormal metabolism. Rickets tends to present with skeletal deformities, while osteomalacia tends to present with fractures.

- **Pyogenic osteomyelitis** produces local symptoms accompanied by fever and is commonly due to *S. aureus* that may reach bone via blood, direct inoculation, or spread from nearby infection. Complications include ischemic necrosis of bone, sequestrum formation, fracture, intraosseous abscess, secondary amyloidosis, sinus tract formation and (rarely) osteogenic sarcoma. Tuberculous osteomyelitis is a rare but very destructive and difficult-to-treat complication of TB.

- **Avascular necrosis of bone** (particularly common in the femoral head) is an ischemic necrosis of bone and bone marrow (predisposing to osteoarthritis and fractures). It can be idiopathic or occur secondary to trauma, steroid use, sickle cell anemia, among others.

(continued)

Chapter Summary (cont'd)

- **Hypertrophic osteoarthropathy** may complicate other diseases (bronchogenic carcinoma, chronic lung disease, cyanotic congenital heart disease, and IBD). It is caused by periosteal new bone formation with pain and swelling of the ends of long bones, notably in wrists, fingers, ankles, knees, or elbows.

- **Osteitis fibrosa cystica** is the name for the generalized bone resorption with accompanying histologic changes seen in hyperparathyroidism; hemorrhage and fibrosis within the bone may produce "brown tumors."

- **Osgood-Schlatter disease** is a common cause of knee pain in adolescents.

- **Fibrous dysplasia** usually occurs in children and young adults, and presents with painful swelling, deformity, or pathologic fracture of the involved bone. Multiple bone involvement may be associated with **Albright syndrome**.

- Benign tumors of bone include:

  - Osteoma (skull, may be associated with Gardner syndrome)
  - Osteoid osteoma (tibia or femur of older children to young adults)
  - Osteoblastoma (vertebrae)
  - Osteochondroma (long bones of adolescent boys, bony outgrowth with cartilage cap; may be hereditary syndrome if multiple)
  - Enchondroma (cartilage in medullary cavity; may be part of Ollier disease or Maffucci syndrome if multiple)
  - Giant cell tumor of the bone; tends to involve the knee of young to middle-aged adults; x-ray shows expanding lytic lesion surrounded by a thin rim of bone possibly resembling a "soap bubble"

- **Osteosarcoma** is the most common primary malignant tumor of bone.

  - Often causes a large mass of the knee in teenagers or young adults
  - May be associated with familial retinoblastoma
  - Has characteristic x-ray pattern with periosteal elevation (Codman triangle), "sunburst" pattern, and bone destruction

- **Chondrosarcoma** tends to cause an enlarging mass of pelvis, spine, or shoulder in middle-aged individuals (male > female); it may arise *de novo* or secondary to a preexisting enchondroma, exostosis, or Paget disease.

- **Ewing sarcoma** is an aggressive (yet often responsive to therapy) malignant neoplasm of small, undifferentiated cells which develops within the marrow cavity of femur, pelvis, and tibia of children and teenagers.

- **Metastases to bone** are more common than primary bone tumors; common primary sites include prostate, breast, lung, thyroid, and kidney.

Joint Pathology 27

Learning Objectives

❏ Solve problems concerning osteoarthritis, rheumatoid arthritis, and seronegative spondyloarthropathies

❏ Describe arthritis related to crystal deposition, infectious arthritis, and neuropathic arthropathy (Charcot joint)

OSTEOARTHRITIS

Osteoarthritis (OA) (degenerative joint disease) is joint degeneration with loss of articular cartilage, with no to minimal inflammation. It is the most common form of arthritis. Risk increases with age; OA affects at least 1 joint in 80% of people age >70.

Clinically, there is an insidious onset of joint stiffness; deep, aching joint pain, which worsens with repetitive motion; decreased range of motion; crepitus; and joint effusions and swelling. Osteophytes may cause nerve compression. X-ray studies show narrowing of the joint space due to loss of cartilage; osteosclerosis and bone cysts; and osteophytes (osteophytic lipping).

The pathogenesis involves both biomechanical factors (aging or wear and tear of articular cartilage) and biochemical factors (chondrocyte injury and abnormal collagen activity). Predisposing factors include obesity, previous joint injury, ochronosis, diabetes, and hemarthrosis.

OA affects weight-bearing joints (knees, hips, and spine), often with asymmetrical involvement.

- There is degeneration and loss of articular cartilage with eburnation (exposed bone becomes polished) and subchondral bone sclerosis.

- The changes may include subchondral bone cysts, loose bodies (joint mice), which are free-floating fragments of cartilage and bone, and osteophytes (bone spurs), which are reactive bony outgrowths.

- **Heberden nodes** are osteophytes at the distal interphalangeal (DIP) joints, while **Bouchard nodes** are osteophytes at the proximal interphalangeal (PIP) joints.

Osteoarthritis vs RA

Osteoarthritis	RA
"Wear and tear"	Systemic autoimmune disease (+) Rheumatoid factor (+) Rheumatoid nodules
Degeneration of articular cartilage	Synovial proliferation
Knees and hands (DIP) in women; hips in men	Hands (PIP) and feet
Asymmetrical	Symmetrical and migratory

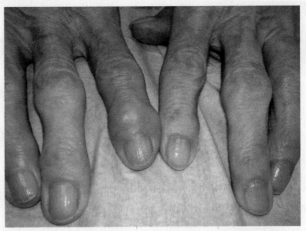

© commons.wikimedia.org.

Figure 27-1. Heberden (Distal Interphalangeal Joint) and
Bouchard (Proximal Interphalangeal Joint) Nodes in Patient with Osteoarthritis

RHEUMATOID ARTHRITIS

Rheumatoid arthritis (RA) is a systemic, chronic, inflammatory disease character-ized by progressive arthritis, production of rheumatoid factor, and extra-articular manifestations. It affects females 4x more than men, with highest incidence at ages 20–50. Some cases have a genetic predisposition (HLA-DR4 and -DR1).

RA is thought to be caused by an autoimmune reaction triggered by an infectious agent in a genetically susceptible individual.

RA most commonly affects the hand, wrist, knee, and ankle joints, and the involve-ment tends to be symmetrical. There is often morning stiffness which improves with activity.

- There is typically fusiform swelling, redness, and warmth of the proximal interphalangeal (PIP) joint.

- X-ray studies show juxta-articular osteoporosis and bone erosions; joint effu-sion may also be present.

- RA causes a diffuse proliferative synovitis, pannus formation (proliferation of the synovium and granulation tissue over the articular cartilage of the joint), fibrous and bony ankylosis (joint fusion), and joint deformities. Joint deformities can include:

    ◦ Radial deviation of the wrist and ulnar deviation of the fingers

    ◦ Swan neck deformity (hyperextension of PIP joint and flexion of DIP joint

    ◦ Boutonniere deformity (flexion of PIP and extension of DIP joints)

- Baker cysts (synovial cysts in the popliteal fossa) may be present.

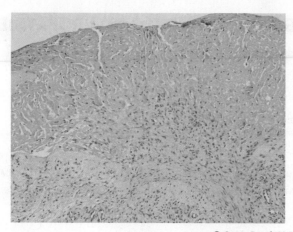

© Gregg Barré, M.D.
Used with permission.

Figure 27-2. Pannus Formation (Rheumatoid Arthritis)

Lab studies show elevated sedimentation rate and hypergammaglobulinemia. Rheumatoid factor (RF) is an autoantibody (usually IgM) against the Fc fragment of IgG; it is present in 80% of cases. RF may circulate and form immune complexes, and titer of RF correlates with the severity of the arthritis and prognosis.

- Extra-articular manifestations may be prominent. Systemic symptoms include low-grade fever, malaise, fatigue, lymphadenopathy, and weakness. Arteries may show acute necrotizing vasculitis due to circulating antigen-antibody complexes.

- Rheumatoid nodules, subcutaneous skin nodules, are present in 25% of cases. They are usually found on extensor surfaces of the forearms and elbows, but can also be found in the heart valves, lung, pleura, pericardium, and spleen. They are composed of central fibrinoid necrosis surrounded by epithelioid macrophages, lymphocytes, and granulation tissue.

- **Sjögren syndrome** may be present in 15%. In **Felty syndrome**, RA accompanies splenomegaly and neutropenia. In **Caplan syndrome**, RA is associated with pneumoconiosis.

- Secondary amyloidosis may also complicate RA.

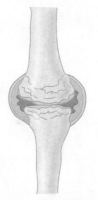

Rheumatoid Arthritis

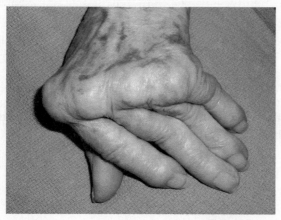

© Richard P. Usatine, M.D.
Used with permission.

Figure 27-3. Ulnar Deviation at the Metacarpophalangeal
Joints in Advanced Rheumatoid Arthritis

SERONEGATIVE SPONDYLOARTHROPATHIES

Clinical Correlate

Complete fusion of the spine can occur in ankylosing spondylitis and can cause complete rigidity of the spine. The resulting condition is known as **bamboo spine**, which can be seen on x-ray.

Seronegative spondyloarthropathies are a group of disorders characterized by the following:

- Rheumatoid factor seronegativity
- Involvement of the sacroiliac joints
- Association with HLA-B27

Ankylosing spondylitis occurs predominantly in young men with HLA-B27 (90% of cases); usually involves the sacroiliac joints and spine; and may be associated with inflammatory bowel disease.

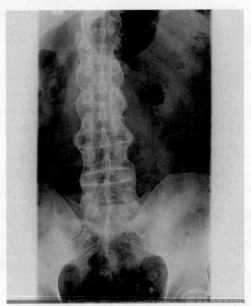

© Daniel W. Gabier, Naval Medical Center Portsmouth.
Used with permission.

Figure 27-4. Ankylosing Spondylitis Can Cause Fusion of Vertebrae, Leading to a "Bamboo Spine"

Reactive arthritis is characterized by a classic triad of conjunctivitis, urethritis, and arthritis. The arthritis affects the ankles and knees. It affects males more than females, with onset age 20s–30s. Onset often follows a venereal disease or bacillary dysentery.

Enteropathic arthritis occurs in 10–20% of patients with inflammatory bowel disease.

Psoriatic arthritis affects 5–10% of patients with psoriasis; is often a mild and slowly progressive arthritis, with pathology similar to RA.

ARTHRITIS RELATED TO CRYSTAL DEPOSITION

In **gout**, hyperuricemia and the deposition of monosodium urate crystals in joints will result in recurrent bouts of acute arthritis. The hyperuricemia can be caused by overproduction or underexcretion of uric acid.

- **Primary gout** (90%) is idiopathic, affects males more than females, and is typically seen in older men.

- **Secondary gout** (10%) is seen with excessive cell breakdown (chemotherapy), decreased renal excretion (drugs), and Lesch-Nyhan syndrome.

Gout affects the great toe (podagra, characterized by an exquisitely painful, inflamed big toe), ankle, heel, and wrist.

Joint aspiration shows birefringent, needle-shaped uric acid crystals and numerous neutrophils. **Tophi** are deposits of crystals surrounded by inflammation. Skin ulceration and destruction of adjacent joints may occur. Complications include joint destruction and deformity, uric acid renal calculi, and renal failure. Treatment is NSAIDs, colchicine, probenecid, and allopurinol.

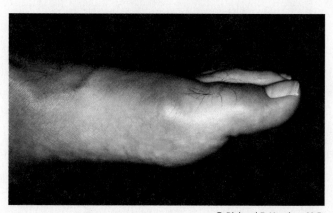

© Richard P. Usatine, M.D.
Used with permission.

Figure 27-5. Gout

Pseudogout (chondrocalcinosis) is deposition of calcium pyrophosphate crystals in joints, leading to inflammation. Affected patients are usually age >50. The knee joint is most commonly involved. Aspiration of the joint demonstrates positively birefringent (weak), rhomboid-shaped crystals. Pseudogout is associated with many metabolic diseases (e.g., diabetes, hypothyroidism, ochronosis), and it may mimic OA or RA.

INFECTIOUS ARTHRITIS

Suppurative arthritis may result from seeding of the joint during bacteremia. Other routes include spread from an adjacent site of infection and direct inoculation. Infecting organisms include gonococci, *Staphylococcus, Streptococcus, H. influenzae*, and gram-negative bacilli.

Suppurative arthritis causes a tender, painful, swollen, and erythematous joint. Large joints (knee, hip, shoulder) are most often infected, and the arthritis is usually

---

Bridge to Biochemistry

Uric acid is the end product of purine metabolism.

In a Nutshell

Lesch-Nyhan Syndrome

- X-linked recessive
- Deficiency of hypoxanthine-guanine phosphoribosyl-transferase (HPRT)
- Cognitive impairment
- Dystonia
- Self-mutilating behaviors
- Hyperuricemia

In a Nutshell

In the presence of pseudogout age <50, suspect one of these metabolic abnormalities (4H):

- Hemachromatosis
- Hyperparathyroidism
- Hypophosphatemia
- Hypomagnesemia

monoarticular. Joint aspiration shows cloudy synovial fluid that clots readily and has a high neutrophil count. Gram stain and culture are positive in 50–70% of cases. Treatment is rapid intervention with antibiotics to prevent permanent joint damage.

Lyme disease is caused by the spirochete *Borrelia burgdorferi*. The disease is arthropod-borne, spread by deer ticks (*Ixodes dammini*). Symptoms are skin rash (erythema chronicum migrans), and migratory arthritis involving the knees, shoulders, and elbows. The histology of the arthritic joint is similar to RA. Lyme disease can also have CNS and cardiac involvement. Serologic tests may remain negative until infection has been present for several weeks.

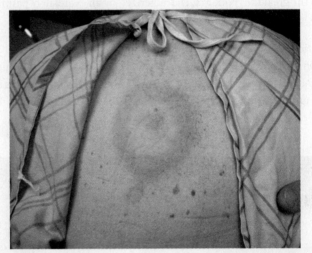

© Richard P. Usatine, M.D.
Used with permission.

Figure 27-6. Large Targetoid Lesion of Erythema Chronicum Migrans Considered Pathognomonic of Lyme Disease

NEUROPATHIC ARTHROPATHY (CHARCOT JOINT)

Charcot joint refers to joint damage secondary to impaired joint innervation (neuropathy), leading to an inability to sense pain. The damage also leads to destruction of joint surfaces, debris in joints, deformity, and dislocations.

Different **underlying neurologic diseases** tend to affect different joints.

- Diabetes mellitus (most common cause) tends to damage the tarsometatarsal joint in the midfoot.
- Syringomyelia (cavity in spinal cord) tends to damage the shoulder, elbow, and wrist joints.
- Tabes dorsalis (neurosyphilis) tends to damage the hip, knee, and ankle joints.

Chapter Summary

- **Degenerative joint disease** is an important cause of chronic joint pain in the elderly populations; it most seriously affects the weight-bearing joints and is related to destruction of the articular cartilage as a result of "wear and tear." Reactive bony spurs (osteophytes, called Heberden nodes if they involve the DIP joints, and Bouchard nodes if they involve the PIP joints) and free-floating fragments of cartilage or bone (joint mice) may contribute to the joint pathology.

- **Rheumatoid arthritis** (RA) is a systemic, chronic, inflammatory, autoimmune disease primarily of the hands, wrists, knees, and ankle joints of middle-aged women. It is characterized by progressive arthritis, production of rheumatoid factor, genetic predisposition (HLA-DR4 and -DR1), morning stiffness that improves with activity, pannus formation within the joint, and rheumatoid nodules. It often coexists with other diseases including Sjögren syndrome and pneumoconiosis (Caplan syndrome). RA is a defining feature of Felty syndrome. Some RA patients develop secondary amyloidosis.

- The **seronegative spondyloarthropathies** (all associated with HLA-B27) include ankylosing spondylitis (young men, sacroiliac joints and spine, association with IBD), reactive arthritis (young men, history of venereal disease or bacillary dysentery, ankles and knees, conjunctivitis, urethritis), enteropathic arthritis (patients with IBD), and psoriatic arthritis (rash and joint pain).

- **Gout** is an arthritis that classically involves the great toe (also may affect ankle, heel, wrist) as a result of hyperuricemia (primary or secondary due to chemotherapy, renal disease, or Lesch-Nyhan syndrome) leading to deposition of monosodium urate crystals in joints (negatively birefringent, needle-shaped crystals) and subcutaneous tissues (tophi). **Pseudogout** (chondrocalcinosis) results from the deposition of calcium pyrophosphate crystals (positively birefringent, rhomboid shaped) and commonly involves the knee of older adults.

- **Suppurative arthritis** typically causes tender, erythematous swelling of a single large joint (primarily knee, hip, and shoulder) as a result of bacterial infection (gonococci, *Staphylococcus*, *Streptococcus*, *H. influenzae*, and gram-negative bacilli) that has usually reached the joint through a hematogenous route.

- **Lyme disease** causes a migratory arthritis (clinically and histologically similar to RA) due to the spirochete *Borrelia burgdorferi*, which is spread by the deer tick *Ixodes dammini*. The arthritis is often preceded by a migratory rash (erythema chronicum migrans) and may be accompanied or followed by CNS and cardiac involvement.

- **Neuropathic arthropathy** is joint damage secondary to impaired joint innervation (neuropathy) leading to inability to sense pain. Examples of neurologic disease that cause this entity are diabetes mellitus, syringomyelia, and tabes dorsalis.

Skeletal Muscle and Peripheral Nerve Pathology

Learning Objectives

❑ Demonstrate understanding of inflammatory myopathies and neuropathies

❑ Describe the mechanism of action of myasthenic syndromes

❑ Explain information related to muscular dystrophy

❑ Solve problems concerning soft tissue and peripheral nerve tumors

Type I (red) skeletal muscle is used in postural weight bearing. It produces a slow twitch as a result of aerobic metabolism of fatty acids.

Type II (white) skeletal muscle is used for purposeful movement. It produces a fast twitch as a result of anaerobic glycolysis of glycogen.

Note

Skeletal muscle fiber type is determined by innervation.

Table 28-1. Type I (Slow-Twitch) Versus Type II (Fast-Twitch) Muscles

	Type I	Type II
Twitch rate	Slow twitch	Fast twitch
Function	Postural weight bearing Sustained tension	Purposeful movement Short, quick bursts
Metabolism	Aerobic (Krebs cycle)	Anaerobic (glycolysis)
Energy source	Fatty acids	Glycogen
Mitochondria	Many	Few
Color	Red	White
Fatigue	Slow fatigue	Rapid fatigue

INFLAMMATORY MYOPATHIES

Polymyositis is an autoimmune disease seen in adults. It presents with bilateral proximal muscle weakness. Microscopic exam demonstrates endomysial lymphocytic inflammation (mostly cytotoxic T8) and skeletal muscle fiber degeneration and regeneration. Patients respond to immunosuppression.

Dermatomyositis is a connective tissue disorder involving inflammation of skeletal muscle and skin. It can affect both children and adults. It presents with bilateral proximal muscle weakness, skin rash of the upper eyelids, and periorbital edema.

Clinical Correlate

Anti-tRNA synthetase antibodies such as the anti-Jo-1 antibody are known to be highly specific for inflammatory myopathies.

Microscopic exam demonstrates perimysial and vascular lymphocytic inflammation, perifascicular fiber atrophy, and skeletal muscle fiber degeneration and regeneration. Adult patients are at increased risk of lung, colon, breast, and gynecologic cancers.

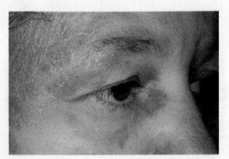

© Richard P. Usatine, M.D.
Used with permission.

Figure 28-1. Periorbital Heliotrope Rash of Dermatomyositis

Inclusion body myositis affects adults age >50, causing slowly progressive, asymmetrical, distal muscle weakness. Light microscopy demonstrates autophagic vacuoles and inclusion bodies in addition to inflammation and necrosis. The disease is refractory to immunosuppressive therapy.

MYASTHENIC SYNDROMES

Myasthenia gravis is an autoimmune disease characterized by autoantibodies against the acetylcholine (ACh) receptor of the neuromuscular junction, resulting in muscular weakness predominantly affecting the facial muscles. Females are affected more frequently than males.

- Extraocular muscle weakness may lead to ptosis and diplopia; the weakness worsens with repeated contractions.

- Respiratory muscle involvement may lead to death.

- There is an association with thymic hyperplasia and thymomas.

Treatment is anticholinesterase agents, steroids, and thymectomy.

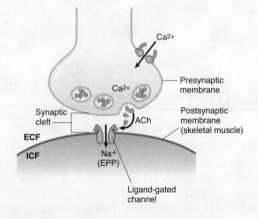

Figure 28-2. Neuromuscular Transmission

Lambert-Eaton myasthenic syndrome frequently arises before a diagnosis of cancer is made, often in cases of small cell lung cancer. Patients report dry mouth and proximal muscle weakness. Autoantibodies are directed against presynaptic calcium channels of the neuromuscular junction. Treatment is immunotherapy and cancer treatment, if indicated.

MUSCULAR DYSTROPHY

Duchenne muscular dystrophy is a recessive X-linked form of muscular dystrophy leading to rapid progression of muscle degeneration. It is the most common and severe form of muscular dystrophy. The affected gene is the dystrophin gene on the X chromosome (Xp21); dystrophin protein is an important muscle structural protein, and mutation results in a virtual absence of the dystrophin protein.

Affected boys are normal at birth but have onset of symptoms by age 5. Clinical features include:

- Progressive muscular weakness

- Calf pseudohypertrophy

- Proximal weakness of shoulder and pelvic girdles

- Possible heart failure and arrhythmias

- Respiratory insufficiency and pulmonary infections as a result of decreased mucociliary clearance

Lab studies show elevated serum creatine kinase. Muscle biopsy shows muscle fibers of various sizes; necrosis, degeneration, and regeneration of fibers; fibrosis; and fatty infiltration. Immunostains show decreased dystrophin protein. Diagnosis can also be confirmed with genetic testing.

Becker muscular dystrophy is a recessive X-linked inherited disorder leading to slowly progressive muscle weakness of the legs and pelvis.

- Less severe than Duchenne

- Not as common as Duchenne

- Has a later onset than Duchenne, with variable progression

- Mutation produces an altered dystrophin protein

- Cardiac involvement is rare, and patients can have relatively normal lifespan

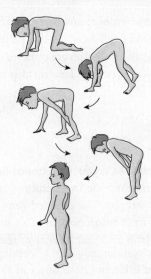

Note the characteristic pattern of rising from the floor using a sequence of hand pushes

Figure 28-3. Gower Sign in Duchenne Muscular Dystrophy

INFLAMMATORY NEUROPATHY

Guillain-Barré syndrome is an autoimmune disease leading to the destruction of Schwann cells and peripheral nerve demyelination. Clinically, it is preceded by a viral illness. Muscular weakness occurs with an ascending paralysis, accompanied by loss of deep tendon reflexes. Diagnosis can be established with nerve conduction studies; lumbar puncture shows elevated protein.

Microscopic examination demonstrates inflammation and demyelination of peripheral nerves and spinal nerve roots, resulting in muscular weakness. Guillain-Barré syndrome is fatal in 5% of cases because of respiratory paralysis. Treatment is plasmapheresis and immunoglobulin therapy.

SOFT TISSUE AND PERIPHERAL NERVE TUMORS

Lipoma is a benign adipose tissue tumor that most often arises in subcutaneous tissue of trunk, neck, or proximal extremities. It is the most common benign soft tissue tumor. The tumor is usually more of a cosmetic problem than a medical one. Microscopically, it is composed of mature fat cells but can contain other mesenchymal elements.

Liposarcoma is a malignant adipose tissue tumor that most often arises in the thigh or retroperitoneum. It is the most common adult sarcoma. It is distinguished from lipoma by the presence of **lipoblasts**. Grossly, it tends to be larger than lipoma, and the cut surface shows fibrous bands. Microscopically, well-differentiated liposarcoma consists of mature fat with varying numbers of hyperchromatic spindle cells and multivacuolated lipoblasts. Metastases are rare but retroperitoneal tumors tend to recur.

Dermatofibroma is a benign dermal spindle cell proliferation that most often arises in the extremities. A small, red nodule is seen, which is tender and mobile on examination.

Fibromatosis is a non-neoplastic proliferative connective tissue disorder that can histologically resemble a sarcoma. Fibrous tissue infiltrates muscle or other tissue, and may cause a mass lesion. The cut surface is trabeculated. Microscopically, bundles of fibroblasts and collagen are seen.

- **Superficial fibromatoses** arise from fascia or aponeuroses. Palmar fibromatosis is the most common type. Penile fibromatosis is known as Peyronie's disease.

- **Deep fibromatoses** (desmoids) occur in extraabdominal sites (children) and abdominal wall and extraabdominal sites (adults). Abdominal desmoids often occur in women within a year of pregnancy. They may also follow surgery or trauma. Intraabdominal fibromatosis is commonly associated with Gardner syndrome (*see* Gastrointestinal Tract Pathology, chapter 16).

Fibrosarcoma is a malignant fibrous tumor, commonly seen on the thigh and upper limb. It may arise spontaneously or after therapeutic/accidental irradiation. Microscopically, there are uniform spindle cells with a "herringbone" pattern. Metastases are hematogenous, often to the lung.

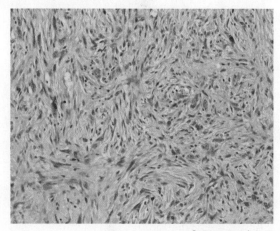

© Gregg Barré, M.D.
Used with permission.

Figure 28-4. Fibrosarcoma

Undifferentiated pleomorphic sarcoma (previously known as malignant fibrous histiocytoma) is a large multilobulated tumor seen in the extremities and retroperitoneum of older adults. Microscopically, they may have a storiform (cartwheel-like) pattern. They recur and metastasize.

Rhabdomyoma (*See* Female Genital and Cardiac Pathology, chapters 22 and 13.)

Embryonal rhabdomyosarcoma (*See* Female Genital chapter.)

Leiomyoma is a benign smooth muscle tumor most often seen in the uterus (*see* Female Genital chapter) and gastrointestinal tract. Less often it is seen in skin, and only rarely in deep soft tissue.

Leiomyosarcoma of soft tissue is less common than its counterpart in the gastrointestinal tract and uterus (*see* Female Genital chapter). In soft tissue, it usually arises in the retroperitoneum of older women.

Grossly, the tumor is fleshy and white with hemorrhage and necrosis. Microscopically, the tumor nuclei are blunt ended ("cigar-shaped"). Longitudinal striations can be seen with Masson trichrome staining. The tumor is highly aggressive in the retroperitoneum, where complete resection may not be possible.

Synovial sarcoma occurs in young adults. The knee is a common location. The gross appearance is variable but calcification is common. Microscopically, tumors may be biphasic (epithelial and spindle cells) or monophasic (spindle cell or epithelial).

Benign peripheral nerve sheath tumors

- **Schwannoma** is an encapsulated nerve sheath tumor with alternating Antoni A and B areas (*see* Central Nervous System, chapter 20). There is an association with NF2.

- **Neurofibroma** is nonencapsulated and may have a solitary, diffuse, or plexiform pattern. Microscopically, neoplastic cells are interspersed among wavy, loose or dense collagen bundles. There is an association with NF1 (*see* Genetic Disorders, chapter 6).

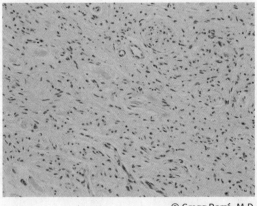

© Gregg Barré, M.D.
Used with permission.

Figure 28-5. Neurofibroma

Malignant peripheral nerve sheath tumor may arise from neurofibromas or *de novo* in a peripheral nerve. It typically occurs in young adults in major nerve trunks (sciatic nerve, brachial plexus, and sacral plexus). Microscopically, it resembles fibrosarcoma. Recurrence and distant metastases are common.

Chapter Summary

- **Type I (red) skeletal muscle** is used in postural weight bearing; it produces a slow twitch as a result of aerobic metabolism of fatty acids. **Type II (white)** is used for purposeful movement; it produces a fast twitch as a result of anaerobic glycolysis of glycogen.

- **Inflammatory myopathies** include polymyositis (adults, bilateral proximal muscle weakness, cytotoxic T8 lymphocytes, and skeletal muscle degeneration and regeneration), dermatomyositis (children or adults with bilateral proximal muscle weakness; periorbital edema with skin rash of eyelids; perifascicular fiber atrophy with lymphocytic infiltrates; and increased risk of cancer), and inclusion body myositis (older adults with asymmetrical distal muscle weakness and autophagic vacuoles and inclusion bodies on microscopy).

- Myasthenic syndromes include:

  - **Myasthenia gravis**: autoantibody attack on muscle acetylcholine receptor, sometimes related to thymic disease, produces muscle weakness that worsens with muscle use

  - **Lambert-Eaton myasthenic syndrome**: paraneoplastic syndrome of small cell carcinoma of lung with autoantibodies against calcium channels, produces proximal muscle weakness that improves with muscle use

- Muscular dystrophies include:

  - **Duchenne muscular dystrophy**: X-linked abnormality of the muscle structural protein dystrophin causes progressive muscular weakness related to muscle necrosis and degeneration; begins by age 5, initially involving shoulder and pelvic girdles

  - **Becker muscular dystrophy**: less common, milder variant of Duchenne with relatively normal lifespan

  - **Guillain-Barré syndrome**: inflammatory neuropathy that typically follows a viral illness and may lead to respiratory failure and paralysis as a result of inflammation and demyelination of peripheral nerves and spinal nerve roots.

- **Benign soft tissue tumors** include lipomas, dermatofibromas, fibromatosis, rhabdomyomas, and leiomyomas.

- **Malignant soft tissue tumors** include liposarcoma, fibrosarcoma, embryonal rhabdomyosarcoma, leiomyosarcoma, undifferentiated pleomorphic sarcoma, and synovial sarcoma.

- **Benign peripheral nerve sheath tumors** include schwannoma and neurofibroma. **Malignant peripheral nerve sheath tumors** may arise from neurofibromas or *de novo* in a peripheral nerve.

Index

pulmonary, 137–139
soft tissue, 294–296
thyroid, 261–262
tumor suppressor genes, 77–78
urinary bladder, 157
Nephritic syndrome, 145, 146–148
Nephritis, tubulointerstitial, 150–151
Nephronophthisis-medullary cystic disease, 145
Nephropathy
diabetic, 267
urate, 151
Nephrosclerosis, benign, 153
Nephrotic syndrome, 145, 149
Nephrotoxic acute tubular necrosis, 151
Nerve sheath tumors, peripheral, 296
Neural tube defects, 202–203
Neuritic plaques, Alzheimer disease, 207
Neurocognitive disorder, HIV-associated, 198
Neurodegenerative disorders, 202, 205
Neuroectodermal tumors, 209
Neuroendocrine tumors, pancreatic, 176
Neuroepithelial tissue tumors, 209–211
Neurofibrillary tangles, Alzheimer disease, 207
Neurofibroma, 296
S100 staining, 76
Neurofibromatosis types 1 & 2, 50–51
Neurogenic shock, 38
Neuromuscular transmission, myasthenia gravis, 292
Neuropathic arthropathy, 288
Neuropathy
diabetic, 267
inflammatory, 294
Neutrophils
acute inflammation, 15, 16–18
leukocytosis (neutrophilia), 217
Nevi, 82
Nevocellular nevus, 82
Nevus flammeus nuchae, 107
Newborn
hemolytic disease of, 184
physiologic jaundice of, 184
respiratory distress syndrome, 133
Niemann-Pick disease, 48
Nipple, Paget disease of, 246, 247
Nitroblue tetrazolium, acute inflammation, 18
Nodular glomerulosclerosis, 150
Nodular hyperplasia, liver, 191
Nodular sclerosis, 224
Non-Hodgkin lymphoma
in AIDS, 64
testicular, 255
Nonalcoholic fatty liver disease, 190
Nonatopic asthma, 131
Nonbacterial thrombotic endocarditis (NBTE), 116
Nonfunctional adenoma, pituitary, 263
Nonspecific interstitial pneumonia, 133
Nonspecific lymphadenitis, acute/chronic, 219

Nontropical sprue, 166
Normocytic anemias, 95–98
classification, 92
Nutritional imbalance, cellular injury, 5

O

Obesity, 5
Obstruction/resorption atelectasis, 125
Obstructive pulmonary disease, 130–132
restrictive pulmonary disease vs., 129–130
Occlusions, thrombolic/embolic, 199
Occupation-associated diseases
asthma, 131
pneumoconioses, 134–135
pneumonia, 134–135
Oligodendroglioma, 211
Oligohydramnios sequence, 143
Oliguria, glomerular disease, 145
Oncocytomas, kidney, 154
Oncogenes, carcinogenesis, 73–74
Oncogenic viruses, cancer risk, 73
Oncotic pressure, pulmonary edema, 136
Opportunistic infections, in AIDS patients, 63
Opsonins, inflammation, 18
Optochin-resistant *Viridans streptococci*, 116
Orchitis, 252
Organs
manifestations of shock, 38
sarcoidosis, 128
systemic lupus erythematosus, 59
tissue repair, 26
tuberculosis dissemination, 127
vasculitides, 104
Orthopnea, congestive heart failure, 114
Osgood-Schlatter disease, 277
Osler-Weber-Rendu syndrome, 169
Osmotic fragility test, hemolytic anemia, 98
Osteitis deformans, 273
Osteitis fibrosa cystica, 50, 262, 276–277
Osteoarthritis, 283–284
Osteoarthropathy, hypertrophic, 277
pulmonary involvement, 139
Osteoblastoma, 277
Osteoblasts, 271
Osteochondroma, 277
Osteoclastoma, 278
Osteoclasts, 271
Osteocytes, 271
Osteogenesis imperfecta, 49, 272
Osteoid osteoma, 277
Osteoma, 277
Osteomalacia, 275
Osteomyelitis, 275–276
tuberculous, 276
Osteopetrosis, 272–273
Osteoporosis, 273–274
Osteosarcoma, 279
Ovarian tumors, 238–239
epithelial, 238
germ cell, 238
origins, 239
sex chord-stromal, 238–239

Ovary, 237–239
cancer, 234
tumors. *See* Ovarian tumors
Ovotesticular disorder, 45–46
Oxygen-dependent/oxygen-independent killing, acute inflammation, 18

P

Paget disease
of bone, 273
extramammary disease of the vulva, 232
mammary, 247
of nipple, 246
Pain, mediators, 19
Panacinar emphysema, 130
Pancoast tumor, 138
Pancreas
agenesis, 175
carcinoma, 177
congenital anomalies, 175
inflammation, 175–176
tumors, 176–177
Pancreatic divisum, 175
Pancreatic neuroendocrine tumors, 176–177
Pancreatitis
acute, 175–176
amylase/lipase, 8
chronic, 176
Panencephalitis, subacute sclerosing, 197
Panhypopituitarism, 263
Pannus formation, rheumatoid arthritis, 284, 285
Papanicolaou (Pap) test, 234, 238
Papillary carcinoma, thyroid, 261
Papillary hidradenoma, 232
Papillary precursors, urinary bladder cancer, 157
Papillary renal cell carcinoma, 155
Papilloma, intraductal, 245
Pappenheimer bodies, red blood cells, 91
Para-aortic lymph nodes, 252
Paradoxical emboli, 120
Paraneoplastic syndromes, pulmonary, 139
Paraspinal nerve tumors, 211
Parathyroid glands, 262
Parenchymal abscesses, 151
Parkinson disease (PD), 205
Parkinson syndrome, 205
Paroxysmal nocturnal hemoglobinuria, 98
Partial mole, 240
Partial thromboplastin time (PTT)
bleeding disorders, 34
liver disease, 185
Parvovirus
hereditary spherocytosis, 98
sickle cell anemia, 97
Passive hyperemia, 30
Patau syndrome, 42–43
Patchy atelectasis, 125
Patent ductus arteriosus (PDA), 119, 120
Pathogenesis, 1
Pathogens, cellular injury, 5

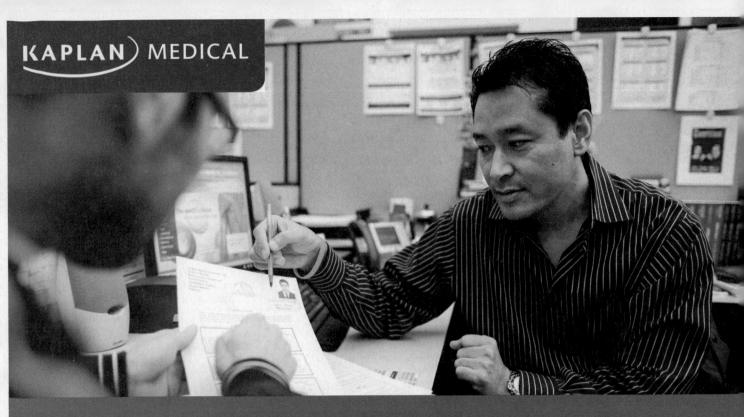

Improve your odds of matching.
Meet your medical advisor: your personal coach to USMLE® and the Match™.

Behind each champion, you will find a great coach. Schedule a complimentary 30-minute session with a medical advisor and connect with them via Skype, on the phone or in person.

You'll discuss your:
- personalized study plan
- Qbank and NBME® performance
- exam readiness
- residency application timeline

Our medical advisors know every exam and every part of the medical residency application process. They will help you understand every step you'll take on the road to residency.

Don't delay. Request your free med advising appointment today.
Visit **kaplanmedical.com/freeadvising**